The AOTA
Practice
Guidelines
Series

Occupational Therapy
Practice Guidelines *for*

Adults With Traumatic Brain Injury

Kathleen Golisz, OTR, OTD
Associate Professor
Occupational Therapy Graduate Program
Mercy College
Dobbs Ferry, NY

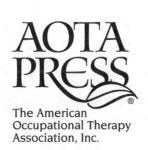

AOTA
PRESS ®

The American
Occupational Therapy
Association, Inc.

Centennial Vision

We envision that occupational therapy is a powerful, widely recognized, science-driven, and evidence-based profession with a globally connected and diverse workforce meeting society's occupational needs.

Vision Statement

AOTA advances occupational therapy as the pre-eminent profession in promoting the health, productivity, and quality of life of individuals and society through the therapeutic application of occupation.

Mission Statement

The American Occupational Therapy Association advances the quality, availability, use, and support of occupational therapy through standard-setting, advocacy, education, and research on behalf of its members and the public.

AOTA Staff

Frederick P. Somers, *Executive Director*
Christopher M. Bluhm, *Chief Operating Officer*

Chris Davis, *Director, AOTA Press*
Ashley Hofmann, *Production Editor*
Victoria Davis, *Editorial Assistant*

Beth Ledford, *Director, Marketing and Member Communications*
Emily Harlow, *Technology Marketing Specialist*
Jennifer Folden, *Marketing Specialist*

The American Occupational Therapy Association, Inc.
4720 Montgomery Lane
Bethesda, MD 20814
Phone: 301-652-AOTA (2682)
TDD: 800-377-8555
Fax: 301-652-7711
www.aota.org

To order: 1-877-404-AOTA (2682)

© 2009 by the American Occupational Therapy Association, Inc.
All rights reserved.
No parts of this book may be reproduced in whole or in part by any means without permission.
Printed in the United States of America.

Disclaimers

This publication is designed to provide accurate and authoritative information in regard to the subject matter covered. It is sold or distributed with the understanding that the publisher is not engaged in rendering legal, accounting, or other professional service. If legal advice or other expert assistance is required, the services of a competent professional person should be sought.
—*From the Declaration of Principles jointly adopted by the American Bar Association and a Committee of Publishers and Associations*

It is the objective of the American Occupational Therapy Association to be a forum for free expression and interchange of ideas. The opinions expressed by the contributors to this work are their own and not necessarily those of the American Occupational Therapy Association.

ISBN-10: 1-56900-258-4
ISBN-13: 978-1-56900-258-2
Library of Congress Control Number: 2009926125

Design by Sarah Ely and Mike Melletz
Composition by Maryland Composition, White Plains, MD
Printing by Automated Graphics Systems, White Plains, MD

Citation: Golisz, K. (2009). *Occupational therapy practice guidelines for adults with traumatic brain injury.* Bethesda, MD: AOTA Press.

Contents

Appendixes

Acknowledgments

Many people contributed to the development and production of this document and deserve a heartfelt thank you. First are the clients with traumatic brain injury and their families with whom I have been honored to work over the years. The learning and motivation to improve was not only their goal but also my personal goal as a clinician.

Deborah Lieberman, AOTA Practice Guidelines Series Editor, and Marian Arbesman, consultant to AOTA's Evidence-Based Practice Project, were untiring in their support, guidance, and feedback throughout this process. I appreciate their mentorship.

Catherine Trombly Latham completed the earlier review of the evidence and was gracious to allow us to include it in this document. I appreciate the thoughtful comments of all the reviewers—Claire Mulry, Melissa Oliver, Shawn Phipps, Mary Vining Radomski, Doug Simmons, and Catherine Trombly Latham—as well as those of Dr. Ruth Meyers, who reviewed earlier drafts of the document.

Finally, thanks to my family and colleagues for their patience and support during the many hours of work devoted to this task.

■ ■ ■

Introduction

Purpose and Use of This Publication

Practice guidelines have been widely developed in response to the health care reform movement in the United States. Such guidelines can be a useful tool for improving the quality of health care, enhancing consumer satisfaction, promoting appropriate use of services, and reducing costs. The American Occupational Therapy Association (AOTA), which represents nearly 148,000 occupational therapists, occupational therapy assistants (see Appendix A), and students of occupational therapy, is committed to providing information to support decision making that promotes a high-quality health care system that is affordable and accessible to all.

Using an evidence-based perspective and key concepts from the second edition of the *Occupational Therapy Practice Framework: Domain and Process* (AOTA, 2008b), this guideline provides an overview of the occupational therapy process for individuals with traumatic brain injury (TBI). It defines the occupational therapy domain and process and interventions that occur within the boundaries of acceptable practice. This guideline does not discuss all possible methods of care, and although it does recommend some specific methods of care, the occupational therapist makes the ultimate judgment regarding the appropriateness of a given intervention in light of a specific person's circumstances, needs, and available evidence to support the intervention.

It is the intention of AOTA, through this publication, to help occupational therapists and occupational therapy assistants, as well as the individuals who manage, reimburse, or set policy regarding occupational therapy services, understand the contribution of occupational therapy in treating adults with TBI. This guideline also can serve as a reference for health care professionals, health care facility managers, education and health care regulators, third-party payers, and managed care organizations. Selected diagnostic and billing code information for evaluations and interventions is provided in Appendix B.

This document may be used in any of the following ways:

- To assist occupational therapists and occupational therapy assistants in communicating about their services to external audiences
- To assist other health care practitioners, case managers, families and caregivers, and health care facility managers in determining whether referral for occupational therapy services would be appropriate
- To assist third-party payers in determining the medical necessity for occupational therapy
- To assist health and education planning teams in determining the need for occupational therapy
- To assist legislators, third-party payers, and administrators in understanding the professional education, training, and skills of occupational therapists and occupational therapy assistants
- To assist program developers, administrators, legislators, and third-party payers in understanding the scope of occupational therapy services
- To assist program evaluators and policy analysts in this practice area in determining outcome measures for analyzing the effectiveness of occupational therapy intervention
- To assist policy, education, and health care benefit analysts in understanding the appropriateness of occupational therapy services for TBI
- To assist policymakers, legislators, and organizations in understanding the contribution occupational therapy can make in program development and health care reform for persons with TBI
- To assist occupational therapy educators in designing appropriate curricula that incorporate the role of occupational therapy with TBI.

The introduction to this guideline continues with a brief discussion of the domain and process of occupational therapy. This discussion is followed by a detailed description of the occupational therapy process for TBI, including a summary of evidence from the literature regarding best practices with people who have sustained a TBI. Finally, Appendix C contains a description of evidence-based practice as it relates to occupational therapy and the process used to conduct the evidence-based practice review related to TBI, additional information about occupational therapists and occupational therapy assistants, and other resources related to this topic. All studies identified by the review, including those not specifically described in this section, are summarized in the evidence tables in Appendix D. Readers are encouraged to read the full articles for more details.

Domain and Process of Occupational Therapy

Occupational therapists' expertise lies in their knowledge of occupation and of how engaging in occupations can be used to support health and participation in home, school, the workplace, and community life (AOTA, 2008b).

In 2008, the AOTA Representative Assembly adopted the *Occupational Therapy Practice Framework: Domain and Process, 2nd Edition*. Informed by the first edition of the *Occupational Therapy Practice Framework: Domain and Process* (AOTA, 2002), the previous *Uniform Terminology for Occupational Therapy* (AOTA, 1979, 1989, 1994), and the World Health Organization's *International Classification of Functioning, Disability, and Health* (*ICF;* WHO, 2001), the *Framework* outlines the profession's domain and the process of service delivery within this domain.

Domain

A profession's *domain* articulates its sphere of knowledge, societal contribution, and intellectual or scientific activity. The occupational therapy profession's domain centers on helping others participate in daily life activities. The broad term that the profession uses to describe daily life activities is *occupation*. As outlined in the *Framework*, occupational therapists and occupational therapy assistants[1] work collaboratively with people, organizations, and populations (clients) to engage in everyday activities or occupations that they want and need to do in a manner that supports health and participation (see Figure 1). Using occupational engagement as both the desired outcome of intervention and the intervention itself, occupational therapy practitioners are skilled at viewing the subjective and objective aspects of performance and at understanding occupation simultaneously from this dual, yet holistic, perspective. The overarching mission to support health and participation in life through engagement in occupations circumscribes the profession's domain and emphasizes the important ways in which environmental and life circumstances influence the manner in which people carry out their occupations. Key aspects of the domain of occupational therapy are defined in Figure 2.

Process

Many professions use the process of evaluating, intervening, and targeting outcomes that is outlined in the *Framework*. Occupational therapy's application of this process is made unique, however, by its focus on occupation (see Figure 3). The process of occupational therapy service delivery typically begins with the occupational profile, an assessment of the client's occupational needs, problems, and concerns, and the analysis of occupational performance, which includes the skills, patterns, contexts and environments, activity demands, and client factors that contribute to or impede the client's satisfaction with

---

[1] *Occupational therapists* are responsible for all aspects of occupational therapy service delivery and are accountable for the safety and effectiveness of the occupational therapy service delivery process. *Occupational therapy assistants* deliver occupational therapy services under the supervision of and in partnership with an occupational therapist (AOTA, 2004).

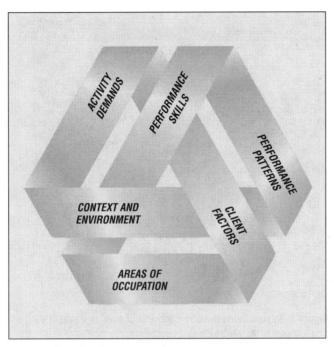

Figure 1. Domain of occupational therapy.

Source. American Occupational Therapy Association. (2008). Occupational therapy practice framework: Domain and process (2nd ed., p. 627). *American Journal of Occupational Therapy, 62,* 625–683. Used with permission.

his or her ability to engage in valued daily life activities. Therapists then plan and implement intervention using a variety of approaches and methods in which occupa-tion is both the means and ends (Trombly, 1995). Occu-pational therapists continually assess the effectiveness of the intervention and the client's progress toward targeted

AREAS OF OCCUPATION	CLIENT FACTORS	PERFORMANCE SKILLS	PERFORMANCE PATTERNS	CONTEXT AND ENVIRONMENT	ACTIVITY DEMANDS
Activities of Daily Living (ADL)*	Values, Beliefs, and Spirituality	Sensory Perceptual Skills	Habits	Cultural	Objects Used and Their Properties
Instrumental Activities of Daily Living (IADL)	Body Functions	Motor and Praxis Skills	Routines	Personal	Space Demands
Rest and Sleep	Body Structures	Emotional Regulation Skills	Roles	Physical	Social Demands
Education		Cognitive Skills	Rituals	Social	Sequencing and Timing
Work		Communication and Social Skills		Temporal	Required Actions
Play				Virtual	Required Body Functions
Leisure					Required Body Structures
Social Participation					
*Also referred to as *basic activities of daily living (BADL)* or *personal activities of daily living (PADL)*.*					

Figure 2. Aspects of occupational therapy's domain.

Source. American Occupational Therapy Association. (2008). Occupational therapy practice framework: Domain and process (2nd ed., p. 628). *American Journal of Occupational Therapy, 62,* 625–683. Used with permission.

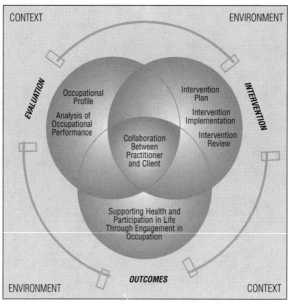

Figure 3. Occupational therapy's process of service delivery as applied within the profession's domain.

Source. American Occupational Therapy Association. (2008). Occupational therapy practice framework: Domain and process (2nd ed., p. 627). *American Journal of Occupational Therapy, 62,* 625–683. Used with permission.

outcomes. The intervention review informs decisions to continue or discontinue intervention and to make referrals to other agencies or professionals.

Current occupational therapy practice with clients with TBI is largely based on the knowledge and clinical judgment of the treating therapist, due to limited evidence supporting the effectiveness of any particular intervention. The intervention review process, based upon careful observation of client response to intervention and tracking and analysis of client progress, can contribute to the science of TBI intervention by providing replicable case examples. Therapists select outcome measures that are valid, reliable, and appropriately sensitive to the client's occupational performance, satisfaction, adaptation, role competence, health and wellness, prevention, self-advocacy, quality of life, and *occupational justice* (i.e., access to and opportunities for participation in the full range of meaningful and enriching occupations afforded to others within the community to satisfy personal, health, and societal needs [adapted from Townsend & Wilcock, 2004]).

Occupational therapy outcome goals may be restorative or compensatory. *Restorative intervention*

seeks to change internal factors in a person that affect performance in areas of occupation. Intervention focuses on attaining restorative goals when the person shows potential and desire for change in body functions, performance skills, or patterns of performance. Restorative intervention includes the use of selected therapeutic procedures designed to promote recovery or change in body functions, such as muscle strength or cognitive ability. Restorative intervention also includes therapeutic practice to improve performance skills and performance patterns. *Compensatory interventions* include adaptations to activity demands and the performance environment that enable a person to resume performance of valued occupations even when deficits in body functions, performance skills, or performance patterns are not amenable to change. Compensatory intervention approaches also involve teaching the client skills and strategies that enable him or her to use preserved abilities to "work around" impairments. By modifying the task demands, pattern of performance, or environment, the client with TBI may be able to continue to engage in valued occupations.

Traumatic Brain Injury— Definition and Epidemiology

Acquired brain injury (ABI) is a broad term that describes a variety of traumatic and nontraumatic injuries that can occur to the brain after birth. *Traumatically acquired brain injuries (TBI)* are caused by a traumatic event such as a car accident, physical assault, explosive concussion, or work- or leisure-related injury. Nontraumatic acquired brain injuries can result from an internal brain disorder such as a stroke or vascular event, infection or toxin, tumor, or metabolic event. While individuals with nontraumatic brain injuries can have similar symptoms to those with traumatic injuries, and some authors use the terms *ABI* and *TBI* interchangeably, this document will focus on occupational therapy services for individuals with TBI.

The Brain Injury Association of America (n.d.) defines *TBI* as

> an insult to the brain, not of a degenerative or congenital nature but caused by an external physical force, that may produce a diminished or altered state of consciousness, which results in an impairment of cognitive abilities or physical functioning. It can also result in the disturbance of behavioral or emotional functioning. These impairments may be either temporary or permanent and cause partial or total functional disability or psychosocial maladjustment.

Changes in Incidence

A combination of prevention awareness (e.g., decreased driving while intoxicated, increased seat belt and child safety seat use) and advances in motor vehicle design (e.g., passive-restraint seat belts and airbags) has decreased TBI incidence (Pintar, Yoganandan, & Gennarelli, 2000; Stewart, Girotti, Nikore, & Williamson, 2003), yet vehicle crashes continue to be the leading cause of hospitalization and TBI-associated deaths among women and children younger than age 15 years (Centers for Disease Control and Prevention [CDC], 1999). Despite airbag deployment and seat belt use, recent trends in the popularity of certain passenger vehicles appear to have caused a shift in the type and severity of injuries observed in motor vehicle crashes (Mayrose & Jehle, 2002) for both front- and side-impact crashes between sedans and sport utility vehicles (SUVs), vans, or light trucks. The greater mass, hood height, and width of SUVs, vans, and light trucks compared with sedans appears to account for the increased incidence of severe TBI, thorax and intrathoracic organ injuries, and face lacerations (Siegel et al., 2001).

Intentional TBI (i.e., injury from a firearm or blunt object) typically involves drug or alcohol use (Wagner, Sasser, Hammond, Wiercisiewski, & Alexander, 2000) and is the leading cause of TBI-related deaths and severe injury since 1990, especially for young men. People at risk for intentional violence-related TBI from gunshot wounds and blunt trauma from assault are typically young (i.e., 15 to 24 years old) men from minority (i.e., black, Hispanic, other nonwhite ethnicity) and low-income (Hanks et al., 2003) populations.

Nonintentional TBI can occur from a variety of normal daily activities. Falls are the leading cause of TBI-associated death and disability in people ages 65 or older, due to physiological changes associated with aging, use of certain medications, and impaired balance and lower-extremity function (CDC, 1999).

Some work settings, such as those requiring the use of motor vehicles and machines, or elevated work stations such as roofing, logging, and forestry, pose a greater risk of TBI, although a brain injury can occur in almost any work setting (CDC, 1999).

TBI has been termed the "signature injury" of recent military conflicts in Iraq and Afghanistan. The sex and age distribution of military personnel falls within the general "at-risk" population for TBI, and the nature of military occupations, even during peacetime, carry higher-than-average risk for TBI (Ivins et al., 2003). Despite improved body armor and helmet technology, combat considerably increases the rate of TBI. Many soldiers receive brain injuries from gunshots or blasts from improvised explosive devices (IEDs). Improved survival rates, increased awareness of the consequences of TBI, and increased surveillance for TBI by military medical personnel have resulted in more diagnoses of brain injury, including mild TBI, than in past military conflicts. While statistics on the mortality and morbidity patterns from the Iraq and Afghanistan wars are years away, the Department of Veterans Affairs estimates that the incidence of TBI from the current Middle East conflicts will far exceed the 20% seen in surviving combat casualties from 1990s Operation Desert Storm (Schwab, Warden, Lux, Shupenko, & Zitnay, 2007).

Many of the returning soldiers who sustained a brain injury present with complex comorbidities or polytrauma, including amputations, burns, vision and hearing loss, and posttraumatic stress disorder (PTSD; Sayer et al., 2008). The Department of Defense and Department of Veterans Affairs have collaborated with civilian partners to form a multisite medical care, clinical research, and education center called the Defense and Veterans Brain Injury Center (DVBIC). The DVBIC aims to provide case management, services, and support to military personnel with TBI and their families (Sigford, 2008). Occupational therapy services are a recognized component of this coordinated TBI program (Friedemann-Sánchez, Sayer, & Pickett, 2008; Ivins et al., 2003).

Classification of Injuries

Brain injuries can be classified as closed- or open-penetrating based on whether the skull and brain matter was breached by some object (e.g., bone, bullets, fragments from an object) and temporally classified as primary or secondary based upon whether the brain injury occurred at the time of the traumatic incident or as a result of secondary brain events resulting from the initial injury (Graham, 1999).

Falls, motor vehicle crashes, and battlefield blasts from bombs can cause rapid oscillating movement of the brain within the skull and bruised and torn brain tissue and blood vessels, resulting in a *closed* TBI. These *primary* focal brain injuries, or *coup contrecoup* injuries, typically occur at the frontal and temporal lobes as a result of the irregular interior skull features in those areas (Book, 2002; Frosch, Anthony, & DeGirolami, 2005; Graham, 1999). Contrecoup bruising can occur in the opposite pole (e.g., occipital lobe), but such bruises are less severe because of the smoother surface of the skull. Straining and shearing of axons throughout the white matter of the brain, accompanied by petechial hemorrhages, result in diffuse axonal injuries (Graham, 1999; Smith, Meaney, & Shull, 2003; Sohlberg & Mateer, 2001). *Open*-penetrating injuries, when the dura mater is torn and the brain substance is exposed (Graham, 1999), are associated with high rates of medical complications (Black et al., 2002). *Secondary* brain injuries occur after the initial neural injury and result from the series of physiological events (e.g., edema, hematoma, hydrocephalus, brain herniation, anoxia, local infarcts) that happen when the brain is injured.

Neurological rehabilitation programs providing services to clients with TBI also may include clients with nontraumatically acquired brain injuries. Clients who have sustained cerebral anoxia and hypoxic brain damage (e.g., from near drowning, smoke asphyxiation, cardiac arrest), aneurysms and arterial–venous malformations, tumors, exposure to toxic substances (e.g., carbon monoxide poisoning, drug overdose), or brain infections (e.g., meningitis, encephalitis) all may present with similar clinical symptoms and rehabilitative needs.

Overview of Resulting Signs and Symptoms

Individuals who sustain a TBI can present with a range of physical, cognitive, and behavioral symptoms based on the areas of their brain that sustained the damage. Physical impairments can include hemiplegia if the brain sustained a focal injury, ataxia, incoordination, or apraxia. Comorbidities such as peripheral nerve injuries and bony fractures also can occur from the events resulting in the brain injury (e.g., car crash). Cognitive symptoms such as impairments in attention, memory, perception, or executive functions may present lifelong challenges for individuals with TBI. Behavioral symptoms including disinhibition, impulsivity, and emotional lability can strain personal relationships and the ability for the individual with TBI to socially participate within his or her community.

The National Center for Injury Prevention and Control (NCIPC) estimates that approximately 5.3 million Americans have experienced a TBI severe enough to require a lifelong need for help to perform activities of daily living (CDC, 2003). Although most clients with TBI who receive occupational therapy intervention are classified as having severe injuries, many people with mild TBI (MTBI) may only be seen in emergency departments. Although these individuals with MTBI may lack any obvious physical signs of injury, they can experience persistent cognitive or behavioral problems that may be responsive to rehabilitation (Evans, 1996; McAllister & Arciniegas, 2002).

There is no universally accepted definition of MTBI, although the NCIPC conceptually defines MTBI as any period of observed or self-reported loss of consciousness lasting less than 30 minutes, dysfunctional memory for the time around the injury, and observed signs of neurological or neuropsychological dysfunction (e.g., seizure, headache, dizziness, irritability; Iverson, Lange, Gaetz, & Zasler, 2007). Clients with uncomplicated MTBI (e.g., no visible brain abnormality on CT scan) may perform poorly on neuropsychological tests initially, but for the majority of individuals, the symptoms are self-limiting and follow a predictable recovery course. There is a group of patients who sustained MTBI who present with a poor long-term outcome and complaints of symptoms labeled a *post-concussion syndrome*. This "miserable minority" (Ruff, Camenzuli, & Mueller, 1996) may benefit from comprehensive intervention programs that couple educational information with short-term cognitive and supportive therapy (Paniak, Toller-Lobe, Durand, & Nagy, 1998; Paniak, Toller-Lobe, Reynolds, Melnyk, & Nagy, 2000).

The occupational therapy evaluation and intervention described in these guidelines are more appropriate to the client who sustains a more severe brain injury.

■ ■ ■

Occupational Therapy Process for Adults With Traumatic Brain Injury

Traumatic brain injury (TBI) often is referred to as the "silent epidemic" because the cognitive and emotional impairments resulting from the injury are not always apparent to the general public (Rutland-Brown, Langlois, Thomas, & Xi, 2006). Current criteria for reimbursement of medical rehabilitation services are more focused on functional limitations resulting from motor impairments than from cognitive and behavioral impairments (Katz, Zasler, & Zafonte, 2007). This contributes to difficulties providing coordinated and comprehensive evaluation and rehabilitation addressing the multitude of underlying impairments that can lead to the functional impairments.

While strong evidence exists that more-intensive multidisciplinary rehabilitation is associated with earlier functional gains (Cope & Hall, 1982; High, Roebuck-Spencer, Sander, Struchen, & Sherer, 2006; Mackay, Bernstein, Chapman, Morgan, & Milazzo, 1992; Mysiw, Fugate, & Clinchot, 2007; Sirois, Lavoie, & Dionne, 2004; Zhu, Poon, Chan, & Chan, 2007), the balance between the cost-effectiveness (i.e., length of hospitalization) and intensity of rehabilitation has not been determined. The chronic and evolving nature of TBI makes it difficult to determine the optimal amount of intervention an individual will need at the initiation of services (Teasell et al., 2007). Because many factors contribute to length of stay, and these factors have not been controlled in the existing studies (only a small percentage of studies use a randomized controlled study design), there is only moderate evidence that inten-

sive rehabilitation leads to shorter hospitalizations and reduced costs, although more-intensive rehabilitation is strongly linked to earlier functional gains (Turner-Stokes, Disler, Nair, & Wade, 2005).

TBI typically occurs during later stages of adolescence or early adulthood, disrupting periods of life that involve educational and social development, employment, marital and family relationships, and adult independence (Katz et al., 2007). The extended natural history and lifelong impairments and limitations associated with TBI may permanently change the individual's ability to engage in meaningful occupations and participate in valued roles within his or her community (CDC, 1999). Transportation, government policies, attitudes, and the natural environment also may present barriers for individuals with TBI, preventing them from fully participating in their communities and society (Fraas, Balz, & DeGrauw, 2007; Whiteneck, Gerhart, & Cusick, 2004). Occupational therapists may focus on direct service to individual clients with TBI or may work to support social policies, actions, and laws that allow all individuals with TBI to engage in occupations that provide purpose and meaning in their lives (AOTA, 2008b).

Individuals who have sustained a TBI often have physical and cognitive limitations that require rehabilitation services from occupational therapy practitioners.[2] Because of the wide variety of pathophysiological impairments, severities, and problems that can occur as a result of the brain injury, occupational

---

[2]When the term *occupational therapy practitioner* is used in this document, it refers to *occupational therapists* and *occupational therapy assistants* (AOTA, 2006).

therapists who work with clients who have sustained TBIs utilize every intervention strategy learned in their educational preparation—biomechanical, neurological, and psychosocial, often combining restorative and compensatory intervention approaches to address clients' valued activities and occupations.

Stages of Recovery

As a group, people who sustain a TBI and survive the initial acute care phase of care experience long-term disability regardless of the severity of the injury, requiring more postinjury hospitalizations, greater lengths of stay, and greater physician claim rates compared to the general population (Cameron, Purdie, Kliewer, & McClure, 2008). Individuals who sustain a TBI may receive occupational therapy intervention in a variety of settings for various lengths of time. A client's movement through the rehabilitative system may not be linear due to individual needs and regional availability of TBI-related services. Even after the initial brain injury and rehabilitation phases, periodic short-term rehabilitation may be necessary as the client faces new challenges in his or her community, where existing

intervention strategies need modification to support independence and participation. An example of such a situation would be a teenage client who returned to high school following a TBI who functions well within the supported learning and home living environments but requires short-term outpatient occupational therapy services to assist in the transition to college studies and dorm living. The client's existing cognitive strategies and environmental supports may require modification for the new task demands and environmental challenges. This same client may require additional short-term occupational therapy services when making the transition from college life to independent community living and employment.

The Rancho Level of Cognitive Functioning Scale (LCFS; Hagen, Malkmus, & Durham, 1972) is commonly used to describe recovery of cognitive and behavioral functioning in individuals with TBI. The original 8-level scale, expanded by Hagen (1998) to 10 levels (see Table 1), describes clients ranging from those with an absence of purposeful responses (e.g., coma) through those with community levels of recovery and ability to display purposeful and appropriate behaviors. This document is organized according to

Table 1. Rancho Los Amigos Levels of Cognitive Functioning

Rancho Cognitive Level	Cognitive, Behavioral, Psychosocial, and Functional Characteristics
Level I: No Response Total assistance	▪ Complete absence of observable change in behavior when presented with visual, auditory, tactile, proprioceptive, vestibular, or painful stimuli
Level II: Generalized Response Total assistance	▪ Demonstrates generalized reflex response to painful stimuli ▪ Responds to repeated auditory stimuli with increased or decreased activity ▪ Responds to external stimuli with generalized physiological changes, gross body movement, and/or nonpurposeful vocalization ▪ Responses noted above may be the same regardless of type and location of stimulation ▪ Responses may be significantly delayed
Level III: Localized Response Total assistance	▪ Demonstrates withdrawal or vocalization to painful stimuli ▪ Turns toward or away from auditory stimuli ▪ Blinks when strong light crosses visual field ▪ Visually follows moving object passed within visual field ▪ Responds to discomfort by pulling tubes or restraints ▪ Responds inconsistently to simple commands ▪ Responses directly related to type of stimulus ▪ May respond to some people (especially family and friends) but not to others

Table 1. Rancho Los Amigos Levels of Cognitive Functioning *(cont.)*

Rancho Cognitive Level	Cognitive, Behavioral, Psychosocial, and Functional Characteristics
Level IV: Confused/Agitated Maximal assistance	▪ Alert and in heightened state of activity ▪ Purposeful attempts to crawl out of bed or remove restraints or tubes ▪ May perform motor activities such as sitting, reaching, and walking, but without any apparent purpose or upon another's request ▪ Very brief and usually nonpurposeful moments of sustained, alternating, and divided attention ▪ Absent short-term memory ▪ May cry or scream out of proportion to stimulus even after its removal ▪ May exhibit aggressive or flight behavior ▪ Mood may swing from euphoric to hostile with no apparent relationship to environmental events ▪ Unable to cooperate with treatment efforts ▪ Verbalizations frequently are incoherent or inappropriate to activity or environment
Level V: Confused, Inappropriate, Nonagitated Maximal assistance	▪ Alert, not agitated, but may wander randomly or with a vague intention of going home ▪ May become agitated in response to external stimulation or lack of environmental structure ▪ Not oriented to person, place, or time ▪ Frequent brief periods of nonpurposeful sustained attention ▪ Severely impaired recent memory, with confusion of past and present in reaction to ongoing activity ▪ Absent goal-directed problem-solving and self-monitoring behavior ▪ Often demonstrates inappropriate use of objects without external direction ▪ May be able to perform previously learned tasks when structure and cues are provided ▪ Unable to learn new information ▪ Able to respond appropriately to simple commands fairly consistently with external structures and cues ▪ Responses to simple commands without external structure are random and nonpurposeful in relation to command ▪ Able to converse on a social, automatic level for brief periods of time when provided external structure and cues ▪ Verbalizations about present events become inappropriate and confabulatory when external structure and cues are not provided
Level VI: Confused, Appropriate Moderate assistance	▪ Inconsistently oriented to person, time, and place ▪ Able to attend to highly familiar tasks in nondistracting environment for 30 minutes with moderate redirection ▪ More depth and detail of remote memory than of recent memory ▪ Vague recognition of some staff ▪ Able to use assistive memory aid with maximum assistance ▪ Emerging awareness of appropriate response to self, family, and basic needs ▪ Moderate assistance needed to resolve barriers (problem solve) to task completion ▪ Supervised for old learning (e.g., self-care) ▪ Shows carry-over for relearned familiar tasks (e.g., self-care) ▪ Maximum assistance for new learning with little or no carry-over ▪ Unaware of impairments, disabilities, and safety risks ▪ Consistently follows simple directions ▪ Verbal expressions appropriate in highly familiar and structured situations
Level VII: Automatic-Appropriate Minimal assistance for routine daily living skills	▪ Consistently oriented to person and place within highly familiar environments; moderate assistance for orientation to time ▪ Able to attend to highly familiar tasks in a nondistracting environment for at least 30 minutes with minimal assistance to complete tasks ▪ Able to use assistive memory devices with minimal assistance ▪ Minimal supervision for new learning; demonstrates carry-over of new learning ▪ Initiates and carries out steps to complete familiar personal and household routines, but has shallow recall of what he or she has been doing ▪ Able to monitor accuracy and completeness of each step in routine personal and household activities of daily living (ADLs) and modify plan with minimal assistance ▪ Superficial awareness of his or her condition but unaware of specific impairments and disabilities and the limits they place on his or her ability to safely, accurately, and completely carry out household, community, work, and leisure tasks

(continued)

Table 1. Rancho Los Amigos Levels of Cognitive Functioning *(cont.)*

Rancho Cognitive Level	Cognitive, Behavioral, Psychosocial, and Functional Characteristics
Level VII: Automatic-Appropriate *(cont.)*	<ul><li>Unrealistic planning; unable to think about consequences of a decision or action</li><li>Overestimates abilities</li><li>Unaware of others' needs and feelings; unable to recognize inappropriate social interaction behavior</li><li>Oppositional or uncooperative</li></ul>
Level VIII: Purposeful and Appropriate Standby assistance for routine daily living skills	<ul><li>Consistently oriented to person, place, and time</li><li>Independently attends to and completes familiar tasks for 1 hour in a distracting environment</li><li>Able to recall and integrate past and recent events</li><li>Uses assistive memory devices to recall daily schedule, create to-do lists, and record critical information for later use with standby assistance</li><li>Initiates and carries out steps to complete familiar personal, household, community, work, and leisure routines with standby assistance; can modify the plan when needed with minimal assistance</li><li>Requires no assistance once new tasks or activities are learned</li><li>Aware of and acknowledges impairments and disabilities when they interfere with task completion, but requires standby assistance to take appropriate corrective action</li><li>Thinks about consequences of a decision or action with minimal assistance</li><li>Overestimates or underestimates abilities</li><li>Acknowledges others' needs and feelings and responds appropriately with minimal assistance</li><li>Depressed, irritable; low tolerance for frustration; easily angered and argumentative</li><li>Self-centered</li><li>Uncharacteristically dependent or independent</li><li>Able to recognize and acknowledge inappropriate social interaction behavior while it is occurring; takes corrective action with minimal assistance</li></ul>
Level IX: Purposeful and Appropriate Standby assistance on request for daily living skills	<ul><li>Independently shifts back and forth between tasks and completes them accurately for at least 2 consecutive hours</li><li>Uses assistive memory devices to recall daily schedule, create to-do lists, and record critical information for later use with assistance when requested</li><li>When asked, initiates and carries out steps to complete familiar personal, household, work, and leisure tasks independently; completes unfamiliar personal, household, work, and leisure tasks with assistance</li><li>Aware of and acknowledges impairments and disabilities when they interfere with task completion and takes appropriate corrective action; requires standby assistance to anticipate a problem before it occurs and take action to avoid it</li><li>When asked, able to think about consequences of decisions or actions with assistance</li><li>Accurately estimates abilities but requires standby assistance to adjust to task demands</li><li>Acknowledges others' needs and feelings and responds appropriately with standby assistance</li><li>May continue to be depressed</li><li>May be easily irritable</li><li>May have low tolerance for frustration</li><li>Able to self-monitor appropriateness of social interaction with standby assistance</li></ul>
Level X: Purposeful and Appropriate Modified independent	<ul><li>Able to handle multiple tasks simultaneously in all environments but may require periodic breaks</li><li>Able to independently procure, create, and maintain own assistive memory devices</li><li>Independently initiates and carries out steps to complete familiar and unfamiliar personal, household, community, work, and leisure tasks; may require more than the usual amount of time or compensatory strategies to complete them</li><li>Anticipates impact of impairments and disabilities on ability to complete ADLs and takes action to avoid problems before they occur; may require more than the usual amount of time or compensatory strategies</li><li>Able to think independently about consequences of decisions or actions but may require more than the usual amount of time or compensatory strategies to select the appropriate decision or action</li><li>Accurately estimates abilities and independently adjusts to task demands</li><li>Able to recognize the needs and feelings of others and automatically respond in an appropriate manner</li><li>May be periodically depressed</li><li>Irritability and low tolerance for frustration when sick, fatigued, or under emotional stress</li><li>Social interaction behavior is consistently appropriate</li></ul>

Source. Adapted from *Rancho Los Amigos Levels of Cognitive Functioning* (3rd ed.), by C. Hagen, 1998, Downey, CA: Los Amigos Research and Educational Institute. Copyright © 1998 by the Los Amigos Research and Educational Institute. Adapted with permission.

three general stages of recovery from a TBI on the basis of the LCFS:

- The coma stage immediately following the brain injury (LCFS Levels I–III)
- The acute rehabilitation stage (LCFS Levels IV–VI), and
- The community stage (LCFS Levels VII–X).

Occupational therapy evaluation and intervention will vary on the basis of a client's stage and pattern of recovery from TBI, the intervention setting, the environment in which the individual with TBI resides, and the extent of neurological and other impairments resulting from the traumatic event. In addition, each person's individual goals and interests will influence the occupational therapy process significantly. Occupational therapists working with clients recovering from TBI expand the focus of their intervention from skilled intervention focused on prevention of potential complications due to existing impairments to include more client-centered, occupation-based goals as clients emerge from coma and are able to share desired outcomes. Collaboration with family members is crucial, as clients with memory and other cognitive impairments may have limited insight into how their present level of functioning might limit engagement in previously valued roles and occupations.

Many, but not all, individuals who sustain a TBI experience a coma for several days or weeks. During the coma stage of recovery, the client typically is hospitalized in an intensive care unit (ICU), a designated TBI unit, or a neurological unit. The focus of occupational therapy intervention is on improving underlying client factors, preventing secondary impairments to create a positive potential for improved occupational performance upon return of alertness and awareness, and restoring motor and cognitive function. As clients emerge from coma, they experience a vegetative state consisting of spontaneous eye opening and sleep–wake cycles. Although a few clients remain permanently vegetative, most individuals with TBI move into a minimally conscious state with inconsistent ability to follow commands and no reliable interactive communication (Giacino, Katz, & Schiff, 2007).

As clients enter the rehabilitation stage of recovery, they typically reside temporarily at a rehabilitation facility or a subacute facility, where they participate in an integrated program of rehabilitation therapies. The initial goals of preventing development of secondary impairments and maximizing recovery continue during rehabilitation with the addition of two important foci:

- Promoting performance skills and activity patterns within the parameters of reemerging motor and cognitive function
- Promoting safe and independent task performance within the parameters and constraints of available recovery.

The community stage of recovery begins with discharge from an inpatient rehabilitation program and may continue for years after the injury. The client initially may participate in continued rehabilitation services in a day program or outpatient setting. Many clients with TBI can function safely in their own homes and communities but need periodic rehabilitation even after the completion of outpatient services when faced with transitions to new roles or environments requiring adaptation of strategies, skills, and time use patterns to meet the new challenges. Some clients, many years after their injury, reach a phase of acceptance of the physical and cognitive changes resulting from the injury and seek focused rehabilitation services to improve their quality of life and ability to cope with the changes in life roles and occupations. Other clients with TBI living in the community may need lifelong support and supervision to structure their daily activities and use of time.

Occupational therapists may provide community-based intervention for individuals with TBI in settings such as the client's home, outpatient rehabilitation programs, community reentry programs, comprehensive day treatment programs, residential community reintegration programs, neurobehavioral programs, supported living programs, independent living centers, clubhouse programs, school-based educational programs, and vocational rehabilitation programs. Occupational therapists working in some of these environments may provide more group (Dahlberg et al., 2007) or population-based interventions using a consultative service delivery model. Finally, some clients with TBI with more limited recovery or family resources may be discharged to long-term nursing homes, not always equipped to manage a younger client, where they strive to maintain independent activity performance and meaningful role engagement within a supported environment.

Boxes 1–3 present case studies illustrating the occupational therapy evaluation and intervention process with clients in the various stages of recovery.

Referral

A referral for occupational therapy services for individuals with TBI is appropriate at many phases of recovery. During initial hospitalization after the injury, a referral generated by a physician typically requests rehabilitative services, including occupational therapy, to provide preventive intervention such as positioning in the bed and wheelchair, splinting or serial casting, range of motion (ROM) of the limbs, and possibly sensory stimulation. Early evaluation and intervention

---

Box 1. Case Study: Coma Stage of Recovery

Ben, a 17-year-old with an adventurous spirit, never backed down from a challenge. When dared to try to ski a double black diamond course that exceeded his skiing skills, Ben accepted and took the chair lift to the top of the slope with his three friends who were more experienced skiers. No one wore a helmet—it just wasn't cool. Halfway down the slope, Ben lost control and skied off course, hitting a tree. When his friends went to his aid, they found Ben unconscious with blood coming from his nose and ears. He had skin abrasions and a growing lump on his forehead. One of Ben's friends called the ski patrol at the lodge, and within 3 minutes, 2 members of the patrol arrived. The rescue skiers, who had recently completed an outdoor emergency training course, took Ben's vital signs and were concerned that he might have sustained a brain injury. They immediately called for additional aid and an ambulance to transport Ben to the hospital once they got him down the mountain in a rescue litter.

Ben was admitted to the neurotrauma ICU of the regional trauma center. He underwent a craniotomy to evacuate a frontotemporal hematoma and place a ventriculo–peritoneal pressure gauge to monitor and treat his elevated intracranial pressure. Two days after surgery, Ben was in a coma with a Glasgow Coma Scale (GCS; Jennett & Bond, 1975) score of 5. His neurologist referred him for occupational therapy and physical therapy.

Peter, an occupational therapist with experience treating individuals with TBI, went to see Ben on the third day of his hospitalization. He noted Ben's left arm was pulled in tight to his chest with the elbow bent (i.e., decorticate position) and that Ben had endotracheal and nasogastric tubes in place to ensure adequate ventilation and nutrition. Ben's parents were sitting by his bed, and although his mother was speaking to him and rubbing his arm, Ben's eyes were closed, and he was unresponsive. Peter spent a few minutes explaining occupational therapy and the purpose of his initial visit. Because Ben was unable to participate in an occupational profile interview, Peter asked Ben's parents to tell him how Ben spent a typical day before his injury, the things he liked and disliked, and his leisure interests. Peter also gave Ben's parents a checklist of descriptive words to gain insight into Ben's personality and personal values and suggested items that the family could bring in from home that would be helpful to the rehabilitation team (e.g., photos of family and friends with labels on the back, a favorite T-shirt, audiotapes of his favorite music).

Due to Ben's state of unconsciousness, Peter's evaluation was limited to PROM, muscle tone (documenting the posturing of his left arm), and Ben's ability to respond to basic stimulation such as touch and auditory commands. Peter charted Ben's responses to stimulation on the Coma Recovery Scale–Revised (CRS–R; Giacino, Kalmar, & Whyte, 2004). Ben's initial score on the CRS–R was a 2 out of a possible 23 points because he showed only a flexion withdrawal to noxious stimuli on both upper extremities.

by the rehabilitation team, including the occupational therapist, is recommended shortly after admission to the acute hospital setting (Katz et al., 2007). Transfer to a rehabilitation unit or facility will depend upon the patient's medical stability, level of dependency, safety, and need for further rehabilitation in an inpatient setting. If acute inpatient rehabilitation is recommended, a referral from a neurologist or physiatrist will request comprehensive evaluation and intervention from multiple members of the rehabilitation team, including occupational therapy. Occupational therapy's unique focus on engagement in valued occupations and roles to promote recovery and participation in one's home and community are an integral component of interdisciplinary rehabilitative services provided in a variety of facility and community-based treatment programs.

During the first 2 weeks of Ben's hospitalization, when he remained in a coma, Peter focused his occupational therapy intervention on preventing secondary physical changes, such as tissue contractures and loss of ROM, as well as a trial of a coma stimulation program. Peter monitored Ben's vital signs for any physiological changes that might indicate a response to the stimuli or require him to stop the session. Peter provided twice-daily PROM and sensory stimulation and began a serial casting program for Ben's left elbow to try to decrease the flexor tone and his posturing in the decorticate position. Peter left the initial cast on for 3 days, then changed the cast every 5 days, consistently gaining approximately 7 to 10 degrees of PROM with each cast change. Because Ben's parents were frequently present when he treated Ben, Peter instructed them in how to provide PROM to Ben's limbs and how to structure basic coma stimulation techniques. Peter also used these sessions to educate them about what the next few weeks or months of Ben's recovery might entail. He encouraged Ben's parents to contact the local chapter of the Brain Injury Association for additional information and support.

At the beginning of the third week that Ben was in the ICU, Peter noticed increased responses to sensory stimulation. By the end of the week, Ben would inconsistently track his parents in the room, raise his right arm to reach for his mother's hand, and turn his head toward the recorder playing a tape of his favorite band. Peter charted the frequency and consistency of Ben's responses on the CRS–R grid, and his score had improved to 11/23. During Ben's fourth week in the ICU, the neurologist and neurosurgeon felt that Ben's status had stabilized, and he was transferred to a room on the inpatient rehabilitation floor of the trauma center, where Peter continued as his therapist. Ben's GCS was now a 12, his CRS–R was 18/23, and the team scored him as Rancho Los Amigos Level III. Although no longer in coma, Ben was considered minimally responsive.

On the rehabilitation floor of the trauma center, Ben continued to show purposeful responses to environmental stimuli with increasing consistency. Peter continued to focus the occupational therapy intervention on restoring Ben's underlying client factors (i.e., mental, sensory, neuromusculoskeletal, and movement-related functions) and performance of basic self-care activities (e.g., personal hygiene and grooming, upper-extremity dressing, feeding) while addressing his sensory and perceptual, motor and praxis, cognitive, and communication and social skills.

Jamie, the physical therapist, and Peter cotreated Ben on many occasions. Jamie helped support Ben to sit on a therapy mat while Peter had Ben perform simple, purposeful motor acts (e.g., throwing a softball, reaching for photos of friends, lifting his head to look at his mother or father, pressing a large switch connected to a recorder to hear his favorite music). They also provided Ben with a tilt-in-space wheelchair with a head rest, lap tray, and inserts to help maintain his trunk balance. During his individual sessions with Ben, Peter tried to incorporate simple, purposeful activities, such as picking up a ringing telephone, washing his face and brushing his hair, and lifting a cup to his mouth. Peter continued with the serial casting program for his left elbow. Five weeks after his injury, Ben's tracheotomy was removed, and he was transferred to the rehabilitation hospital. He was demonstrating behaviors consistent with Rancho Los Amigos Level III to IV (agitation).

Box 2. Case Study: Acute Rehabilitation Stage of Recovery

Adam, a 21-year-old Army sergeant stationed in Iraq, was on patrol near Fallujah when an IED exploded near his vehicle. Despite wearing a Kevlar helmet and body armor, the force of the blast caused serious nerve and muscle damage to his right arm and a TBI. After Adam was stabilized by a field combat medic, he was medically evacuated, first to a combat surgical hospital in Balad and then to one in Baghdad, where he underwent neurosurgery to relieve his increased intracranial pressure and remove shrapnel from his right arm. The next day Adam was flown to Landstuhl Regional Medical Center in Germany and 1 week later was transported to the Walter Reed Army Medical Center in Washington, DC, for an evaluation. After a few days at Walter Reed, Adam was admitted to the Polytrauma Rehabilitation Center at the Hunter Holmes McGuire Richmond VA Medical Center for assessment and treatment. At the time of his admission to McGuire, Adam had emerged from a coma that had lasted 5 days.

Julie, an occupational therapist working in the Polytrauma Rehabilitation Center at McGuire, was informed by the physiatrist that a new patient was admitted that morning and that he had written a consult (i.e., referral) for occupational therapy to evaluate and treat. Julie reviewed Adam's chart and noted that Adam had a fiberglass cast on his right forearm and multiple shrapnel wounds both on his right shoulder and face. Seeing no particular precautions, but noting that according to the documentation, Adam appeared to be entering the agitated phase of recovery (i.e., Rancho Los Amigos Level IV), Julie entered his room cautiously and quietly.

Adam was in his bed rocking back and forth, pulling at his bed covers and grabbing the side rails. Julie introduced herself to Adam and his wife Stacie. Adam spoke loudly, inappropriately complimenting Julie, saying, "You're cute, but I'm married." Julie explained that during the next few days she would be evaluating what Adam could do for himself, and they would begin working on his ability to independently engage in self-care tasks and other home, work, and community tasks. Julie asked Adam if she could take a look at his cast and how far he could move his hand and shoulder. Adam had minimal active extension of his fingers, and the PROM of his shoulder was limited in all planes of motion. As Julie neared the end of his shoulder range, Adam cursed loudly at her, stating that his arm hurt. His wife was embarrassed at his language and apologized to Julie. Julie attempted to complete an occupational profile but found that Adam's restlessness and limited ability to attend to requests made gathering information difficult. Julie knew that her ability to administer formalized assessments would be limited by Adam's agitation, but she administered the brief Test of Orientation for Rehabilitation Patients (Dietz, Beeman, & Thorn, 1993).

Adam was disoriented to personal situation (i.e., cause of hospitalization, length of deployment in Iraq), time (day of week, time of day, month, year), place (he thought he was at a hospital in Iraq), and temporal continuity. Adam was in a state of posttraumatic amnesia (PTA); he had no recollections of conversations shortly after they occurred.

Because Adam's wife Stacie was present, Julie used the opportunity to gather background information for the occupational profile. Adam and Stacie were presently stationed at Fort Bragg in North Carolina, but Stacie was staying with friends near McGuire. Julie asked Stacie to provide information about their base housing by drawing plans of each room with the furniture placement. Stacie said she would do her best to draw their home's layout and asked if she could have a friend at Fort Bragg videotape their home. Julie assured her that this information would be helpful to the team and mentioned that it would be helpful if Stacie's friend at Fort Bragg also could send personal videotapes of Adam engaged in everyday activities. This would enable the rehabilitation team to see Adam's normal movement patterns and interaction style. Julie invited Stacie to join the occupational therapy treatment sessions when she could and to give her a call whenever she had questions. Julie also informed Stacie that there was a brain injury support group that met at the hospital on a monthly basis and that she might find it helpful to attend and get support from other families.

The next morning Julie and one of the unit nurses performed the self-care portions of the FIM™ (Granger, Hamilton, Linacre, Heinemann, & Wright, 1993) to contribute to the team's score. Adam required moderate assistance (scores of 3) for grooming and self-feeding and maximal assistance (scores of 2) for dressing and toileting. Julie felt that Adam's agitation was the primary interfering factor at present. Although Adam showed evidence of impaired motor and cognitive skills, his agitation made it difficult for him to benefit from cueing. Julie recommended that nursing staff members help Adam perform self-care tasks at present rather than begin occupational therapy training in the use of adaptive equipment, as Adam's agitation would limit his ability to learn compensatory strategies. Along with the rest of the team, Julie monitored Adam's agitated behaviors using the Agitated Behavior Scale (Corrigan, 1989) during her sessions. She found that providing cues to redirect Adam's attention during periods of agitation appeared to calm him. The team knew that because Adam had no recall of the events leading to the blast or the several days prior to the blast, there was only a small chance his cognitive and personality changes might be the result of posttraumatic stress disorder (PTSD; Sayer et al., 2008). However, because Adam had served 10 months in Iraq prior to receiving his injury and seen several periods of action, he would be closely monitored for PTSD.

During his third week in the McGuire Polytrauma Rehabilitation Center, Adam's PTA began to clear as noted on the Galveston Orientation and Amnesia Test (Levin, O'Donnell, & Grossman, 1979). Adam showed some day-to-day memory but needed multiple cues to recall details of the previous day. His attention continued to be limited, and Julie felt that this significantly affected his memory. Adam demonstrated retrograde amnesia for approximately 1 month prior to his injury and was unable to recall any of the events of the explosion causing his injury. During the week, Julie completed a formalized evaluation of Adam's cognitive and perceptual skills using the Brief Test of Head Injury (Helm-Estabrooks & Hotz, 1991). Adam demonstrated moderate impairments in attention and memory. Adam's awareness of his motor and cognitive impairments was limited to a vague sense that something was wrong, but he was unable to anticipate or judge the difficulty of tasks or his need for assistance. Consequently, his safety was impaired by this lack of awareness and a tendency to be impulsive. Julie compared her findings from the occupational therapy–based cognitive–perceptual evaluations with those conducted by the speech–language pathologist and neuropsychologist to identify Adam's strengths and challenges and patterns to his performance.

Over the next few weeks, Adam continued to show steady improvements. Functionally, he was able to perform basic self-care activities with minimal assistance and moderate cues to sequence dressing and perform morning grooming. During morning self-care activities, Adam made errors (e.g., missing portions of his face when shaving, putting on his shirt inside out without realizing it, putting on his pants prior to his underwear) that appeared related to his impulsivity and lack of attention to details. Julie administered the Assessment of Motor and Process Skills (Fisher, 1993a, 1993b) to gather additional information on Adam's motor and process skills, and she also administered the Canadian Occupational Performance Measure (COPM; Law et al., 1998) to identify the things that Adam wanted or needed to be able to do upon discharge (this information was verified with Stacie because Adam's awareness was still impaired). Specific cognitive skills of attention and memory were evaluated with the Test of Everyday Attention (TEA; Robertson, Ward, Ridgeway, & Nimmo-Smith, 1994) and the Rivermead Behavioral Memory Test–Extended (RBMT–E; Wilson, Clare, Baddeley, Watson, & Tate, 1998). Adam displayed difficulty on all subtests of the TEA (i.e., selective visual and auditory attention, sustained attention, switching attention, divided attention), and although he scored below average on all areas of the RBMT–E, he performed better on tasks that required recognition than on those that required recall. Adam did not appear to use any type of strategies to help him remember information as demonstrated on his performance on the Contextual Memory Test (CMT; Toglia, 1993). On the CMT, Adam scored 6 on both the immediate and delayed recall. He reported that he did not use any particular strategy (e.g., he did not use the context of the restaurant setting to recall items from the restaurant image page) and stated, "I just looked at them." When given recognition cues, he was able to identify correctly 14 of the original 20 items.

(continued)

Box 2. Case Study: Acute Rehabilitation Stage of Recovery *(cont.)*

Adam needed a contact guard to walk because of his impaired balance. Julie discussed modifications to Stacie and Adam's bathrooms and arranged for the delivery of a tub bench and the installation of grab bars in the home prior to Adam's discharge. The cast was removed from Adam's right forearm, and Julie began a ROM and strengthening program as the full extent of the muscle and nerve damage was noted. Adam wore a dynamic hand splint during the day to assist his finger extension and a resting hand splint at night. Julie monitored Adam's motor progress using a dynamometer and pinch meter, along with tests of coordination and hand function (e.g., lifting up different size objects, holding and moving objects, picking up small objects). During functional tasks, such as brushing his hair or shaving his face, Adam frequently switched to using his nondominant left hand out of frustration.

During Adam's fourth week in the rehabilitation hospital, the polytrauma team social worker asked Stacie to complete the Family Needs Questionnaire (Kreutzer & Marwitz, 1989) to ensure that the team addressed her need for health information, emotional support, instrumental support, professional support, community support network, and her level of involvement with Adam's care. Julie and the rest of the team continued to address Stacie's identified needs during family meetings with her and during the treatment sessions she observed.

Julie also used occupation-based interventions with Adam, such as shopping online for music to load onto his iPod,™ performing simple budgeting tasks, folding laundry, making his bed, emptying the dishwasher, and cooking simple meals in the mock apartment set up in the hospital's occupational therapy department. Together they began to explore how Adam could use his PDA to assist his memory. Julie and the other members of the rehabilitation team asked Adam to bring in particular items from his room, to ask his wife and other team members certain questions, and to remember to ask his therapists for particular items at different points in the day. Adam was coached to enter these items into his PDA to cue his recall. They also role-played different scenarios in which entering data into the device would be helpful.

Although Adam was showing improved motor and cognitive skills, he continued to show impaired patterns of performance and needed cues to complete self-care tasks at appropriate times and to establish the performance of these tasks as routine. After 5 weeks as an inpatient in McGuire, Adam was discharged home to Fort Bragg to continue rehabilitation as an outpatient at a rehabilitation facility near the base. On the discharge administration of the FIM, Adam scored as "modified independent" (i.e., score of 6) on the self-care, mobility, and locomotion items of the FIM. He scored as "minimal assistance" (i.e., score of 4) to "supervision" (i.e., score of 5) on the social adjustment/cooperation, cognitive/problem solving, and communication items.

Individuals with TBI who reside in the community in either independent or supportive environments may request referral to intermittent occupational therapy services for a variety of reasons over the long course of recovery:

- A client, previously in a minimally conscious state, may display increased alertness and ability to produce goal-directed volitional behaviors, thus warranting evaluation to determine the ability of occupational therapy intervention to reduce disability and improve quality of life (McMillan & Herbert, 2004; Sbordone, Liter, & Pettler-Jennings, 1995).

- A client with fairly good motor and cognitive recovery may need to develop skills and abilities in performing new tasks because of changes in his or her environment or transitions in life roles. Examples include learning to drive a car, learning to manage the demands of attending college, adapting existing cognitive strategies in a transition from school to employment, adjusting to a new role of spouse or parent (see Box 3), or learning new technology to aid compensation for memory or other residual cognitive impairments.

- Continued motor recovery may necessitate short-term intervention to learn how to use new adaptive equipment for mobility and upper-extremity function (e.g., improvement from wheelchair-level performance of activities to standing or walking) or to adjust existing adaptive equipment to meet changes in body structure or function (e.g., splinting after muscle release surgery or intervention for joint contracture).
- Gradual improvements in cognitive–behavioral impairments may continue long after the acute rehabilitation phase of recovery. Comprehensive occupational therapy evaluation of cognitive and motor skills and functional task performance can determine the client's ability to benefit from cognitive strategy training or task and environmental modification to improve independence in the home and community. Often, the true degree of cognitive impairments is not noted until clients with TBI are discharged to the home and community and face completing complex daily activities within their natural environments. Corrigan, Whiteneck, and Mellick (2004) found that 34% of individuals discharged from acute care hospitals after rehabilitation for TBI expressed a desire for help improving their cognition, 28% for managing stress, and 23% for managing their finances.
- Clients with TBI and social communication impairments, who experience social isolation and limited participation in their communities, may benefit from group intervention focused on pragmatic communication skills, including cognitive abilities, self-monitoring of social interactions, awareness of social rules and boundaries, and emotional control. Intervention, even 1 year after the TBI, can improve overall social integration in work, school, and leisure environments and improve the client's life satisfaction (Dahlberg et al., 2007).

Shortened lengths of stay in acute care and acute rehabilitative care result in a greater demand for outpatient and community rehabilitative services, as well as a greater burden on the family of the individual with TBI (Hawkins, Lewis, & Medeiros, 2005). Postacute rehabilitation has been shown to be effective in improving functional outcome after TBI, even for persons who have reached stable neurologic recovery at 12 or more months postinjury (Coetzer & Rushe, 2005; High et al., 2006; Parish & Oddy, 2007). Families of individuals with TBI identify the need for periodic access to short-term rehabilitation services and long-term life planning during the ongoing recovery from TBI to assist both themselves and the individual with TBI to adjust to the behavioral, cognitive, and mobility impairments that limit independence and participation as an active member of the community (Rotondi, Sinkule, Balzer, Harris, & Moldovan, 2007). Routine periodic evaluation of the individual with TBI should be a component of all rehabilitative services for clients with TBI to ensure that those clients demonstrating change, whether an improvement or decline in status, have appropriate intervention to sustain their ability to engage in meaningful occupations or adjust their daily routines and care. Reduction in disability and improvement in quality of life may be possible.

Evaluation

Occupational therapists perform evaluations in collaboration with the client and target information specific to the desired outcomes. The two elements of the occupational therapy evaluation are (a) the occupational profile and (b) the analysis of occupational performance (AOTA, 2008b). Occupational therapists working with clients with TBI may use standardized and nonstandardized assessments that are specifically designed for use with people with TBI. Occupational therapists should validate clinical observations with data from standardized assessments. Consistent use of standardized assessments across the continuum of care settings during the recovery process enhances continuity of care and allows for retrospective analysis of client outcomes, contributing to the evidence supporting

Box 3. Case Study: Community Stage of Recovery

Dana sustained a TBI in a motor vehicle accident at the age of 25. She participated in the full spectrum of rehabilitative programs after emerging from her coma, including a transitional living program. For the past 2 years she has lived in her community with support from her family to manage new challenges. At the age of 29, Dana married and gave birth to a son within the year. Her family observed that Dana was struggling to adapt her existing strategies for dealing with her residual cognitive impairments (e.g., memory and executive functions). The new challenges of being a spouse and mother appeared to overwhelm her, and her family became concerned for her safety and the baby's safety. Her physician made a referral for occupational therapy to provide an evaluation and intervention focused on improving Dana's IADLs and ability to fulfill the activities she wanted and needed to do as a new wife and mother. Sue, an occupational therapist from a home health agency, set up an appointment to visit Dana in her home during the hour that is typically her son's naptime.

During the first session, Sue asked Dana to describe her typical day and the difficulties she was having. Sue used the Canadian Occupational Performance Measure (COPM; Law et al., 1998) to identify the key areas that were concerning Dana. Sue also used the Mayo–Portland Adaptability Inventory (MPAI–4; Malec, 2005) to gain a broader picture of Dana's ability, adjustment, and participation since her TBI. Because Dana described issues that were related to memory and executive functions, Sue also decided to administer the Contextual Memory Test (Toglia, 1993) and the Profile of Executive Control System (PRO-EX; Branswell et al., 1992) using a task that required Dana to investigate local "Mommy and Me" groups using a computer and phone book. On the COPM, Dana identified 3 areas of her daily tasks with which she was dissatisfied with her performance: completing all her errands in a logical sequence (she reported she frequently forgot items or errands and had to make multiple trips to town), finding time during the day to practice her yoga, and having dinner ready when her husband got home. Sue asked Dana for her interpretation of the safety risks that were reported by her mother and husband. Dana described having twice left the oven on after taking out a roast or dessert she had made for dinner. She credited the incident to fatigue and distraction from the baby crying. Overall, Dana felt she was safe, just overwhelmed to the point that she was confused at times and forgetting tasks.

Sue had Dana completed a modified time configuration assessment to see the pattern of Dana's daily tasks. As with most new mothers, Dana's daily tasks appeared to revolve around her son's needs. Dana had a schedule of daily tasks that she had been following since her discharge from the transitional living center, but the schedule didn't incorporate the tasks of her new role of mother. Dana was proficient in using a memory notebook for personal appointments but reported that she often was confused when she saw her notes indicating a doctor's appointment, as she wasn't sure whether the appointment was for her or her son. Since her injury, Dana had been doing a daily yoga routine each morning just after waking but found that in the morning rush of caring for her son, she hasn't had the time. She reported missing this quiet time to get her head together and to stretch out her muscles and joints. Dana felt the lack of physical exercise was affecting her balance and fatigue level.

Sue visited Dana for several sessions to adapt and develop organizational strategies, modify her external memory aids to incorporate her new life tasks, and help Dana achieve a pattern of her daily life tasks that included some time for herself. Together, Dana and Sue identified a community-based group for new mothers that incorporated yoga with the baby. Dana attended several sessions with her son and reported that she was beginning to perform her daily yoga and used the activity as play time with her son. She reported that the group activity at the local community center also offered emotional support and new friendships. She found names of teenage babysitters in the area and had already used one of the sitters to care for her son one evening so she and her husband could reconnect with the local brain injury support group.

Sue and Dana adapted her daily schedule to have color-coded columns for both her and her son so she could see times in the day when she could focus on completing tasks for herself or household chores. Sue arranged one of her sessions with Dana for a time when her husband Mike and mother could attend. Dana, with the assistance of Sue, explained how she needed their assistance to schedule reminders into her memory notebook and on the wall calendar of family events. Both Mike and Dana's mother agreed to schedule some time during the week when Dana could run errands without her son so she would have less distractions. Sue assisted Dana in making checklists on the computer for typical grocery items needed and typical errands completed when in town.

After 6 weekly sessions, Sue felt Dana had achieved the goals that they had initially established. She told Dana that she was going to discontinue her occupational therapy services at this time, but if new challenges presented difficulty and Dana needed Sue's assistance in meeting the challenges, she should contact her. Sue informed Dana that even if the insurance company was unable to pay for periodic occupational therapy services, Sue was available for private-pay home-based services.

practice. Table 2 provides a brief overview of selected commonly used TBI assessments. More detailed information on many of these TBI-based assessments may be found online at the Center for Outcomes Measurement in Brain Injury (COMBI, 2000).

Occupational Profile

The purpose of the occupational profile is to determine who the client or clients are, identify their needs or concerns, and ascertain how these concerns affect engagement in occupational performance. Information for the occupational profile is gathered through formal and informal interviews with the client and significant others. Conversations with the client help the occupational therapist gain perspective of how the client spent his or her time; what activities the client wants or needs to do; and how the environment in which the client lives, works, and plays supports or hinders occupational engagement. During the initial phases of recovery from TBI, when the client may experience disorders of consciousness or significant confusion and impaired awareness, the occupational therapist may need to take a broad perspective of the client that includes the family, friends, and colleagues and seek information from these people about the occupations and activities in which the client engaged prior to the injury, in addition to his or her typical patterns of performance. Family videotapes of the client engaging in typical occupations

and activities can provide the therapist with insight into the client's mannerisms and personality. Once the client is cognitively capable of contributing personal information, the occupational therapist can informally and formally gather information for the occupational profile during one or more sessions and verify the accuracy of information previously gathered from family and close friends. Developing the occupational profile involves the following steps:

- *Identify the client or clients.*
- *Determine why the client is seeking services.*
  Through interviews or checklists, the occupational therapist assists the client in identifying the current concerns relative to the areas of occupation and performance. This is a critical part of the evaluation and may be revisited throughout the recovery process as the client gains greater insight and experiences physical and cognitive changes resulting in a new or different request for focused intervention. Assessments such as the Canadian Occupational Performance Measure (COPM; Law et al., 1998) may be helpful in setting client-centered goals for occupational performance (Jenkinson, Ownsworth, & Shum, 2007; Phipps & Richardson, 2007; Trombly, Radomski, & Davis, 1998); however, clients experiencing impaired awareness may not be cognizant of changes in their functioning and thus may have difficulty identifying and prioritizing areas that

Table 2. Common Assessments Used by Occupational Therapists With Clients With Traumatic Brain Injury

Assessments Commonly Used During the Coma Phase of Recovery (Rancho Los Amigos Levels I–III)	
Assessments typically focus on state of consciousness and WHO ICF areas of impairments.	
Assessment	**Intended Purpose**
Coma/Near Coma Scale [CNC] (Rappaport, Dougherty, & Kelting, 1992)	An expansion of the levels of the Disability Rating Scale to 5 levels of minimally responsive patients. It is sensitive to small changes in auditory, response to command, visual, olfactory, tactile, pain, and vocalization stimulation. A valid and reliable measure for recognizing low-level patients most likely to respond to further rehabilitation care, justifying ongoing intensive rehabilitation, and preventing premature transfer to lower levels of care.
Coma Recovery Scale–Revised [CRS–R] (Giacino, Kalmar, & Whyte, 2004)	The scale is used to monitor patients with disorders of consciousness. 23 items in the areas of arousal/attention, auditory function, motor function, oromotor/verbal ability, and communication are arranged hierarchically to represent 4 levels of responsiveness: (1) generalized, (2) localized, (3) emergent, and (4) cognitively mediated. Specific stimuli are administered to elicit specific responses, and a patient is given credit for specific responses only if it is the behaviorally defined response for that stimulus. Information obtained can assist with differential diagnosis and treatment planning.
Full Outline of UnResponsiveness [FOUR Scale] (Wijdicks, Bamlet, Maramattom, Manno, & McClelland, 2005)	Consists of four components (eye, motor, brain stem, and respiration) assigned a score of 0 to 4. A score of 4 points would represent a *normal functioning* in each category, while a score of 0 indicates *nonfunctioning*. Developed to address limitations of the GCS in assessing verbal scores in intubated patients and lack of testing brain stem reflexes. Can further distinguish patients with lower GCS scores.
Glasgow Coma Scale [GCS] (Teasdale & Jennett, 1974)	Three ordered subscales (eye opening, motor, and verbal responses) used to serially assess initial severity of brain dysfunction and improvement or deterioration in consciousness level. Overall scores range from 3 to 15, with scores of 8 or less indicating coma.
Western Neurosensory Stimulation Profile [WNSSP] (Ansell & Keenan, 1989)	33-item assessment developed to objectively measure arousal and attention; expressive communication; and response to auditory, visual, tactile, and olfactory stimulation in patients emerging from states of unconsciousness post–severe TBI. Several levels of response are scored, with spontaneous and prompt responses receiving higher scores than cued and delayed ones.

Assessments Commonly Used During the Acute Rehabilitation Phase of Recovery (Rancho Los Amigos Levels IV–VI)	
Assessments typically focus on motor and cognitive skills and WHO ICF areas of impairments and activity limitations.	
Assessment	**Intended Purpose**
Action Research Arm Test [ARAT] (Carroll, 1965; Lyle, 1981)	Measurement of arm motor function using four subtests: grasp (lift up different-size objects), grip (hold and move objects), pinch (pick up small objects), and gross movement (hand to mouth). Developed for use with the patients with stroke population, but also appropriate for use with patients with TBI.
Agitated Behavior Scale [ABS] (Corrigan, 1989)	Reliable and valid serial assessment of the presence and degree of agitation during the acute phase of recovery from TBI.
Assessment of Motor and Process Skills [AMPS] (Fisher, 1993a, 1993b)	Observational measure of the quality of a person's performance of functional tasks. The quality of the person's activities of daily living (ADL) performance is assessed by rating the effort, efficiency, safety, and independence of 16 motor and 20 process skill items. Requires therapist certification to administer.
Brain Injury Visual Assessment Battery for Adults [biVABA] (Warren, 1998)	Quick and reliable standardized assessment of visual processing ability that focuses on identification of the functional limitations resulting from a TBI-related visual impairment to guide treatment planning and identify rehabilitation potential.
Brief Test of Head Injury [BTHI] (Helm-Estabrooks & Hotz, 1991)	Brief and efficient measure of cognitive, linguistic, and communicative abilities of clients with TBI that can track recovery patterns due to sensitivity to small performance changes.

Table 2. Common Assessments Used by Occupational Therapists With Clients With Traumatic Brain Injury *(cont.)*

Assessment	Intended Purpose
COGNISTAT [Neurobehavioral Cognitive Status Screening Examination] (Kiernan, Mueller, & Langston, 1983)	Brief screening of cognitive dysfunction for use in neurosurgical units. Provides profile scores for each of the domains assessed (language constructions, memory, calculations, reasoning, attention, level of consciousness, orientation). Initial test item in each domain is at a near-normal level of difficulty with subsequent items provided only if initial item is failed.
Cognitive Log [Cog-Log] (Alderson, Novack, & Dowler, 2003)	Brief 10-item bedside assessment of general cognitive abilities, including orientation, concentration, memory, and executive skills. Intended for serial use to identify change in gross cognitive status.
Confusion Assessment Protocol [CAP] (Sherer, Nakase-Thompson, Yablon, & Gontkovsky, 2005)	Combination of objective measures of orientation and cognition and clinician ratings of other symptoms of early confusion after TBI. Contains elements of the GOAT, the ABS, the Delirium Rating Scale–Revised (Trzepacz et al., 2001), the Cognitive Test for Delirium (Hart et al., 1996), and the attentional subtest from the Toronto Test of Acute Recovery from TBI attentional subtest (Stuss et al., 1999). Observational subscales address (1) disorientation, (2) cognitive impairment, (3) restlessness, (4) fluctuation in presentation, (5) night-time sleep disturbance, (6) decreased daytime level of arousal, and (7) psychotic-type symptoms.
Family Needs Questionnaire [FNQ] (Kreutzer & Marwitz, 1989)	40-item questionnaire that explores the needs of family members during acute rehabilitation for TBI, seeking their perception of the importance of the needs and the extent to which each need has been met. Needs are analyzed in categories of health information, emotional support, instrumental support, professional support, community support network, and involvement with care.
Fugl-Meyer Assessment [FMA] (Fugl-Meyer, Jääskö, Leyman, Olsson, & Steglind, 1975)	Developed for use with individuals who sustain stroke, the FMA also has been used to assess recovery of motor impairments (i.e., motor performance, balance, sensation, range of movement, pain) in individuals with TBI.
Functional Independence Measure [FIM™] (Granger, Hamilton, Linacre, Heinemann, & Wright, 1993).	18-item, commonly used measurement rating patient functional performance in the areas of self-care, sphincter control, transfers, locomotion, communication, and social cognition on a 7-level scale of disability from "total assist" to "complete independence."
Galveston Orientation and Amnesia Test [GOAT] (Levin, O'Donnell, & Grossman, 1979)	Evaluates cognition serially during the subacute stage of recovery from TBI, measuring orientation to person, place, and time, and recall of events before (retrograde amnesia) and after (anterograde amnesia) the injury. The total GOAT score is obtained by deducting error points from 100. Two consecutive GOAT scores ≥76 are considered an indication that the client has emerged from posttraumatic amnesia.
Kohlman Evaluation of Living Skills [KELS] (Kohlman-Thomson, 1992)	Assesses 17 basic living skills administered in 5 main areas (self-care, safety and health, money management, transportation and telephone, and work and leisure) by interview and task performance. Items are scored as independent or needs assistance.
Lowenstein Occupational Therapy Cognitive Assessment [LOTCA] (Katz, Itzkopvich, Elazar, Averbuch, & Rahmani, 1990)	Standardized, reliable, and valid battery provides baseline data to evaluate cognitive–perceptual abilities and disabilities and assists in developing and evaluating treatment goals.
Modified Ashworth Scale (Bohannon & Smith, 1987)	Commonly used assessment of tone and spasticity using deep tendon reflexes.
Motor-Free Visual Perception Test [MVPT–3] (Colarusso, & Hammill, 2002)	Measures visual–perceptual ability (matching, figure-ground, closure, visual memory, and form discrimination) without reliance on client's motor skills.
Orientation Log [O-Log] (Jackson, Novack, & Dowler, 1998)	10-item serial assessment of orientation to time, place, and circumstances in acute rehabilitation population. Two consecutive O-Log scores ≥25 are considered an indication that the client has emerged from posttraumatic amnesia.

(continued)

Table 2. Common Assessments Used by Occupational Therapists With Clients With Traumatic Brain Injury (cont.)

Assessment	Intended Purpose
Overt Aggression Scale–Modified for Neurorehabilitation [OAS–MNR] (Alderman, Knight, & Morgan, 1997)	A 16-item scale that looks at agitated behavior in four categories: verbal aggression, physical aggression against objects, physical aggression against self, and physical aggression directed at others. Giles and Mohr (2007) developed a reliable extended version of the OAS–MNR.
Test of Orientation for Rehabilitation Patients [TORP] (Dietz, Beeman, & Thorn, 1993)	Criterion-referenced test of orientation to person and personal situation, place, time, schedule, and temporal continuity that can be administered to screen or monitor patient progress. Contains 46 items that can be posed as an open-ended or auditory recognition task.

Assessments Commonly Used During the Community Phase of Recovery (Rancho Los Amigos Levels VII–X)
Assessments typically focus on higher cognitive skills and WHO ICF areas of activity limitations and participation restrictions.

Assessment	Intended Purpose
Awareness Questionnaire [AQ] (Sherer, Bergloff, Boake, High, & Levin, 1998)	Client, family member/significant other, and a clinician independently compare the client's self-awareness of ability to perform various tasks after the TBI to before the injury using a 5-point scale ranging from *much worse* to *much better.*
Behavioural Assessment of the Dysexecutive Syndrome [BADS] (Wilson, Alderman, Burgess, Emslie, & Evans, 1996)	Measures executive function and higher-level cognitive functions with 6 subtests and a 20-item questionnaire that samples the range of real-world problems commonly associated with executive dysfunction. Parallel versions allow for measuring outcome.
Behavior Rating Inventory of Executive Function–Adult Version [Brief–A] (Roth, Isquith, & Gioia, 2005)	A standardized rating scale designed to measure the range of behavioral manifestations of executive function. Compares the client's personal perception of difficulties with those of a parent, spouse, child, or friend.
Brain Injury Community Rehabilitation Outcome–39 [BICRO–39] (Powell, Beckers, & Greenwood, 1998)	39 items structured into 8 domains (personal care, mobility, self-organization, partner/child contact, parent/sibling contact, socializing, productive employment, psychological well-being). All items are rated on a 6-point scale, with some domains rating frequency and other domains rating degree of assistance. Total scores range from 0–195, with lower scores representing better outcome.
Canadian Occupational Performance Measure [COPM] (Law, Baptiste, McColl, Carswell, Polatajko, & Pollock, 1998)	Client-centered, occupation-based assessment in which the client identifies personal goals in areas of occupation (self-care, productivity, and leisure), rating his or her perceived performance and satisfaction with each occupation on a scale of 1 to 10.
Community Integration Questionnaire [CIQ] (Willer, Ottenbacher, & Coad, 1994)	Developed for the TBI Model Systems program, this 15-item questionnaire assesses home integration, social integration, and productivity in employment, volunteer work, or school. It can be administered in person or via telephone to either the individual with TBI or a proxy.
Contextual Memory Test [CMT] (Toglia, 1993)	Evaluates awareness of memory capabilities, knowledge of and spontaneous use of strategies for memory (recall and recognition), and immediate and delayed visual memory. Also has a recognition component.
Craig Handicap Assessment and Reporting Technique [CHART] (Mellick, Walker, Brooks, & Whiteneck, 1999; Whiteneck, Charlifue, Gerhart, Overhosler, & Richardson, 1992)	32 items measure the degree to which impairments and disabilities result in handicaps in the years after initial rehabilitation in the areas of physical independence, cognitive independence, mobility, occupation, social integration, and economic self-sufficiency. Multiple measurements over time can provide insight into adaptation and adjustment to the TBI. A 19-item short form (CHART–SF) is also available.

Table 2. Common Assessments Used by Occupational Therapists With Clients With Traumatic Brain Injury
(cont.)

Assessment	Intended Purpose
Craig Hospital Inventory of Environmental Factors [CHIEF] (Whiteneck, Harrison-Felix, Mellick, Brooks, Charlifue, & Gerhart, 2004)	Assesses the frequency and magnitude of the impact that physical, social, and political environments have as barriers or facilitators to full participation in the community. The 25 items fall under 5 domains (policies, physical and structural, work and school, attitudes and support, services and assistance). Multiple measurements over time can provide insight into adaptation to the TBI and changes in environmental barriers. A 12-item short form (CHIEF–SF) is also available.
Executive Function Route Finding Task [EFRT] (Boyd & Sautter, 1993)	Flexible test requiring the client to find his or her way from a starting point to a predetermined location within the building, and the route must include at least 5 choice points and 1 floor-level change. The client is required to provide his or her own plan and structure and modify it according to feedback from the environment. Performance is measured on a 4-point scale that rates understanding the task, seeking information, remembering instructions, detecting errors, correcting errors, and ability to stick with the task (or task behavior).
Functional Assessment Measure [FAM] (Hall, 1997)	Expansion of the FIM to include 12 items related to community functioning (e.g., car transfers, employability, adjustment to limitations, swallowing function). Used in conjunction with the FIM as the FIM+FAM.
Independent Living Scales [ILS] (Loeb, 1996)	Measures competence in IADLs, including memory, orientation, managing money, managing home and transportation, health and safety, and social adjustment.
Mayo–Portland Adaptability Inventory [MPAI–4] (Malec, 2005)	35-item inventory designed to assist in the evaluation of people during the community phase of recovery from TBI. Items representing typically experienced physical, cognitive, emotional, behavioral, and social problems post-TBI are analyzed on three indices: ability, adjustment, and participation.
Motor Assessment Scale [MAS] (Carr, Shepherd, Nordholm, & Lynne, 1985)	Although this performance-based scale was developed as a means of assessing everyday motor function in patients with stroke, the MAS can provide useful information for the post-TBI population who are experiencing hemiplegia.
Multiple Errands Test [MET] (Shallice & Burgess, 1991)	Ecologically valid measure of executive functioning requiring nonroutine, problem solving, planning, organization, and initiation. The original version is completed in a community shopping area. The MET Hospital Version [MET–HV] can be completed within a hospital environment (Knight, Alderman, & Burgess, 2002).
Neurobehavioral Functioning Inventory [NFI] (Kreutzer, Seel, & Marwitz, 1999)	A 76-item inventory that collects information on a wide variety of behaviors and symptoms commonly encountered in daily living and their frequency and change over time. Identical versions completed by family members and the person with TBI are compared to identify differing perceptions. Often used to evaluate health-related quality of life post-TBI.
OT-ADL Neurobehavioral Evaluation [A-ONE] (Arnadottir, 1990)	Uses activity analysis to relate the results of an occupational therapy ADL evaluation to specific neurobehavioral impairments and to generate a hypothesis about the localization of cerebral dysfunction.
Patient Competency Rating Scale [PCRS] (Prigatano & Altman, 1990)	Evaluates *self-awareness,* defined as the ability to judge current strengths and weaknesses. Client and caregivers independently rate, on a 5-point scale, how easy or difficult it is to carry out each of 30 specific activities. Discrepancies between the client and caregiver's ratings indicate impaired self-awareness. A modified and shortened version of the PCRS–NR is available for use with patients on an acute neurorehabilitation unit (Borgaro & Prigatano, 2003).
Profile of Executive Control System [PRO-EX] (Branswell et al., 1992)	Observational rating scale of behaviors associated with the executive control system: goal selection, planning and sequencing, initiation, time sense, awareness of impairments, and self-monitoring. Observations made while the client performs an unstructured activity (e.g., organizing contents of a desk drawer, finding out how to register to vote).
Revised Observed Tasks of Daily Living [OTDL–R] (Diehl, Willis, & Schaie, 1995)	Behavioral test of everyday problem solving includes nine tasks, representing medication use, telephone use, and financial management.

(continued)

Table 2. Common Assessments Used by Occupational Therapists With Clients With Traumatic Brain Injury (cont.)

Assessment	Intended Purpose
Rivermead Behavioral Memory Test–Extended Version [RBMT–E] (Wilson, Clare, Baddeley, Watson, & Tate, 1998)	Predicts everyday memory tasks that will be difficult. Tests both visual (mainly recognition) and verbal memory (mainly recall). The RMBT–E has two parallel versions to allow re-assessment.
Supervision Rating Scale [SRS] (Boake, 1996)	Rates the level of supervision required on a 13-point scale divided into categories of independent, overnight supervision, part-time supervision, full-time indirect supervision, and full-time direct supervision.
Test of Everyday Attention [TEA] (Robertson, Ward, Ridgeway, & Nimmo-Smith, 1994)	Evaluates three aspects of attention in higher-level clients: selective attention, sustained attention, and attentional switching. Eight subtests use familiar, everyday materials, such as map and telephone book searching, counting elevator beeps on tape, visual elevator floor counting, and lottery ticket reviews. Three parallel versions allow for easy retesting for change.
Toglia Category Assessment [TCA] (Toglia, 1994)	Dynamic assessment of category flexibility that uses 16 plastic utensils of different sizes and colors. Deductive reasoning component consists of a questioning activity that investigates the client's ability to formulate and test different hypotheses, switching of conceptual sets, and problem solving.
Vocational Independence Scale [VIS] (Malec, Buffington, Moessner, & Degiorgio, 2000)	Classifies individual's employment status on a 5-point scale: 1 = *unemployed;* 2 = *sheltered* (work in a sheltered workshop); 3 = *supported* (community-based work with permanent supports or less than 15 hours per week OR volunteer work); 4 = *transitional* (community-based work, at least 15 hours/week, with temporary supports, such as job coach, reduced hours OR enrollment in an educational or training program); 5 = *competitively employed in the community* at least 15 hours per week without external supports.

Assessments Commonly Used Throughout the Phases of Recovery
These assessments may be administered serially throughout recovery to track progress.

Assessment	Intended Purpose
Barthel Index (Mahoney & Barthel, 1965)	Assessment of functional status in 10 ADLs. Scores range from 0–100, with higher scores indicating greater independence.
Caregiver Strain Index (Robinson, 1983)	13-item measure of strain related to provision of care to an individual with disability. Items are divided into employment, financial, physical, social, and time domains. A positive screen (7 or more items rated positively) indicates a greater level of strain and the need for more in-depth assessment and possible intervention.
Disability Rating Scale [DRS] (Rappaport, 2005; Rappaport, Hall, Hopkins, & Belleza, 1982)	Eight-item scale that covers arousability, awareness, responsivity, cognitive ability for self-care activities, dependence on others, and psychosocial adaptability. Covers all three WHO *ICF* categories (i.e., impairments, activity limitations, and participation restrictions) to track individuals with TBI from coma to community. Scores range between 0 and 30, with higher scores reflecting greater disability.
Glasgow Outcome Scale–Extended [GOS–E] (Wilson, Pettigrew, & Teasdale, 1998)	Used to categorize outcome from TBI into one of 8 broad hierarchical categories: dead, vegetative state, lower severe disability, upper severe disability, lower moderate disability, upper moderate disability, lower good recovery, and upper good recovery. Good interrater reliability and content validity have been demonstrated.
Role Checklist (Oakley, Kielhofner, Barris, & Reichler, 1986)	Designed to obtain information on client's perceptions of his or her participation in 10 occupational roles throughout his or her life (e.g., held role in the past, current, or future) and the value they place on those occupational roles. Patterns of role engagement are interpreted and validated with the client.
Sickness Impact Profile [SIP] (Gilson et al., 1975)	Self- or interviewer-administered, behaviorally based measure of health status. 136 everyday activities are divided into 12 categories (sleep and rest, emotional behavior, body care and movement, home management, mobility, social interaction, ambulation, alertness behavior, communication, work, recreation and pastimes, and eating).

might benefit from rehabilitative intervention. In addition, self-ratings of satisfaction on the COPM in community-dwelling individuals may be correlated with anxiety level, suggesting that results should be interpreted in the context of other outcome indicators (Jenkinson et al., 2007).

- *Identify the areas of occupation that are successful and the areas that are causing problems or risks.* On the basis of the client's current concerns, the occupational therapist identifies possible motor, cognitive, and behavioral impairments and environmental barriers and supports related to occupational performance.
- *Discuss significant aspects of the client's occupational history.* Significant aspects can include life experiences (e.g., medical interventions, employment history, vocational preferences), occupational roles, interests, and previous patterns of engagement in occupations that provide meaning to the client's life. These experiences may shape how the person deals with everyday routines and occupations. Familiar and often routine occupations can provide a source of structure during confusional states in the early stage of recovery.
- *Determine the client's priorities and desired outcomes.* At various points in the provision of occupational therapy services, the occupational therapist and the client and/or family will discuss and prioritize outcomes so that the therapist's evaluation and intervention will match the client's/family's desired outcomes. Early in recovery, the client and family may be unable to share their hopes and desires for the client's future, as the traumatic events surrounding the injury leave them functioning in a state of crisis. Lack of awareness of the typically protracted length of recovery from TBI also may limit the client's and family's abilities to envision the future. As the client progresses through the various stages of recovery, the occupational therapist should revisit the priorities and desired outcomes with the client and family. Adjustment to both the temporary and permanent impairments resulting from the TBI and the functional limitations may result in

the client and family changing the focus of their priorities and desired outcomes. The occupational therapist may need to refer the client to additional professionals to achieve some of the desired outcomes.

Analysis of Occupational Performance

Information from the occupational profile is used by the occupational therapist to focus on the specific areas of occupation and the context and environment in which the client will live and function. During the early phases of recovery, an occupational therapist may not be able to focus on occupational performance because the client's ability to engage in purposeful and goal-directed behavior is limited by coma or confusional states. During this period of rehabilitation, the occupational therapist may address underlying impairments that have the potential to interfere with occupational performance upon the return of mental alertness and purposeful behavior. When the occupational therapist is able to analyze occupational performance, the following steps are generally included:

- Observe the client as he or she performs the occupations in the natural or least-restrictive environment (when possible), and note the effectiveness of the client's performance skills (e.g., motor and praxis, sensory–perceptual, cognitive, emotional regulation, communication and social) and performance patterns (e.g., habits, routines, rituals, roles).
- Select specific assessments and evaluation methods that will identify and measure the factors related to the specific aspects of the domain that may be influencing the client's performance. These assessments may focus on the client's body structures and functions, activity performance, or community participation. See Table 2 for examples of selected assessments.
- Interpret the assessment data to identify what supports or hinders performance.
- Develop or refine a hypothesis regarding the client's performance (i.e., identify underlying impairments or performance skill limitations that may be influencing occupational performance

in multiple areas, such as memory impairments affecting morning hygiene, home management tasks, work tasks, and social interaction).

- Develop goals in collaboration with the client and possibly the family that address the client's desired outcomes.
- Identify potential intervention approaches, guided by best practice and the evidence, and discuss them with the client and/or family.
- Document the evaluation process and communicate the results to the appropriate team members and community agencies.

Areas of Occupation

Evaluation of various areas of occupation relevant to the client's age and previous lifestyle are performed as the client emerges from coma and is able to perform activities of daily living (ADLs) and instrumental activities of daily living (IADLs). Because individuals often experience TBI at a young age (CDC, 2006; Katz et al., 2007) and can live for many years after the injury (Brown et al., 2004; Shavelle, Strauss, Day, & Ojdana, 2007), clients may need periodic reevaluation of their rehabilitative needs throughout life as developmental changes occur and they assume new roles involving new areas of occupation (Poole et al., 2007). See Box 3 for an example of a client with new rehabilitative needs several years after the brain injury.

Occupational therapists may elect to use an evaluation approach that focuses on possible impairments affecting performance of functional tasks (labeled a *bottom-up evaluation* by some occupational therapists) or a evaluation approach that begins by analyzing the roles of the individual with TBI and the areas of occupation that encompass the client's typical day (labeled a *top-down evaluation* by some occupational therapists). In the top-down evaluation approach, deeper analysis of underlying impairments contributing to activity limitations and participation restrictions are explored only if difficulty is observed during performance of the actual occupation. Using a bottom-up approach, the occupational therapist focuses on the client's impairments and generic abilities and makes inferences as to how these might affect performance in present

and future occupations. The choice of evaluation approach is partially influenced by the client's ability to engage actively in the evaluation process. During the evaluation process, the occupational therapist may move between a top-down and bottom-up approach, depending on the phase of recovery and the client's expressed desired outcomes. An occupational therapist evaluating a client emerging from coma may choose to employ a bottom-up approach due to the client's limited ability to engage actively in the evaluation process, whereas an occupational therapist first meeting a client in a community setting more typically would engage in a top-down evaluation process focused on the client's performance skills and occupational roles. Occupational therapists are skilled at analyzing the interaction among the underlying skills possessed by the client, the demands of the activity on these skills, and the barriers or supports offered by the environment in which the activity is performed.

Performance Skills

The evaluation of individuals with TBI includes overt and subtle factors that may affect performance. *Performance skills*, the observable elements of action of an occupation, can be subdivided into motor and praxis, sensory–perceptual, cognitive processing, emotional regulatory, and communication and social skills. Individuals who sustain a TBI may present with deficits in any or all of these performance skills. Motor and praxis deficits such as spasticity, ataxia, apraxia, balance and vestibular disorders, and weakness and deconditioning are common in clients with TBI (Kane, 2006; Sullivan, 2007) and interfere with the performance of many desired occupations, including self-care, work, and leisure.

The most disabling impairments following TBI, whether the injury is mild or severe, are cognitive (Blundon & Smits, 2000; Cicerone et al., 2000). Cognitive deficits include disturbed *executive function* (defined as those integrative processes that determine goal-directed and purposeful behavior and are superordinate in the orderly execution of daily life functions [Cicerone et al., 2000] and include reasoning, planning, concept formation, mental flexibility, aspects of attention and awareness, and purposeful behavior [McDonald, Flashman, & Saykin, 2002]); *attention* (e.g., processing speed, focused attention, divided attention); and/or *prospective memory* (the ability to remember to do things at the appropriate time [Raskin & Sohlberg, 1996]). Ninety-five percent of rehabilitation facilities serving persons with TBI provide some form of cognitive rehabilitation, including combinations of individual, group, and community-based therapies (Cicerone et al., 2000). As part of these rehabilitation programs, occupational therapists use various interventions to remediate these impairments or compensate for their effects on occupational performance (Blundon & Smits, 2000; Wade & Troy, 2001). Occupational therapists devote extensive time to cognitive rehabilitation interventions to diminish activity limitations and participation restrictions in individuals with TBI.

Emotional regulatory, communication, and social skills deficits may contribute to difficulties in social interactions and community participation and often are cited as common contributors to caregiver distress and family dysfunction (Ergh, Rapport, Coleman, & Hanks, 2002; Fraas et al., 2007). Neurobehavioral changes associated with TBI are broad due to the diffuse nature of the injury. Difficulties controlling behavior (e.g., aggression, impulsivity, apathy) or emotions (e.g., irritability, moodiness, apathy) can affect interpersonal communication and relationships (Ashman, Gordon, Cantor, & Hibbard, 2006). Comorbid psychiatric disorders such as anxiety, depression, mania, psychosis, posttraumatic stress disorders, and substance abuse, often combined with cognitive skills deficits, can make full integration back into the community a challenge for individuals with TBI and their families. Occupational therapists, along with other members of the rehabilitation team, should evaluate the neurobehavioral changes that may be contributing to limitations in safe activity performance in the home and community using behavioral checklists such as the Neurobehavioral Functioning Inventory (Kreutzer et al., 1999) and encourage families and caregivers of individuals with TBI to seek emotional support through the regional brain injury support groups.

Client Factors

Client factors are the underlying abilities, values, beliefs, and spirituality; body functions; and body structures that affect the individual's occupational performance. Clients with TBI may experience both primary and secondary impairments as a result of the injury. Due to the traumatic nature of the event leading to the brain injury, they also may experience impairments in multiple body structures and body functions. Common primary impairments are motor paralysis, sensory loss, and cognitive impairments. Early in the rehabilitation process with clients in coma or emerging from coma, the occupational therapist must adopt a bottom-up evaluation approach and assess body structures and functions to determine current potential for improvement and the risk for secondary impairments if these factors are not addressed. Secondary impairments, such as joint contractures or heterotopic ossifications, can present future obstacles to the client's abilities, skills, and performance of valued activities. Most of these assessment procedures require specialized training, which is a core component in occupational therapy education.

The occupational therapist evaluates neuromusculoskeletal and movement-related functions such as joint ROM, muscle length and tone, reflex function, postural alignment, limb edema, and skin integrity to identify problems early and implement intervention to prevent further decline. Loss of ROM and joint contractures due to joint injury, abnormal muscle tone, prolonged immobility, or *heterotopic ossification* (*HO;* an abnormal deposition of bone tissue in the soft tissue surrounding joints) can be seen in the coma and acute care phases of recovery (Kane, 2006; McNeny, 2006).

TBI can impair the skilled coordination of the muscles and nerves that are involved in the ability to safely eat and swallow food and liquids. In addition, neurobehavioral cognitive impairments of impulsivity, impaired attention, and poor initiation can contribute to an increased risk of aspiration during eating. Neurogenic dysphagia (difficulty eating and swallowing due to a neurological disease or injury) is a frequent complication following TBI that can be a contributing factor in the mortality and morbidity of patients (Cope

& Hall, 1982; Halper, Cherney, Cichowski, & Zhang, 1999; Langmore, 1991; Terré & Mearin, 2007). In acute rehabilitation settings, occupational therapists are members of the rehabilitation team that provides evaluation and intervention to prevent aspiration during feeding. They may assist in videofluoroscopic evaluations and bedside evaluations of feeding and swallowing. Together with colleagues in speech–language pathology, occupational therapists may provide feeding programs that modify the texture and consistency of the food and liquids and oral–motor skill exercises to strengthen the muscles and nerves involved in feeding and swallowing, as well as ensure proper positioning of the client during feeding (Avery-Smith, 1996; Avery-Smith & Dellarosa, 1994).

During the coma phase of recovery, the entire rehabilitation team is attentive to the client's behavior during sensory stimulation activities to observe for possible sensory impairments in the senses of touch, temperature, taste, sound, and sight (e.g., cranial nerve injuries). In collaboration with other rehabilitation team members, the occupational therapist evaluates sensory functions in the areas of vision and peripheral senses as the client emerges from coma and is able to consistently respond to yes-or-no questions. Visual impairments, frequently described by the client as headache, dizziness, inability to concentrate, blurred or double vision, fatigue, light sensitivity, and an inability to read (Kane, 2006), should be evaluated in collaboration with ophthalmologists, neuro-ophthalmologists, and optometrists specializing in vision therapy to determine the contribution of the visual impairments to functional and mobility skills.

Occupational therapists, with their holistic approach to care of individuals with TBI, also consider the influence of the client's values, beliefs, and spirituality on the recovery process. These client factors can hold the key to the client's motivation to engage in the therapy process and resilience to work toward regaining independence in those occupations and roles that provided meaning to the individual's life. For example, a therapist can use a client's strong belief in one's personal ability to affect change in one's life and a com-

mitment to resuming a valued family role to motivate the client to work on related client-centered goals in the occupational therapy rehabilitation program.

Although multiple rehabilitation team members may evaluate some aspects of global and specific mental functions, occupational therapists provide a unique contribution to the understanding of the link between cognition and occupational performance (Toglia, Golisz, & Goverover, 2008). Training in analyzing the demands of the activity and environment in which the activity is performed provides the occupational therapist with a holistic perspective of the effect of cognitive impairments on ADLs, IADLs, rest and sleep, education, work, leisure, and social participation of the individual with TBI.

Performance Patterns

Performance patterns are "behaviors related to daily life activities that are habitual or routine" (AOTA, 2008b); they include habits, routines, rituals, and roles. In the acute rehabilitation phase of recovery, when confusion and memory impairments are most evident, individuals with TBI may have difficulty recalling habits, organizing and sequencing routines, and fulfilling their previous life roles. Obsessional symptoms also may be seen as rigidity in one's routines and structure of the environment (e.g., location of personal possessions). These obsessive-like behaviors may be a premorbid tendency, a result of the injury (e.g., impairments in mental flexibility) or compensation for cognitive impairments (Berthier, Kulisevsky, Gironell, & López, 2001; Coetzer, 2004). Impairments in executive functioning may result in difficulty planning and initiating the performance of routines such as morning hygiene or automatically engaging in behaviors that previously were habitual (e.g., placing keys on a hook by the door). Decreased initiation, flexibility, impulsivity, or perseveration may be observed during performance of routine tasks, requiring dependence upon others to monitor the individual's time engagement in occupations and activities. Individuals with TBI living in the community may not efficiently sequence community errands or schedule appropriate time to complete errands. Although the ability to engage in long-standing, well-learned habits and rituals may be retained after the brain injury, the ability to learn new patterns of performance may require multiple practice sessions and environmental cues.

Community-dwelling clients with TBI may be able to verbally describe an appropriate pattern of daily tasks but display difficulty with the volition, planning, and purposeful components of executive dysfunction (Lezak, Howieson, & Loring, 2004). Clients with executive dysfunction, often resulting from prefrontal lobe injuries (Lezak et al., 2004), may show a disassociation between stated intentions and actions. Once engaged in carrying out a planned action, they may have difficulty being flexible and changing their pattern of performance if challenges or barriers are encountered. For example, a client who goes to the grocery store to purchase a particular item may not automatically purchase an alternative if the desired item is not in stock.

Impairments in the ability to establish patterns of performance often are not fully recognized by family members or rehabilitative therapists until the client is discharged to a less-structured environment that has fewer time-oriented routines. Common home and community tasks that require flexible scheduling to deal with novel and unexpected situations may be challenging for clients with TBI (Burgess et al., 2006; Katz & Hartman-Maeir, 2005).

Disturbances in sleeping patterns, including difficulty falling asleep and frequent or prolonged awakenings throughout the night, have been found to occur in 30% to 70% of individuals after TBI (Clinchot, Bogner, Mysiw, Fugate, & Corrigan, 1998). These symptoms are often underreported by clients and family members and may contribute to exacerbation of cognitive problems that affect daily functioning and rehabilitation outcomes. In a small ($N = 11$) group of individuals with TBI, short-term (i.e., 8 weeks) cognitive–behavioral therapy has been shown to reduce insomnia as well as general and physical fatigue (Ouellet & Morin, 2007).

Contexts

Occupational therapists acknowledge the influence of cultural, personal, temporal, virtual, physical, and social–contextual factors on occupations and activities. Environmental factors that support or inhibit occupational performance of individuals with TBI should be identified throughout the evaluation and intervention process.

Cultural

The *cultural context* includes the customs, beliefs, activity patterns, behavior standards, and expectations accepted by the client and his or her cultural group. These often deep-rooted patterns of performance (e.g., shaking hands when greeting someone, waiting one's turn in a conversation, saying prayers prior to meals) can be tapped into early in the TBI recovery process to provide structure to social interactions and daily activities (Kane, 2006). Occupational therapists provide culturally responsive care by displaying an awareness of and sensitivity to the client's cultural beliefs about health and how culture may influence the client's typical activity patterns and occupations. By engaging in culturally competent care, the occupational therapist will incorporate the individual's values, beliefs, ways of life, and practices into a mutually acceptable treatment plan.

Personal

Personal attributes, such as gender, socioeconomic status, age, and level of education, all factor into the evaluation and intervention process. Because TBI can occur at any point across the lifespan, occupational therapists need to ensure that interpretations from standardized assessments compare the client's performance to a normative sample with similar age and educational levels. Patterns of role performance based on culturally and personally defined expectations should be considered.

Temporal

On a large scale, *temporal context* may refer to the time in a person's lifespan that the injury occurred, such as adolescence or adulthood. Temporal context also refers to the phase of TBI recovery, which influences decisions about choice of evaluation tools and treatment interventions. In the initial phases of recovery, when the client is in or emerging from coma, passive observation-based assessments are used to attempt to identify patterns in the client's behaviors that may be reinforced through external stimulation. Passive evaluation of physical impairments in the client's joints and limbs is also possible during the coma phase of recovery.

As the client's range of behavioral responses expands and alertness and awareness of the environment returns, more standardized assessments can be used along with the observation-based assessments to provide a more holistic and comprehensive evaluation of the client's functioning. Given the long natural recovery period from TBI, the client may need periodic reassessment to identify areas of performance as well as occupations and activities that have the potential for change and should be addressed through continuation or re-initiation of occupational therapy services.

During the early phase of recovery, when the client may be receiving care in a neurosurgical ICU, he or she may experience temporal confusion due to the consistency of the environmental stimuli and the rhythm of care activities. Health care staff need to provide some normalcy to typical daily patterns of activity (e.g., hygiene routines) and sleep–wake cycles (e.g., dimming lights, eliminating extraneous noise). The temporal context should be considered when evaluating the client in a confusional state. *Sundowning,* an increase in confusion often seen in clients with dementia, can also be observed in clients with TBI. As the day progresses and light fades, fatigue levels increase and the client may display more signs of confusion and cognitive impairments. The timing of assessments should consider what, if any, effect the time of day has had on the client's performance.

Physical

As the client transitions through the various rehabilitation phases and settings, the occupational therapist evaluates the *physical environment* for supports and barriers to the client's occupational performance. This becomes most important when the client is preparing to be discharged from the inpatient rehabilitation setting to his or her home and community. Evaluation of the client's home, workplace, and commonly used community locations is needed to engage in collaborative problem solving with the client and family. Physical and motor impairments resulting in the need for mobility and ambulation devices, including ramps, stair glides, and bathroom grab bars, may require modification to the home environment. Residual cognitive impairments also may require organization and modification of the home to cue task performance or minimize the demands on the impaired area. Labeling kitchen and clothing closets, organizing kitchen tools and bathroom grooming products, posting orienting information, or color marking salient environmental features such as the medicine schedule may aid the individual in completing everyday tasks.

Social

The *social environment or context* includes the social network of friends, family, groups, and organizations with which the client has contact. These social relationships carry expectations for interaction, and the individual with TBI and cognitive and neurobehavioral problems may be particularly challenged when functioning within the social environment. Difficulty following the pragmatics or interaction rules of social environments (e.g., an inability to follow conversations, being rude, interrupting people, talking too fast or too slowly) can contribute to social isolation. The occupational therapist and the rehabilitation team may need to explore the client's social network at the time of the injury and the possible network that might exist upon discharge. Some clients may have drifted away from family, leaving the family with little knowledge of the client's preinjury lifestyle (McNeny, 2006). These families may be willing to provide care to the client after discharge, so their expectations for the client to be able to return home upon discharge need to be explored.

Virtual

The *virtual environment* is one in which communication occurs by means of airways or computers and an absence of physical contact. Occupational therapists may need to evaluate the client's previous use of technology to interact in the virtual environment (e.g., use of and expertise in e-mailing and text messaging, conversing in chat rooms). The client's comfort level with the tools of the virtual environment may guide the occupational therapist in selecting possible external memory aids (e.g., whether the client consistently schedule appointments into a personal digital assistant [PDA]).

Activity Demands

Determining whether a client may be able to complete an activity depends not only on the performance skills, performance patterns, and client factors of an individual but also on the demands the activity itself places on the person. The demands of an activity are aspects of the activity that include the tools needed to carry out the activity, the space and social demands required by the activity, and the required actions and performance skills needed to take part in the given activity.

During the early phases of recovery when the client is emerging from coma and inconsistently responds to verbal commands and environmental stimuli, the occupational therapist will identify the parameters of the activity demands in which the client is able to best perform. For example, does the client respond better to auditory than visual stimuli? Does the client respond more accurately when limited stimuli are presented in a structured linear arrangement? As the client enters the agitated phase of recovery, the therapist again will analyze various activities to identify those demands or components of the activities that either increase or decrease the client's agitation and self-stimulatory behavior. Selecting intervention activities that meet the client's current level of functioning and do not overly challenge areas of impairment may assist the client in maintaining a calm behavioral state. For example, the occupational therapist may engage the client in gross

movement tasks that are repetitive in nature (e.g., bouncing a ball), minimizing sequencing and timing activity demands. Or the therapist may minimize the objects, space, and rules to engage in familiar or simple cognitively challenging activities to control the client's level of frustration and potential for agitated behavioral outbursts.

Clients with cognitive impairments from TBI may demonstrate varied performance skills on the basis of the demands of the environment and activity. Clients able to perform structured and predictable functional activities within the rehabilitation setting may experience significant difficulty when attempting similar activities in more complex, unstructured, and unpredictable natural settings of the home and community. Occupational therapists, through their use of activity analysis, can identify the type of activity and environment in which the client can perform at his or her best. During the course of occupational therapy intervention, occupational therapy practitioners grade and vary the activity demands of the selected intervention task, and the environment in which it is performed, to provide the client with a "just-right challenge" to be therapeutic without exceeding his or her current level of skills. As the client improves, the therapist gradually modifies the activities to provide more challenge to the client. Therapists assist the clients in their ability to perform under the current environment and activity demands and also consider how future changes in the environment and activity may challenge the client's skill level. Part of the rehabilitation process may include training the client to identify environmental barriers to performance and how to modify the environment to improve performance (e.g., turning off radio and beginning most challenging task first when studying).

Clients with motor impairments from TBI may need adaptive equipment and environmental modifications to engage in the selected activities (e.g., changes to the tools or utensils used in the activity, reorganization of equipment and supplies in the environment). The occupational therapist carefully analyzes the client's need for adaptive equipment and balances the selected equipment and environmental modifications to the client's cognitive ability to learn new ways of approaching and completing activities.

Considerations in Assessments

It is critical that therapists use their knowledge of assessments and clinical judgment to decide which assessments should be selected for each client at a particular time. This careful selection of assessments provides the most valuable data and eliminates the tendency to bombard the client with excessive assessment demands.

Knowledge of the typical recovery pattern seen after TBI (see Table 1) can help the occupational therapist determine when it is most appropriate to focus on various components of the client's occupational performance and the types of assessments to administer. For example, until the client emerges from the coma and agitated phases of recovery, he or she has very limited ability to tolerate or understand standardized assessments with established protocols and strict scoring criteria. During these recovery phases, observationally based assessments can provide clinically relevant information about the influence of environmental contexts on the client's functioning. Careful documentation of observations may help the occupational therapist and rehabilitation team to see patterns in the client's behavior and hypothesize possible underlying impairments to further evaluate as the client becomes able to engage in more standardized assessments.

Standardized assessments of various performance skills and client factors are routinely administered to establish baseline data at the initiation of occupational therapy services and to provide reliable and valid data for quantitative documentation of clients' progress. Periodic reevaluations determine the client's progress and need for continued treatment. In addition, scores from standardized assessments at the time of discharge from occupational therapy services and periodically during the remainder of the client's life can be used to provide outcome data to assess the effectiveness of intervention, determine the client's readiness for more cognitively and physically demanding occupations (e.g., driving, return to work) or less-structured and

supportive environments, and understand the natural course of recovery from TBI.

Occupational therapists vary their approach to evaluating the individual with TBI, shifting their focus among the broad components of health and functioning defined by the WHO (2001) *ICF* classification of impairments, activity limitations, or participation restrictions (see Table 3 for a comparison of the *ICF* language to the *Framework* language). Initially, when the client is in or emerging from coma, the occupational therapist focuses the evaluation process on underlying impairments and targets intervention to prevent secondary impairments. During the acute rehabilitation stage, the occupational therapist dynamically evaluates all three *ICF* components of health and functioning (i.e., body function and structure, activities, and participation) in a holistic and comprehensive manner. While the occupational therapist may continue to focus on addressing impairments in the client's body structure and/or function (labeled *client factors* in occupational therapy language), evaluation and intervention in the areas of activities and participation are broadened in the occupational therapy perspective to consider the interrelationship of the client's areas of occupation, performance skills, and performance patterns, along with the activity demands, environment, and context. Preparing for discharge from acute rehabilitation to the community, the occupational therapist may again shift the focus of evaluation to the client's ability to participate in meaningful roles and activities within the community, focusing on the fit among the client, the desired areas of occupation, and the environment. Level of participation and activity engagement are strong predictors of life satisfaction after TBI (Pierce & Hanks, 2006).

Assessment Instruments

In selecting the most appropriate type of assessment, an occupational therapist first decides the focus of the assessment, given the client's stage of recovery, and what questions need to be answered. If the therapist needs to determine the presence and severity of impairments, a standardized assessment that compares the client's scores with expected performance within the person's age

Table 3. Comparison of the Terminology of the *International Classification of Functioning, Disability and Health* to the *Occupational Therapy Practice Framework*

Publication	Function	Activities and Participation	Contextual Factors
International Classification of Functioning, Disability and Health (*ICF*; World Health Organization, 2001) Classification of health and health-related domains from body, individual, and societal perspectives by means of two lists: body functions and structure, and domains of activity and participation. Because an individual's functioning and disability occurs in a context, the *ICF* also includes a list of environmental factors.	**Body Function and/ or Structures** Mental; sensory and pain; voice and speech; cardiovascular, haematological, immunological and respiratory systems; digestive, metabolic, and endocrine systems; genitourinary and reproductive; neuromusculo-skeletal and movement-related; skin and related structures *(Impairment: Anomaly, loss, or significant deviation from typical)*	**Activities and Participation** Learning and applying knowledge, general tasks and demands, communication, movement, self-care, domestic life areas, interpersonal interactions, major life areas, community, social and civic life *(Disability defined in terms of activity limitations or participation restrictions)*	**Environmental Factors** Products and technology; natural environment and human-made changes to the environment; support and relationships; attitudes; services, systems, and policies **Personal Factors** Gender, age, other health conditions, coping style, social background, education, profession, past experience, character styles *(Environmental and personal factors may influence the person's functioning.)*
Occupational Therapy Practice Framework (AOTA, 2008b) Developed to articulate occupational therapy's contribution to promoting the health and participation of people, organizations, and populations through engagement in occupation.	**Client Factors** Person (values, beliefs, and spirituality) Body structures Body functions	**Performance in Areas of Occupation** ADLs, IADLs, rest and sleep, education, work, play, leisure, social participation **Performance Skills** Sensory–perceptual, motor and praxis, emotional/regulation, cognitive, communication and social **Performance Patterns** Habits, routines, roles, and rituals *(Performance skills and patterns may be modified by activity demands.)*	**Contexts** Cultural Personal Temporal Virtual **Environments** Physical, social

The Occupational Therapy Practice Framework's *emphasis on occupations and outcomes is not addressed in the* ICF *classification.*

Source. Adapted from "Occupational therapy practice framework: Domain and process (2nd edition)," by the American Occupational Therapy Association, 2008, *American Journal of Occupational Therapy, 62,* pp. 625–688. Copyright © 2002 by the American Occupational Therapy Association. Adapted with permission.

group may be selected. If the therapist needs to understand the effect of impairments on occupational performance, a top-down approach using direct observation of function may provide information on how the cognitive or motor impairments affect functional activity performance or community participation (Toglia et al., 2008). Occupational therapists may select dynamic assessments that emphasize the processes involved in learning and change to gather information to guide treatment planning and intervention (e.g., conditions that increase or decrease display of impairments [Grigorenko & Sternberg, 1998]). Performing evaluations that include all three components of functioning as defined by the *ICF* (i.e., body structures and functions, activities, and participation) enables occupational therapists to compile a comprehensive view on the person's functioning.

Because individuals with TBI may have impairments (e.g., motor, praxis, cognitive) similar to other clients with neurological diagnoses (e.g., multiple sclerosis, stroke), occupational therapists may consider using assessments developed for these populations when evaluating the status of clients with TBI. Some of these assessments may be generic enough in their design to provide valid information regarding the recovery of skills in the individual with TBI; however, the therapist should be cautious, as the validity of these assessments with the TBI population may not have been established. It is preferable that occupational therapists select assessments that have proven efficacy in detecting and quantifying the typical pattern of impairments seen in clients with TBI (see Table 2). Keeping current with the published literature on evaluations of persons with TBI provides important information to guide therapists in selecting specific assessments for individual clients.

Intervention

Occupational therapy intervention with individuals who have sustained a TBI may occur at any point along the continuum of recovery. The intervention, guided by information about the client gathered during the evaluation, incorporates a variety of approaches using preparatory methods (i.e., therapist-selected methods and techniques that prepare the client for occupational performance, such as serial casting or sensory stimulation), purposeful interventions (i.e., specifically selected activities that allow the client to develop skills that enhance occupational engagement, such as role-playing of social situations or practicing grocery shopping in a simulated environment), and occupation-based interventions (i.e., client-directed occupations within context that match identified goals, such as interviewing for a job or preparing a meal for one's family). The focus of intervention may shift among establishing, restoring, or maintaining occupational performance; modifying the environment and/or contexts and activity demands or patterns; promoting health; or preventing further disability and occupational performance problems.

During occupational therapy intervention, therapists make demands on persons with brain injury to learn new strategies and relearn old activities and tasks under new environmental, social, and temporal conditions. Many occupational therapists believe that challenging demands to the brain reorganizes brain function beyond spontaneous recovery, yet evidence supporting the efficacy of common rehabilitation intervention for clients with TBI remains limited and tends to support interventions associated with a compensatory rather than restorative approach, at least in the area of cognitive rehabilitation (Cicerone et al., 2000, 2005).

Investigation regarding the evidence to support the question "Can demands that occupational therapists make on patients actually contribute to recovery of brain organization as well as the recovery of behavior that can be observed?" largely has focused on laboratory research concerning brain recovery. This recovery is considered one of the primary intended effects of therapy provided to individuals who have experienced a change in brain functions secondary to brain trauma. Experimental studies on focal brain injuries in rats have demonstrated that environmental enrichment significantly improves functional outcome, increases dendritic branching and number of dendritic spines in the contralateral cortex, influences expression of many genes, and modifies lesion-induced stem cell differentiation in the hippocampus (Johansson, 2003; Will, Galani, Kelche, & Rosenzweig, 2004). The environmental enrichment gives the rats the opportunity to solve motor problems; that is, they are challenged to learn new ways of behaving and concurrent morphological changes occur in the cortex in response to those demands (Ivanco & Greenough, 2000). The capacity to change seems to be a fundamental characteristic of the nervous system, and when the nervous system changes, there is often correlated behavioral change, such as learning, memory, recovery, and so on (Kolb, 2003).

Few humans with brain injury or stroke have been studied. However, some preliminary functional magnetic resonance imaging (fMRI) studies that have been done on individuals with TBI indicate alterations in the pattern of brain activation, suggesting recruitment of more extensive cortical regions to perform tasks that stress computational resources (Levin, 2003), similar to the effects of enriched environments on the rats' brains. Although there is no direct evidence that challenging demands reorganize brain function beyond spontaneous recovery after TBI, case reports suggest that tasks that require mental manipulation of information or solving novel problems do affect brain organization.

Studies provide tentative evidence to suggest that therapeutic interventions that place challenging demands on the brains of persons with TBI reorganize brain function whether the person is in the acute or chronic stage of recovery (Laatsch, Jobe, Sychra, Lin, & Blend, 1997; Laatsch, Thulborn, Krisky, Shobat, & Sweeney, 2004; Page & Levine, 2003; Scheibel et al., 2003, 2004; Tillerson & Miller, 2002). Interventions that place challenging demands include those that require mental manipulation of information in short-term memory, are nonroutine, involve solving novel problems (e.g., relearning to use a weak limb to accomplish ADLs), or require reallocating attention or selecting a response. In other words, studies suggest that brain reorganization is associated with learning new things and relearning old things in a new way.

Intervention Plan

As a part of the occupational therapy process, the occupational therapist develops an intervention plan that considers the client's goals, values, and beliefs; the client's health and well-being; the client's performance skills and performance patterns; collective influence of the context, environment, activity demands, and client factors on the client's performance; and the context of service delivery in which the intervention is provided (e.g., caregiver expectations, organization's purpose, payer's requirements, or applicable regulations; AOTA, 2008b). The intervention plan outlines and guides the therapist's actions and is based on the best available evidence to meet the identified outcomes (AOTA, 2008b).

Once the occupational therapist has identified targeted goals in collaboration with the client or family, the therapist determines the intervention approach that is best suited to address the goals. Some approaches may be more appropriate at various points in the recovery from TBI (see Table 4) than others. The intervention approaches used by occupational therapy practitioners include

- *Prevent,* an intervention approach designed to address clients with or without disability who are at risk for occupational performance problems (Dunn, McClain, Brown, & Youngstrom, 1998); for example, intervention to prevent development of secondary impairments such as joint contractures during the coma phase of recovery;
- *Establish* and *restore,* an intervention approach designed to change client variables to establish a skill or ability that has not yet developed or to restore a skill or ability that has been impaired (Dunn et al., 1998); for example, restoring hand coordination to engage in functional activities such as cooking;
- *Modify* activity demands and the contexts in which activities are performed to support safe, independent performance of valued activities within the constraints of motor, cognitive, or perceptual limitations;
- *Create* or *promote* a healthy and satisfying lifestyle that includes adherence to medication routine, appropriate diet, appropriate levels of physical activity, and satisfying levels of engagement in social relationships and activities by providing enriched contextual and activity experiences that will enhance performance for all persons in the natural contexts of life (Dunn et al, 1998); and
- *Maintain* performance and health that the individual with TBI has previously regained or that neuropathology has spared.

Occupational therapy practitioners also consider the types of interventions when determining the most effective treatment plan for a given client. The types of interventions include therapeutic use of self; therapeutic use of occupations and

Table 4. Occupational Therapy Intervention Approaches and Examples of Their Use With Clients at Various Levels of Recovery From Traumatic Brain Injury

Intervention Approaches Commonly Used During the Coma Phase of Recovery (Rancho Los Amigos Levels I–III) *Interventions typically focus on state of consciousness and WHO ICF areas of impairments.*	
Intervention Approach	**Sample Occupational Therapy Treatment Activities**
Prevent	▪ *Prevent* loss of muscle length and joint mobility by performing ROM, serial casting, tone-inhibiting techniques, and positioning of patient in the bed and wheelchair. ▪ *Prevent* skin breakdown and postural deformities by providing the client with proper body alignment in tilt-in-space wheelchair with head rest, lap tray, gel seat cushion, and trunk inserts and providing nursing staff with a splint-wearing schedule.
Establish/Restore	▪ *Restore* the client's connection to the external environment by positively reinforcing appropriate behavioral responses to sensory stimulation. ▪ *Restore* the client's ability to follow one-step demands for a motor response in relation to sensory stimulation within 15 seconds of request or stimulus.
Modify	▪ *Modify* environment to vary levels of stimulation and prevent accommodation and attenuation to environmental stimuli (e.g., vary lighting, noise level, visual stimulation, temperature).
Maintain	▪ *Maintain* muscle length and joint mobility by instructing caregivers in routine stretching exercises.
Intervention Approaches Commonly Used During the Acute Rehab Phase of Recovery (Rancho Los Amigos Levels IV–VI) *Interventions typically focus on motor and cognitive skills and WHO ICF areas of impairments and activity limitations.*	
Intervention Approach	**Sample Occupational Therapy Treatment Activities**
Prevent	▪ *Prevent* aspiration during feeding by modifying the food texture and head positioning if the client displays signs of dysphagia.
Establish/Restore	▪ *Establish* the client's ability to release energy constructively during agitated periods by providing structured and familiar activities with minimal challenges to areas of impairments. ▪ *Restore* ability to perform self-care by engaging the client in a daily self-care program of showering, dressing, and grooming, providing verbal and physical cues as needed. ▪ *Restore* normal patterns of movement by engaging the client in various functional motor tasks (e.g., grooming, self-feeding, object manipulation) with gradual increases in the unpredictability and complexity of the contextual and activity demands, providing tactile input to guide and normalize movement patterns. ▪ *Establish* skills to safely and efficiently transfer from wheelchair to various surfaces (e.g., toilet, bed, chair, car). ▪ *Establish* and *restore* cognitive skills by teaching cognitive strategies to improve performance; engage in a variety of activities related to roles, responsibilities, and interests (e.g., financial management, cooking, parenting, leisure pursuits). ▪ *Establish* strategies and new routines to accurately use external memory aids to recall scheduled appointments and events and to take medications. ▪ *Establish* habits to ensure accuracy of work (e.g., self-monitoring of work for errors, timely completion, match with instructions).

activities, which includes preparatory methods, purposeful activity, and occupation-based activity; consultation; and education. Although all types of occupational therapy interventions are used for all approaches, the *therapeutic use of self* (i.e., therapist's use of his or her personality, perception, and judgment; AOTA, 2008b) is an overarching concept that should be considered in each therapeutic interaction. Therapeutic use of self is a vital responsibility of the occupational therapist and occupational therapy assistant, as well as all members of the health care team.

Table 4. Occupational Therapy Intervention Approaches and Examples of Their Use With Clients at Various Levels of Recovery From Traumatic Brain Injury *(cont.)*

Intervention Approach	Sample Occupational Therapy Treatment Activities
Modify	■ *Modify* the client's hospital room to provide environmental cues to minimize confusion and to provide orientation to person, time, and place. ■ *Modify* tasks and environments to enable independence (e.g., provide adaptive equipment to increase independence in ADLs and IADLs, such as checklists for activity sequences and external memory aids).
Maintain	■ *Maintain* the client's postural alignment while sitting by providing structural wheelchair supports. ■ *Maintain* the client's maximum ROM obtained with serial casting by providing resting cast/splint for night wear.

Intervention Approaches Commonly Used During the Community Phase of Recovery (Rancho Los Amigos Levels VII–X) *Interventions typically focus on higher cognitive skills and WHO ICF areas of activity limitations and participation restrictions.*	
Intervention Approach	**Sample Occupational Therapy Treatment Activities**
Prevent	■ *Prevent* development of substance abuse and depression by educating the client about the risks and developing healthy alternative coping strategies. ■ *Prevent* client injury by modifying the home environment to decrease safety risks (e.g., installing grab bars and raised toilet seats, removing throw rugs and potential obstacles, installing automatic turn-off switches for stove burners and safety locks on cabinets).
Establish/Restore	■ *Restore* cognitive and social communication skills by having the client plan and complete a community outing with family and friends; practice social pragmatics in group activities and role-playing. ■ *Establish* daily routines to enable the client to complete desired morning rituals in a timely manner and prevent late arrival at work or school. ■ *Restore* joint mobility and motor function after surgical excision of HO or botulism toxin injections for muscle spasticity. ■ Work with local brain injury support group to *establish* leisure skill program to increase social networks for community-dwelling individuals with TBI.
Modify	■ *Modify* home and community environments to support independent performance of activities. ■ *Modify* daily routines to plan physically and cognitively challenging activities when well rested (e.g., pay bills in the morning when well rested; perform activities requiring fine motor demands when muscles are not fatigued). ■ *Modify* community mobility to accommodate for nondriving status.
Create/Promote	■ *Promote* a healthy lifestyle that includes engagement in occupations that support physical and mental health (e.g., develop exercise program, create list of healthy food and meal selections, identify healthy social activities to foster social relationships). ■ Advocate for development of an accessible, community-based center that *promotes* healthy leisure occupations for all citizens, including those community-dwelling individuals with TBI.
Maintain	■ *Maintain* gains made in ROM achieved by serial casting by wearing resting elbow splint for several hours per day. ■ *Maintain* social support systems in the community by engaging in leisure activities with friends from the local brain injury family group.

Note. Rancho Los Amigos levels taken from Hagen (1998).

Evidence-Based Intervention

The following sections include both an overview of specific interventions and findings from the evidence-based literature of occupational therapy for adults with TBI. A standard process of searching for and reviewing literature related to practice with adults with TBI was utilized and is summarized in Appendix C. The research studies presented here include primarily *Level I* randomized controlled trials (RCTs); *Level II* studies, in which assignment to a treatment or a control group is not randomized (cohort study); and *Level III* studies, which do not have a control group. In this systematic review, if Levels I, II, and III evidence for occupational therapy practice were adequate, then only those levels are used to answer a particular question. If, however, higher-level evidence is lacking and the best evidence provided for occupational therapy specifically is ranked as *Levels IV and V,* then those levels were included. Level IV studies are experimental single-case studies, and Level V evidence includes descriptive case reports. All studies identified by the review, including those not specifically described in this section, are summarized and cited in full in the evidence tables in Appendix D. Readers are encouraged to read the full articles for more details.

Intervention During the Coma Recovery Phase

During the early period of recovery from a TBI, the occupational therapist working with the client in coma typically focuses the intervention on establishing or restoring the client factors or impairments that resulted from the injury. Intervention also focuses on preventing the development of secondary impairments that occur in the period of unconsciousness. Global mental functions, such as level of consciousness and alertness, often are addressed through a program of coma arousal or sensory stimulation.

Sensory Stimulation Programs

Some persons who sustained a TBI continue in a coma or a vegetative state for a prolonged period of time or permanently. Because the senses are the gateways to consciousness, controlled application of sensory stimuli in an organized way is an adjunctive treatment often provided to these patients by occupational therapists (see Kearns, 2005): "Coma stimulation is based on the belief that through systematic stimulation of the reticular activating system (RAS), a change can be brought about that results in a response, thus increasing arousal" (p. 1).

The format of sensory stimulation or coma arousal programs vary greatly in their intensity, sensory modalities stimulated, involvement of family and friends in the application of regulated sensory stimulation, and client criteria for the program. Typically, a sensory stimulation program involves team-coordinated brief therapeutic sessions (e.g., 15 minutes) of application of multimodality sensory stimuli with close observation of the patient for a behavioral response. Observed responses (e.g., gazing toward photo of mother as requested when presented with two photos in vertical orientation) are reinforced with verbal praise and requests for repetition of the behavior. Standardized monitoring and charting of patients' responses enable the rehabilitation team to identify patterns of performance and ensure that multiple modalities are being stimulated.

RCTs, the gold standard of evidence-based investigation, are not easily conducted in the area of coma rehabilitation due to ethical concerns and methodological difficulties in participant recruitment and comparison of the sensory stimulation program to the standard rehabilitative treatment that includes some naturally occurring environmental stimulation. Coma arousal research is heavily dependent on the sensitivity of the instrument used to measure responsiveness. The implications for sensory stimulation efficacy may appear radically different depending on the sensitivity of outcome measures selected and the assessments used to determine level of arousal and awareness. While the beneficial effects of early and aggressive rehabilitative intervention on functional recovery of clients emerging from coma are supported (Cope & Hall, 1982; High et al., 2006; Mackay et al., 1992; Mysiw et al., 2007; Sirois et al., 2004; Zhu et al., 2007), it is questionable if coma arousal programs can actually *shorten* a coma or hasten return of consciousness. The consistent and controlled monitoring of patients' responses that occurs during sensory stimulation programs may, however, enable therapists to identify when clients have emerged naturally from coma and permit therapists to reinforce the client's voluntary and purposeful responses to environmental stimuli.

Research Evidence on Sensory Stimulation

There is a dearth of sound research regarding the effects of sensory stimulation for patients in coma or vegetative state. Lombardi, Taricco, De Tanti, Telaro, and Liberati (2002) surveyed the literature from 1966 to January 2002 and found only three studies that met criteria of being an RCT or a controlled clinical trial. The authors' conclusion was, "There is no reliable evidence to support the effectiveness of multisensory stimulation programs in patients in coma or the vegetative state" (p. 465).

Johnson, Roethig-Johnson, and Richards (1993; Level I) compared the efficacy of a program of multisensory stimulation with usual care for patients with severe diffuse brain injury while they were in the ICU. Fourteen participants were randomly assigned to groups. Stimulation to the 5 senses of the experimental group was provided in random order for 20 minutes per day for a median of 8.1 days. Results were not reported in functional terms. There was no significant difference between groups on heart rate or skin conductance. Only 3-methoxy, 4-hydroxyphenylglycol (a metabolite of norepinephrine degradation) showed a significant difference between groups; it rose in the treated group and fell in the control group. This study gave no unequivocal support for the effectiveness of multisensory stimulation in the acute stage of recovery after severe diffuse TBI.

Mitchell, Bradley, Welch, and Britton (1990; Level II) used a two-group, matched-pairs design to study the efficacy of a coma arousal procedure administered by patients' relatives to 12 persons ages 17 to 40 years for 1 hour, once or twice per day, 6 days per week, for 4 weeks, as compared with the matched group, who received no arousal procedure. They found that the arousal procedure reduced the time in coma by an average of almost 5 days. The training and compliance of the relatives was not reported. The authors did not link this finding to any functional outcome measure.

In their two-group, pretest–posttest study, Davis and Gimenez (2003; Level II) compared auditory sensory stimulation, consisting of various tone frequencies, music, familiar and unfamiliar voice patterns, and simple spoken messages, with routine nursing and rehabilitative care. The intervention group improved significantly more than the control group on the Sensory Stimulation Assessment Measure and the Disability Rating Scale but not on the GCS or the Rancho Los Amigos Cognitive Functioning Scale. They did not find definitive support for an auditory sensory stimulation program but did find a trend toward improvement. They also found that the stimulation program did not compromise cardiac responses or neurological function.

The Level I RCT (Johnson et al., 1993) and one of the Level II studies (Mitchell et al., 1990) included here were two of the three studies included in the systematic review by Lombardi and colleagues (2002). Limitations of those studies include failure to report method of randomization, assessors not blind to assignment, and failure to state how decisions were made regarding the details of treatment (e.g., intensity). The other Level II study (Davis & Gimenez, 2003) did not randomize assignment to group nor report who administered the intervention or assessed the outcome, and all control participants were recruited after the experimental participants.

There is no reliable, clinically relevant evidence to support or rule out the use of controlled sensory stimulation to arouse persons in coma or persistent vegetative state. There is evidence that arousal procedures do not have detrimental effects. There is minimal evidence that arousal procedures may decrease duration of coma and improve recovery as measured by the Disability Rating Scale. Therefore, given the assumption that arousal from coma is the first step on the way to increased occupational performance with continued therapy, incorporating sensory stimulation as an adjunctive intervention into occupational therapy practice may be warranted.

The bottom line is that valid research is needed to verify the effectiveness of sensory stimulation to arouse patients from coma or persistent vegetative state and the effectiveness of familiar and meaningful stimuli over a standard protocol of simulation, as well as to relate the arousal enabled by such an adjunctive therapy to ultimate functional outcome. Continued validation of sensory stimulation programs is needed with RCTs using large sample sizes and looking at both short- and long-term outcomes (Lombardi et al., 2002).

Neuromusculoskeletal Recovery Programs

Occupational therapy intervention for neuromusculoskeletal and movement-related functions after brain injury is focused on either impairments that are a primary consequence of that injury (e.g., impairments in voluntary movement, abnormal tone, balance) or secondary impairments resulting from the immobility or excessive muscle tone, such as contractures of the muscles or joints and diffuse weakness and deconditioning (Sullivan, 2007). At the coma phase of recovery, intervention for neuromuscular motor impairments is generally passive in nature, using more preparatory methods such as passive range of motion (PROM), splinting and serial casting, and positioning in the bed and wheelchair to either establish and restore motor control or prevent the development of secondary joint and muscle contractures. Joint contractures can result in significant limitations in self-care, particularly dressing and hygiene (Mysiw et al., 2007; Sullivan, 2007).

Related Evidence on Motor Recovery

There is moderate evidence (Lannin, Horsley, Herbert, McCluskey, & Cusick, 2003; Level II) that application of nocturnal hand splinting in combination with conventional therapy does not improve ROM, function, or pain control in the spastic hand. Occupational therapists may apply a series of casts to the limbs of patients with brain injury (i.e., applying either a plaster or fiberglass cast to one or multiple joints) to reduce muscle spasticity and foster maintenance of joint ROM by providing prolonged stretch and pressure, along with neutral warmth (Marshall et al., 2007). There is strong (Level I) evidence that serial casting reduces ankle plantar contractures but limited evidence that serial casting reduces upper-extremity contractures due to spasticity

(Marshall et al., 2007). The majority of research using serial casting has focused on lower-extremity joints. An older study by Hill (1994, Level II) used a crossover research design with a small sample of 15 patients alternately assigned to two conditions. Patients showed significantly greater improvements in ROM with casting than when they participated in more traditional therapy for contractures, such as ranging, splinting, and neurophysiological movement reeducation techniques, although there was no apparent correlation between the improved ROM and functional use of the arm. A more recent study (Pohl et al., 2002; Level III) that included upper-extremity joints found a significant improvement in ROM regardless of whether the patient received conventional casting of 5 to 7 days or a shortened period of 1 to 4 days. However, there were significantly fewer complications and discontinuation rates in the group that wore the casts for 1 to 4 days.

Management of Heterotopic Ossifications

Monitoring clients for the development of HO (e.g., observation for an inflammatory reaction, palpable mass, or limited ROM in joints of the limbs) in clients with abnormal tone is important. During the acute inflammatory stage, the occupational therapist should position the patient's involved limb in a functional position and initiate gentle PROM, monitoring the patient for signs of pain (e.g., facial grimace, change in vital signs). Once acute inflammatory signs have subsided, continued mobilization is indicated to maintain range. Resting the joint appears more likely to lead to decreased joint range, whereas continued mobilization may lead to formation of a pseudarthrosis (Banovac & Speed, 2008). Positioning the client in coma in a wheelchair with adequate supports for the head and trunk also can decrease muscle tone, foster increased upright motor control in a functional posture, and improve awareness of stimuli within the environment.

Related Evidence on Heterotopic Ossifications

Cullen, Bayley, Bayona, Hilditch, and Aubut (2007) conducted a Level I systematic review of management of HO following ABI, and identified only a single case study (Level V) that explored the use of a continuous passive motion (CPM) device coupled with conventional physiotherapy as treatment of bilateral HO in the knees. The study suggests that CPM reduces the development of HO in individuals with severe brain injury. Cullen, Bayley, and colleagues (2007) also report limited evidence (Level III) that forceful manipulation under general anesthesia can increase joint range and that surgical excision of HO at the hip, elbow, and knee improves clinical outcomes.

As the client emerges from coma and is able to produce voluntary and purposeful motor responses to demands and environmental stimuli, the occupational therapist attempts to engage the client in more therapeutic use of occupations and activities, focusing on the establishment or restoration of motor and cognitive performance skills.

Intervention During the Acute Rehabilitation Recovery Phase

The acute rehabilitation phase of recovery begins as the client is medically stable and emerging from the coma. Occupational therapists, as part of the rehabilitation team working with clients who have TBI, must address the client's physical, cognitive, communicative, emotional, and spiritual needs while planning for the client's transition to the next setting, whether it is subacute rehabilitation, an outpatient program, or home in the community. Reduced lengths of stay and a reimbursement system focused more on motor recovery than cognitive and neurobehavioral recovery can make justification for the client's need for occupational therapy intervention challenging.

Addressing the Needs of the Patient With Agitation

Clients with TBI often are admitted to an acute rehabilitation hospital when they begin to display signs of entering the phase of agitation (i.e., Rancho Los Amigos Level IV). *Agitation* has been defined as a state of aggression during posttraumatic amnesia in the absence of physical, medical, or psychiatric causes that

may involve a component of *akathisia* (i.e., a constant sensation of inner restlessness; Lombard & Zafonte, 2005), impulsivity, decreased frustration tolerance, disinhibition, and inappropriate social behavior (Kane, 2006). This phase of recovery from TBI encompasses a spectrum of behaviors that fluctuate with changes in situational factors such as environmental stimulation, task demands, and time of day (Lequerica, Rapport, Loeher, Axelrod, Vangel, & Hanks, 2007). Not all clients with TBI experience a period of agitation during their recovery. Agitation is associated with increased length of hospitalization, poorer cognitive and motor function at discharge (Bogner, Corrigan, Fugate, Mysiw, & Clinchot, 2001), and noncompliance with splinting programs (O'Brien & Bailey, 2008). Severity of confusion at 1 month after injury is strongly associated with employment outcome (Nakase-Richardson, Yablon, & Sherer, 2007).

Agitated behavior may limit the client's engagement and progress in rehabilitative therapy (Lequerica et al., 2007); however, occupational therapists may engage clients in structured self-care activities, simple games and activities requiring use of cognitive skills, and simple gross motor activities to expend excess energy and deal with the restlessness or akathisia. Frequent breaks may be needed and treatment sessions may need to be shortened or varied to maintain the client's attention and lessen frustration and potential display of agitated behavior. Although it is difficult to focus on restoring underlying impairments because the client's capacity for new learning is significantly limited by the posttraumatic amnesia that typically accompanies the period of agitation, the occupational therapist can structure tasks and the environment to regulate overstimulation, confusion, and frustration. The therapist also may provide environmental cues to help orient the client during periods of confusion (e.g., wall calendars, clocks, labeled photos of rehabilitative staff, signs indicating the client's room). As the agitation lessens, the cognitive and motor challenges presented to the client gradually can be increased to address underlying impairments.

Addressing Motor Recovery

As the client with TBI emerges from coma and performs more voluntary movement, the occupational therapist begins to address impairments seen within the sensory (i.e., peripheral and cranial nerve function, vision) and neuromusculoskeletal and movement-related systems (i.e., joint and bone integrity, muscle tone, movement functions). Because focal areas of the brain may have been injured during the traumatic event, the clinical presentation of the client's volitional movement may include hemiparesis; hemiplegia; or ataxia with abnormal movement synergies, abnormal tone, and postural instability. Some clients with TBI who appear to have had the motor system spared during the initial injury may display impaired motor speed (Haaland, Temkin, Randahl, & Dikmen, 1994; Incoccia, Formisano, Muscato, Reali, & Zoccolotti, 2004) and weak grip strength (Haaland et al., 1994) or general weakness and deconditioning from a lengthy period of unconsciousness and immobility.

Whereas the greatest improvement in motor recovery is seen between initial evaluation on inpatient admission and 6-month follow-up, persistent neuromotor abnormalities may be observed in more than one-third of individuals with severe TBI 2 years following acute rehabilitation (Walker & Pickett, 2007). Clients with persistent spasticity resulting in joint contractures interfering with performance of functional activities, who have not been successfully managed with more conservative rehabilitation techniques, may be candidates for botulinum toxin A injections (Mayer, Whyte, Wannstedt, & Ellis, 2008), motor point or neural blocks, surgical release of the contracted tissue (Mysiw et al., 2007), or intrathecal bacolfen pump placement. Occupational therapy intervention following these procedures can be helpful to increase functional integration of the limb into daily activities.

Recent research in neurorehabilitation (Nudo & Dancause, 2007) suggests that neuroplasticity after TBI (i.e., regeneration of brain neuronal structures and/or reorganization of the function of neurons in response to injury) may be modified by engagement in motor skill acquisition, learning, and exercise. Occupational therapists apply the principles of practice and feedback, task-specificity, and training intensity when providing intervention focused on motor skill recovery. Two commonly used approaches to address movement related impairments after TBI are motor learning and constraint-induced movement therapy (CIMT).

Motor learning is a process of learning to produce skilled movement that involves practice and experience. Because motor learning, like most learning, involves nonobservable cognitive processes, the observed motor performance suggests that motor learning has occurred. A motor skill is learned truly when it can be retained or transferred to a novel situation. Motor skill learning is a problem-solving thought process in which the patient learns to perform motor skills efficiently and effectively (Sullivan, 2007). Occupational therapists using a motor learning approach set up the therapeutic learning environment, typically the occupational therapy clinic, to promote skill acquisition by varying the tasks and environment to meet the patient's current learning abilities. Controlling the practice conditions, the occupational therapy practitioner may have the client repeatedly practice discrete components of the motor task (e.g., opening a milk carton) or the full sequence of the motor act (e.g., opening the carton and pouring a glass of milk). The practitioner provides the patient with feedback focused on either knowledge of the motor performance (e.g., "You used too much force in your grip") or feedback focused on knowledge of the results (e.g., "Great! You poured the milk and were able to stop the motion before you overfilled the glass"). Much of the theory and research on motor learning is founded on observations of how healthy, able-bodied individuals learn motor skills. There is minimal evidence to confidently recommend particular sequences to applying motor learning principles (i.e., whole vs. part practice, knowledge of results vs. knowledge of performance feedback, repetitive practice of a single task vs. random practice of a variety of tasks) to motor skill acquisition with individuals with

TBI and cognitive and motor impairments (Kane, 2006; Sullivan, 2007).

CIMT, a motor skill intervention approach based on the learning principles of shaping and preventing learned nonuse, was initially designed to increase the use of the impaired arm in chronic stroke patients (Taub, Crago, & Uswatte, 1998). CIMT involves three main components: (1) intensive training of the affected arm, (2) practice to promote transfer of therapeutic gains from the clinical environment to real-world situations, and (3) constraint of the less-affected arm during the entire period of intervention. CIMT programs typically involve several consecutive days (e.g., 10–14) of intervention, during which the less-affected arm is constrained by a splint or sling during waking hours, and functional movements are performed with the hemiparetic arm for up to 6 hours each day (Taub et al., 1998). Variations of the program (e.g., *modified constraint-induced therapy [mCIT],* which involves lessened hours of constraint and guided functional movement sessions or elimination of the constraint element entirely) have been developed to address institutional, therapist, client, and family reservations regarding patient safety and compliance and also practicality and resource utilization during inpatient hospitalizations. The majority of the evidence supporting use of CIMT and mCIT has been completed with the stroke population, but many studies did not distinguish the diagnostic cause of the upper-extremity hemiparesis. Because CIMT is an approach that focuses on remediation of the impairment of hemiparesis, this guideline looks to the literature from the *Occupational Therapy Practice Guidelines for Adults With Stroke* (Sabari, 2008) for their applicability to the population with TBI.

Research Evidence Supporting Motor Interventions

There are a variety of intervention approaches to address motor impairments and performance skill limitations following TBI. Neistadt (1994), in an RCT (Level I), demonstrated that occupational-based functional activities (e.g., meal preparation) may be more effective than remedial activities (e.g., pegboards, puzzles) in improving fine motor coordination in adult men with TBI. Intervention approaches such as CIT that place challenging demands on the reorganization of brain function beyond spontaneous recovery after TBI are supported by only limited evidence (Marshall et al., 2007).

Summary of Levels I–III Evidence on Constraint-Induced Therapy

Although the majority of the evidence supporting use of CIMT has been gathered from clients with stroke, the approach also has been successfully used with clients recovering from TBI (Cho et al., 2005; Page & Levine, 2003; Shaw et al., 2005; Sterr & Freivogel, 2003). Results of the CIMT approach to motor recovery show not only improved quality and speed of movement but also increased spontaneous use of the affected arm in real-world situations as measured by the Motor Activity Log (MAL; Taub, Uswatte, Mark, & Morris, 2006). The MAL uses a structured interview of both the patient and an informant to investigate quality of movement and frequency of use of the affected arm in 28 ADL tasks within the home. Several studies provide Level I evidence (Lin, Wu, Wei, Lee, & Liu, 2007; Page, Levine, Leonard, Szaflarski, & Kissela, 2008; Wu, Chen, Tsai, Lin, & Chou, 2007; Wu, Lin, Chen, Chen, & Hong, 2007) that clients who sustained strokes and participated in mCIMT intervention in addition to traditional occupational therapy intervention made significantly greater improvement (as measured by kinematic analysis, standardized motor scales, and the Functional Independence Measure [FIM™]) than those patients who participated only in traditional occupational therapy intervention. Additional research is needed to study the long-term functional carryover of mCIMT. Although the majority of research on CIMT has been conducted with clients who sustained strokes, both the CIMT and mCIT approaches have been shown to achieve substantial benefits that were not confined to the therapeutic setting for low-functioning clients with TBI who were well beyond spontaneous recovery and had been at a stable level for many months (Page & Levine, 2003;

Sterr & Freivogel, 2003). Treatment with CIMT has shown transfer of movements practiced within the intervention program to real-world settings; however, the documented studies contain small sample sizes and often limited details on the components of the treatment protocols used.

Page and Levine (2003; Level III) examined the effects of mCIT on 3 recruited volunteers who had experienced TBI 1 to 6 years before the study. The participants were able to follow directions and had 10° of metacarpal extension and 20° of wrist extension of the more-affected upper extremity. These requirements are the same as required of stroke patients, the first patients to be treated with this intervention. All 3 participants improved between 5.5 to 14 points in their ability to pinch, grip, and grasp (Action Research Arm Test) and more than 2 points in the amount of use and quality of movement of the more-affected upper extremity (MAL) after 10 weeks of therapy. There was no change on the Wolf Motor Function Test. None of the data were tested statistically. The evidence suggests that mCIT may be effective in improving upper-limb use and function following TBI.

The 25-minute use of the more-affected limb to accomplish valued (patient-chosen) ADLs while the less-affected arm was restrained, along with shaping of behavior, are believed to be the critical therapeutic variables of the program. The strength of the evidence is compromised by the lack of random assignment to condition; small, highly selected samples; lack of information regarding the reliability of outcome measures; questionably adequate outcome measures; no statistical analysis of data; and no information about compliance with the use of the restraint at home. If we can extrapolate from the studies of the effects of CIMT on rat brain reorganization (Tillerson & Miller, 2002), then the demands of CIMT to relearn to use the weak extremity may not only result in behavioral changes but also in neurogenesis as well. Obviously, this question needs to be studied directly.

Intervention Addressing Cognitive Impairments

Interdisciplinary and comprehensive cognitive rehabilitation is an integral component of intervention with individuals who have sustained TBI. Even in those clients with good physical and medical recoveries, cognitive impairments in the area of attention, memory, and executive functions can limit the person's ability to engage in functional, social, and vocational activities. As the client emerges from the agitated phase of recovery and can more actively engage in the rehabilitative process, the occupational therapist begins to address cognitive impairments and the resulting limitations to functional activity performance and social participation more formally. Although the area of cognitive rehabilitation is discussed here under the acute rehabilitation phase, this intervention focus continues long after the client is discharged from inpatient services into the community.

Cognitive Rehabilitation Approaches

Occupational therapists select cognitive rehabilitation intervention approaches that focus on the individual, the task, or the environment, on the basis of an understanding of the client's ability to learn and generalize information (Toglia et al., 2008). When there is potential for change in the client's underlying cognitive impairments, the occupational therapist uses a remedial approach focused on improving and restoring the client's attention, memory, or executive function skills. Using activities that challenge the client's inherent cognitive processes and abilities, the therapist provides opportunities for the client to practice using the skills in controlled therapeutic settings and graded tasks. Remedial approaches are postulated (Luria, 1973) to promote reorganization of functional neural networks within the brain, facilitating recovery of cognitive functions.

Functional approaches, which capitalize on the client's strengths and abilities, shift the focus of intervention from restoring underlying impairments to minimizing their limitations on engagement in activities and participation within the community. Occupational therapists' training in analyzing and adapting activities and environments enables them to consider the cognitive strengths of the person and match compensatory strategies to those abilities. Therapists may modify the clients' environment (e.g., placing cue cards or signs in key locations, labeling closets or drawers to identify their contents) or modify the activity (e.g., pre-selecting and pre-arranging items needed for completion of the task or presenting items for only one step of a task at a time). For clients with limited ability to learn and generalize information, a functional skill training program incorporating vanishing cues and errorless learning in the natural environment may be used (Toglia et al., 2008).

Capitalizing on procedural memory, occupational therapists may teach the client to perform specific activities (e.g., completing morning hygiene, preparing simple snacks, following a medication schedule) that would decrease caregiver burden and provide some level of independence (Giles, 2005; Parish & Oddy, 2007). Clients are trained on the same activity that they are expected to perform in the same environment in which it would be performed.

Because functional skill training is context and activity specific (i.e., not anticipated to generalize), occupational therapists tend to use this approach more in community settings when the client's natural recovery from TBI is expected to have stabilized and the environment is one in which the client lives and functions. Consistent training in the performance of the specific activity leads to the task becoming part of the client's routine and activity patterns. Compensation requires adaptation or modification of the method used to perform a task. Some features of the activity may be enhanced (e.g., placing colored tape on key appliance buttons/switches), whereas other features may be reduced to decrease distractibility (e.g., simplifying task instructions).

Occupational therapists have developed a variety of theories to explain the link between cognitive skills and functional limitations. These theories are reflected in occupational therapy cognitive rehabilitation approaches such as the Cognitive Disabilities Approach (Allen, 1985, 1993), the Cognitive Retraining Module (Averbuch & Katz, 2005), the Multicontext Approach (Toglia, 2005), the Neurofunctional Approach (Giles, 2005), and the Quadriphonic

Approach (Abreu & Peloquin, 2005). Occupational therapists working with clients with cognitive impairments resulting from TBI typically focus their intervention, regardless of the theoretical approach, on the cognitive skills of awareness, attention, memory, and executive functions.

Research Evidence Supporting Cognitive Rehabilitation

The evidence supporting cognitive rehabilitation has recently received significant scrutiny as insurers have questioned its efficacy and their willingness to fund these services. Systematic reviews of research in the area of cognitive rehabilitation have provided recommendations for clinical practice. This review of the evidence will focus on unidisciplinary (i.e., single profession) versus multidisciplinary intervention; treatment intensity; the areas of awareness, attention, memory, and executive function; and teaching methods (e.g., cognitive orthoses, individualized vs. group intervention).

Unidisciplinary Cognitive Rehabilitation

Ho and Bennett (1997; Level III) used a one-group pretest–posttest design to test the efficacy of a cognitive rehabilitation program that appears to have been designed and administered by neuropsychologists. The study had two goals: (1) demonstrate that cognitive functioning, as measured by neuropsychological test scores, would improve following a specific program of remedial and compensatory therapies; and (2) demonstrate that these improvements in neuropsychological scores would reflect improvements in ADLs. The treatment was individualized but always consisted of two parts: formal cognitive remediation and compensatory training to compensate for cognitive deficits within everyday life settings. Frequency varied from 22 to 155 sessions, and duration ranged from 5 to 82 weeks. All neuropsychological test scores improved significantly. Functional performance, as measured by the modified Acimovic–Keatley ADL subtest scores (Acimovic & Keatley, 1991) as well as the total score, also improved significantly. The ADL test measured cognitive and behavioral processes related to ADLs; it did not measure actual occupational performance. There was no significant correlation between neuropsychological measures and ADL ratings. The authors concluded that cognitive rehabilitation that includes both remediation and compensatory strategies is effective. They further concluded that because there was no significant correlation between the neuropsychological test scores and the modified ADL scale scores, the latter may measure aspects of cognitive functioning that are not the same as the aspects of cognitive functioning that are reflected in neuropsychological test scores.

There are several limitations to this study: the lack of a control group; pretest data obtained from historical records, which may indicate, although not stated, that this is a retrospective, not prospective, study; a timing bias—some participants were in treatment for 1½ years, during which procedures and therapists could have changed or spontaneous recovery could have occurred; and failure to report the validity and reliability of the outcome measures. In addition, unlabeled numbers were reported in the tables for outcomes and the exact probability levels were not reported, nor were the sample sizes on which the statistics were calculated, so no effect sizes could be calculated.

Multidisciplinary Cognitive Rehabilitation

Salazar and colleagues (2000; Level I) used a two-group RCT over a 5-year period to evaluate the efficacy of multidisciplinary inpatient cognitive rehabilitation for patients with moderate to severe TBI. A total of 107 active-duty military personnel with moderate to severe closed-head injuries participated in either an 8-week intensive standardized in-hospital cognitive rehabilitation program that included occupational therapy among other disciplines or an 8-week limited standardized home rehabilitation program with weekly telephone support, administered solely by a psychiatric nurse. At 1-year follow-up, there was no significant difference between Groups 1 and 2 in return to employment (90% vs. 94%), fitness for duty (73% vs.

66%), or employment (91% of the hospital group and 93% of the at-home group were working full-time). The authors concluded that the more costly in-hospital rehabilitation was no more effective than the limited at-home rehabilitation.

One limitation of the study is that prestudy power analysis goals were not reached, and poststudy power analysis indicated that the number of participants was one-fifth of that required to achieve significance. This limitation seems moot because the outcome percentages were so similar between groups. The patients were hospitalized at the time of recruitment; therefore, it appears that they were in the acute stage of recovery. If so, and because the measurements were taken 1 year after treatment, we cannot attribute the outcome to the intervention alone. Other explanations, such as spontaneous recovery, implicit learning, or experience, could account for the outcome. A no-treatment control group was needed to control for this.

Braverman and colleagues (1999; Level III) used a one-group pretest–posttest design, as part of a larger RCT, to describe the effects of a multidisciplinary rehabilitation program for active-duty military service members with moderately severe brain injury. In this multidisciplinary program, occupational therapists (sometimes with the co-leadership of other professionals) led a cognitive skills group 50 minutes 3 to 4 times per week; a planning and organization group 30 to 40 minutes 4 times per week; individual therapy 50 minutes 1 to 2 times per week week; work therapy 2 to 3 hours 4 days per week; a work skills group 1½ hours once per week; and community reentry outings several hours per week. At 1-year follow-up, 64 of the participants (95.5%) were able to work or were enrolled in college. Forty-four (66%) remained on active duty or remained fit for duty but were discharged from the military for nonmedical reasons.

The authors concluded that the rehabilitation program demonstrates one successful effort to rehabilitate soldiers with TBI who have potential to return to duty. The study has limitations, however. Specifically, there was no control group, so the outcome may have occurred for a reason other than the intervention, such as spontaneous recovery or implicit learning, or experience because the patients were in the acute stage of recovery (within 90 days of trauma) and the measurements were taken 1 year after treatment. These alternate explanations are plausible. Also, there was no statistical testing of outcome or operational definition, nor description of reliability of the outcome measure.

Mills, Nesbeda, Katz, and Alexander (1992; Level III) used a one-group pretest–posttest design to report functional outcomes of patients with TBI in a structured community-based rehabilitation program that emphasized improvement of the patient's real-life functional abilities (occupational performance) and psychological support. A functional rather than cognitive remedial approach was used. Treatment occurred 6 hours per day, 5 days per week, for 6 weeks. Eight treatment goals were individually established by each patient and family with the team. The disciplines that comprised the team were not identified. Outcome on each goal was rated on a 5-point scale from *independent* to *dependent*. There was a significant improvement in functional evaluation before and after treatment ($p < .05$, $r = .65$). The average overall percentage of treatment goals achieved was 67.5%; range was 25% to 93.7%. The majority of patients ($n = 32$) maintained or improved their overall status in the home (87.5%), community (87.5%), leisure (90%), and vocational function (90%) 6 months after discharge. These gains continued to be maintained or improved at 12 months.

The authors concluded that late treatment aimed at practical real-life goals, and not at specific cognitive deficits, accompanied by psychological support for patients and their families can lead to improved functioning and independence. They further stated that no demographic features, except low education, limited the potential success of this approach. In addition to the lack of control group and lack of detail, one limitation is that there may have been a memory bias regarding maintenance of goal performance because it was evaluated by interviewing the patient and family members, who had to remember immediate past performance.

None of these studies on multidisciplinary intervention contained a control group; however, Turner-Stokes and colleagues (2005; Level I) state that the expanding body of evidence for the effectiveness of multidisciplinary research in other populations, such as clients with stroke, makes it difficult ethically and practically to randomize those with TBI to control groups with no treatment or standard care.

Treatment Intensity

Paniak and colleagues (1998, 2000; both Level I), using a cohort of 119 persons with acute mild TBI (MTBI), studied the immediate (1998) and long-term (2000) effects of *treatment as needed* (TAN), operationally defined as a 3–4-hour neuropsychological and personality assessment and feedback, a consultation with a physical therapist, and further TAN, in addition to that received by a *single-session group*, whose only treatment consisted of meeting with the primary investigator to discuss any concerns about head injury and the contents of a brochure on minor head injury. There was no statistically significant difference between groups on the Community Integration Questionnaire (CIQ) in either study. Occupational status improved significantly over time in the 1998 study, but there was no difference between groups on occupational status or in satisfaction with treatment scores. There was no decline in functioning between the 3- and 12-month evaluations, which were by telephone interview, in either group.

The authors concluded that, when applied within 3 weeks of MTBI, a brief educational and reassurance-oriented intervention is just as effective and as highly patient rated as a potentially more intensive and expensive model. However, the independent variable (amount of therapy) may have been compromised (equalized between groups) because the TAN group reported a median of only 1 further treatment after the initial educational treatment. Another limitation of the study is that no information was given concerning ceiling effects on the CIQ, which are likely in this population.

Cullen, Chundamala, Bayley, and Jutai (2007; Level I) conducted a systematic review on efficacy of rehabilitation interventions for ABI and found moderate evidence that increasing the intensity of rehabilitation reduced length of stay and improved short-term motor recovery and functional outcomes. Therapy intensity was not found to be correlated with improved cognitive outcomes.

Zhu and colleagues (2007; Level I) evaluated the effects of differing levels of treatment intensity on the functional outcomes of 68 patients with moderate to severe TBI at the early posttraumatic stage (up to 6 months postinjury). Patients were randomized to either 4 or 2 hours of therapy per day, including occupational, physical, and speech therapies, for a period of up to 6 months on the basis of individual patient needs. Occupational therapy included functional retraining and psychosocial retraining including social skills. Although there were no differences between the levels of intensity on the FIM and Neurobehavioral Cognitive Status Examination at 3 months, there were significantly more patients in the high- than low-intensity group who achieved a maximum total FIM and Glasgow Outcome Scale (GOS) scores.

The Level I systematic review by Turner-Stokes and colleagues (2005) found that, for patients with moderate to severe TBI, there is strong evidence that more-intensive programs result in earlier functional gains. There is moderate evidence that continued outpatient therapy sustains these early gains.

Awareness and Metacognition

Metacognition refers to the use of clients' knowledge and experiences of their own cognitive processes to guide their engagement in tasks. A lack of awareness (i.e., diminished metacognition) of the functionally relevant effects of cognitive or physical impairments resulting from the TBI can be a barrier to the patient's active engagement in the rehabilitation program. Clients with limited awareness may not put forth adequate or consistent effort in intervention programs focused on motor recovery; see the necessity of compensatory strategies and therefore not initiate their use; or accurately estimate their abilities to independently perform functional tasks, thus compromising their safety

(Goverover, 2004; Toglia & Kirk, 2000). Clients who understand their cognitive challenges may be more effective in using compensatory strategies and have better functional outcomes (Goverover, Johnston, Toglia, & DeLuca, 2007). Clients with TBI consistently report fewer cognitive, motor, and behavioral problems than their families and treating therapists (Abreu et al., 2001; Powell, Machamer, Temkin, & Dikmen, 2001).

Occupational therapists attempt to foster clients' awareness of their abilities and limitations in a supportive yet constructive manner. They may have clients estimate performance prior to engaging in quantifiable tasks, then compare actual performance to the estimate, rate achievement of specific goals (i.e., goal attainment scales), analyze videotapes of themselves performing tasks, use self-monitoring checklists, engage in self-questioning (e.g., "Did I check my work for errors?"; Toglia et al., 2008), or engage in structured journaling at the end of each treatment session to help clients reflect on their activity experiences, identify challenges, and anticipate what they might do differently the next time (Goverover et al., 2007). A trial of awareness training can help distinguish those clients who may be able to generalize compensatory strategies to a variety of situations and those clients who might benefit more from a task-specific functional training approach.

Research Evidence Addressing Awareness Training and Metacognition

Goverover and colleagues (2007; Level I) examined the effects of an awareness training program embedded within IADLs on the self-awareness and functional performance of 20 individuals with ABI (10 clients randomized to intervention and control groups each). Intervention consisted of 6 sessions of self-awareness training during IADLs, while the control group received conventional therapeutic practice during IADLs. The effects of the self-awareness training were measured by clients' scores on the Awareness Questionnaire (AQ), the Assessment of Awareness of Disability, the Self-Regulation Skills Inventory, and the Assessment of Motor and Process Skills (AMPS).

Clients in the self-awareness training group showed significant improvement on IADL performance and self-regulation (i.e., the cognitive aspect of performance) compared with those in the control group. No differences, however, were observed in task-specific self-awareness, general self-awareness, or self-regulation.

Although there was a trend toward participants in the self-awareness training group displaying a better understanding of their difficulties and strengths in specific task performance, the results did not show a statistically significant change. The researchers suggest a larger sample size may have shown significance. The researchers also looked at possible distal effects of the intervention on general self-awareness (using the AQ), actual functional activities (using the AMPS motor score), and reports of community integration (using the CIQ). The lack of statistically significant changes in general self-awareness and community participation were hypothesized to be due to the limited number of intervention sessions, disassociation between general and task-specific awareness, and the use of self-report measures.

Ownsworth and colleagues (2006; Level IV) used a single-case experimental design with multiple baselines across settings to study the effects of a 16-week program of metacognitive contextual intervention with systematic feedback and family education on 1 patient with very severe TBI. The intervention included systematic feedback to target erroneous behavior while the patient performed functional tasks relating to his cooking and paid employment goals. During the 8-week treatment period in the cooking setting, there was a 44% reduction in error frequency. The average error frequency in the maintenance period indicated that the treatment effect was maintained. There was no spontaneous generalization to volunteer work. With specific training, error frequency in the work setting reduced 39%. There was no appreciable improvement in general awareness of deficits. Three weeks after the intervention, the patient gained paid employment with initial use of a job coach (trained by the therapists). After 1 month, the patient no longer

required the job coach due to decreased errors and level of supervision required.

The authors concluded that the study provides preliminary support for metacognitive contextual approach for enhancing self-correction and functional gains for an individual with awareness deficits, but further research is needed. A multiple baseline single-case design provides some weak support for acceptance of a causal relationship between the treatment and the reported outcome; however, in this case, the baseline measure of errors in the cooking setting was descending without treatment, so self-correction may have occurred as a result of practice rather than the feedback intervention. This requires further study.

Landa-Gonzales (2001; Level V), in a report of one case of a person with substantial memory and executive function impairments and poor insight about his functional limitations post-TBI, examined a 6-month multicontextual community reentry occupational therapy program directed at awareness training and compensation for cognitive problems after TBI. Therapy included exploration and use of effective processing strategies, task gradations, and practice of functional activities in multiple, natural contexts. The program lasted for 6 months. The client's awareness level, occupational performance, and satisfaction with performance improved as level of attendant care decreased. On the Kohlman Evaluation of Living Skills, the client needed assistance with 10 skills at baseline but only 3 at discharge (budgeting for food, budgeting monthly income, use of phone book). On the COPM, the client gained 1.5 to 2 points for each performance score and 1.5 to 3 points for each satisfaction score. He predicted task performance more accurately and closer to actual performance. Gains made in treatment were maintained 8 weeks after discharge. The author concluded that training and education using selected processing strategies facilitated improved awareness and occupational performance.

Case reports present interesting ideas but cannot establish the intervention as the cause of change observed, because there are no controls for threats to internal validity. The uniqueness of the subject precludes external validation or generalization to other patients. This case report indicates that further, better-designed study is warranted.

Attention

Multidimensional attentional impairments are common after a TBI and include difficulty sustaining attention, shifting the focus of attention, and processing information rapidly (Cicerone, 2007). Occupational therapists grade intervention activities and control environmental stimuli to provide a "just-right challenge" to the client's attentional capacity by slowly introducing additional stimuli to the task and environment to build the client's ability to work with competing stimuli. For example, the client may initially receive one-to-one treatment in a quiet room with the door closed. Gradually, the therapist will open the door or engage the client in treatment activities within the typically noisier common treatment room. The occupational therapist helps the client understand the conditions that can support or break down attentional skills and apply strategies to control the task and environment to support optimal performance.

Research Evidence on Interventions Focused on Attention

Research examining the efficacy of interventions focused on attentional impairments is complicated by a lack of consensus regarding the definition of attention, use of the same tests to measure different components of attention, repeated use of outcome measures, and significant variability in the intensity of treatment sessions and duration (Rees, Marshall, Hartridge, Mackie, & Weiser, 2007).

Park and Ingles (2001) performed a Level I meta-analysis of 20 studies involving 359 patients concerning the efficacy of current attention rehabilitation after ABI, specifically to determine whether direct-training (remediation of damaged cognitive function through repetitive exercises) and specific-skill programs (development of compensatory alternative ways of performing activities through specific skill training) differ in their effectiveness. The interventions included both auditory and visual exercises. Eighty-three percent of studies specified that the tasks were graduated in difficulty; 77% of the studies indicated that feedback on training performance was provided. The number of training tasks varied, with 50% of studies providing 5 or more tasks. Eighty-nine percent of the programs had a component in which speeded or paced performance was encouraged. In 50% of the studies, treatment was via computer. Mean treatment time was 31 hours.

Park and Ingles concluded that acquired deficits of attention are treatable and that learning that occurs as a function of training is specific and does not generalize to tasks that differ considerably from those used in training. They further concluded that more study is needed in how to best train a person with attentional impairments from a brain injury.

Sohlberg, McLaughlin, Pavese, Heidrich, and Posner (2000; Level I), using a two-group crossover design with random assignment to group, examined *attention process therapy (APT)*, operationally defined as hierarchical organization of tasks that exercise different components of attention: sustained, selective, alternating, and divided, as compared with therapy consisting of brain injury education, supportive listening, and relaxation training on the participants' perceptions (by questionnaire) of the impact of attention deficits on daily living and (by interview) whether the participants noticed any changes in their day-to-day lives that they felt had been due to participating in therapy. The number of changes reported in the interview were significantly greater after APT than education ($p < .05$, $r = .58$). The analysis of the questionnaires indicated significant ($p < .01$) improvements reported over time that were not associated with type of treatment ($p > .65$).

The authors concluded that practice, whether by repeating the assessment tasks or from participating in the training of general processes using APT, improves performance. In the authors' opinion, the significant finding of this study was that for low-vigilance participants, APT resulted in improved attentional skills that generalized to measures that were different from training tasks. The limitations of concern for this study were unequal group characteristics at start of study, despite random assignment to group, and that the experimental treatment was administered at 2½ times the intensity of control treatment.

A more recent systematic review of research evaluating the efficacy of cognitive rehabilitation to improve independence following ABI (Rees et al., 2007; Level I) reports moderate evidence that drills and practice training are not effective for improving attention.

Novack, Caldwell, Duke, Bergquist, and Gage (1996; Level I), using a matched-pairs RCT, studied the effect of a focused attention remediation program versus an unstructured stimulation program (control) on FIM scores. Participants had severe TBI and were in the acute stage of recovery. There was no significant difference between groups at admission. Each treatment was administered for 30 minutes, 5 days per week, for 1 to 15 weeks. The experimental treatment was administered at 2½ times the intensity of the control treatment, an important limitation of the study. There was no significant difference between groups at discharge; however, there was a significant effect for time ($p < .0001$), that is, both groups improved over time, indicating spontaneous recovery may have occurred.

The authors concluded that focused remediation is no more effective than unstructured stimulation in improving the attentional skills of individuals undergoing acute rehabilitation following severe TBI. The FIM, the outcome measure of interest to this review, was introduced halfway through the 3-year study, so it was administered to only 24 out of 44 participants.

Therefore, no causal relationship can be established between the intervention and outcome based on these studies.

A meta-analysis (Park & Ingles, 2001; Level I) and RCTs (Novack et al., 1996; Sohlberg et al., 2000; Level I) confirm that attention deficits of persons with TBI improve with time in the acute stage and with therapy in the chronic stage of recovery. The improvement appears to be limited to tasks similar to training tasks. Whether a focused or hierarchically structured attention program will improve attention performance is equivocal. No particular intervention aimed at improving attention performance in persons with TBI has been supported unequivocally. However, attention performance has been shown to improve, so further research into the most effective intervention methods is warranted.

Memory

Memory deficits are the most common cognitive impairment seen by occupational therapists (Blundon & Smits, 2000) and other rehabilitation professionals who care for patients with TBI. Rehabilitation itself is a learning process requiring memory; thus, clients with TBI and memory impairments may be limited in their ability to adapt to residual impairments without specific interventions aimed at their memory. Early in the recovery from TBI, clients may display posttraumatic amnesia for several days or weeks. During this time they are not encoding or retaining new information, although they may be actively engaged in rehabilitation programs (Eslinger, Zappalà, Chakara, & Barrett, 2007). Clients may display *confabulations* (i.e., filling in memory gaps with imagined stories) or delusions. Although these early memory impairments typically resolve over time, occupational therapists can provide environmental cues to orient the client to personal information and a history of the events leading to the TBI. Therapists also may provide training in the application of specific strategies to enhance encoding of information (e.g., chunking information, rehearsal, creating rhymes and stories with the information, visual imagery) or the retrieval of information (e.g., alphabetical searching, retracing steps, association).

Technology has great potential to help clients with memory impairments be more functionally independent with use of cognitive orthotics or external memory aids. Devices such as alarm watches, PDAs, portable recording devices, and pill boxes with programmable alarms can provide the client with cues to complete time-dependent tasks with more self-sufficiency (McNeny, 2007; Toglia et al., 2008). Occupational therapists train clients in identifying daily situations where use of external memory aids is appropriate, how to program the devices, and how to retrieve information from the devices. Errorless-learning techniques, which capitalize on procedural memory, can be used to train clients with severe memory impairments to consistently use external memory aids. Using role-play situations and homework memory assignments, practitioners provide practice in consistent use of external memory aids. Occupational therapists collaborate with other members of the rehabilitation team to ensure their efforts to address the memory impairments are coordinated and consistent. Independent living requires prospective memory skills (e.g., remembering to pay utility bills by particular dates) and cognitive reminders in PDAs, daily planners, and wall calendars are used by people without brain injury to assist recall, thus making them socially acceptable.

Research Evidence on Interventions Focused on Memory

In an unpublished dissertation, Loya (1999) did a Level I meta-analysis of 14 studies to determine the magnitude and efficacy of memory rehabilitation in individuals with moderate to severe TBI, to identify the most efficacious treatment strategies for improving postinjury memory functioning, and to identify moderating variables that facilitate the rehabilitation process. Interventions were categorized according to three emphases of cognitive rehabilitation: (1) restorative (visualization, mnemonics), (2) compensatory (internal mnemonics, external aids), and (3) environmental adaptation. The author concluded that there was a significant, positive outcome resulting from memory rehabilitation among individuals with TBI. However, analysis of effect size estimates was nonsignificant, which obviated further analyses to rank order treatments by their effectiveness or identify moderator variables. The author concluded that attribution of superiority of one intervention over another could not be justified on the basis of available research.

Rees and colleagues (2007; Level I) found strong evidence in a systematic review that external aids are effective as compensatory strategies for functional day-to-day memory problems and also strong evidence for the use of internal aids such as mnemonics in improving recall for those with mild impairment, but not for those with severe impairment. The evidence is limited, however, that memory training programs and computer-assisted programs are not effective.

Thickpenny-Davis and Barker-Collo (2007; Level I) evaluated the effectiveness of a memory rehabilitation program on impaired memory functioning in 12 adults (10 with TBI, 2 with stroke) randomized to treatment ($n = 6$) or wait-list control ($n = 6$). Participants engaged in 8 learning modules of 1 hour twice per week for 4 weeks that included didactic information about memory and memory strategies, small-group activities, discussion, and inclusion of errorless-learning techniques. Efficacy of the intervention program was measured using before and after performance on the California Verbal Learning Test, Wechsler Memory Scale–Revised–Logical Memory Subtest, Visual Paired Associates; self-report and significant other–report of everyday memory behaviors indicative of memory difficulties; and the use of memory strategies and aids. Participants in the memory intervention group had significant improvement at 1-month follow-up compared to the wait-list control participants on knowledge of memory and memory strategies, use of memory aids and strategies, decreased behaviors indicative of memory impairment, and a positive effect on neuropsychological assessments of memory.

Limitations of the study include a small sample size with participants that had mostly severe TBI, making it difficult to generalize the results to individuals with mild or moderate TBI. In addition, there was a limited length of follow-up.

Cicerone, Mott, Azulay, and Friel (2004; Level II) used a two-group, pretest–posttest nonrandomized design to test the effectiveness of a program of holistic, intensive, cognitive rehabilitation (ICRP) administered by neuropsychologists on community reintegration as compared with conventional rehabilitation for individuals with TBI. The experimental program (ICRP) was administered 5 hours a day, 4 days per week, for 4 months. The control program, standard rehabilitation (SRP), was administered by physical therapists, occupational therapists, speech–language pathologists, and a neuropsychologist 12 to 24 hours per week for 4 months. Both groups showed significant improvement on the CIQ, with the ICRP group exhibiting a significant, but small, treatment effect compared to the SRP group (effect size, η^2 = .10). The SRP participants expressed significantly greater satisfaction with their community functioning on the Quality of Community Integration Questionnaire (nonstandardized) than did the ICRP group (effect size, d = .57).

The authors concluded that intensive, holistic, cognitive rehabilitation (offered by neuropsychologists) is an effective form of rehabilitation, particularly for persons with TBI who have previously been unable to resume community functioning. There is a threat to the validity of that conclusion because the SRP group was significantly more acutely injured than the ICRP group, raising the question of whether neuropsychological rehabilitation is effective or appropriate for persons in the acute phase of recovery. The difference in stage of recovery also would affect the satisfaction with community reintegration, because those in the chronic stage would have more experience and therefore be more aware of their limitations. Intervention contamination may have occurred because both groups were treated in the same facility with no controls reported to prevent comparison of programs and sharing of experiences.

Freeman, Mittenberg, Dicowden, and Bat-ami (1992; Level II) used a two-group pretest–posttest design to investigate the efficacy of memory retraining in patients with TBI using executive and compensatory memory retraining strategies as compared with patients who received no treatment. The experimental treatment consisted of training to remember paragraphs read out loud, with techniques to enhance retention such as note-taking in a memory notebook, self-monitoring skills, prompting from staff, restatement of presented material in the patient's own words, imagery, encouragement from others, asking for clari-

fication, and specific feedback concerning success. The treatment group performed significantly better than the control group at posttest (Paragraph Memory Task), and the effect was strong (p = .02, r = .59).

The authors concluded that the inclusion of memory retraining in cognitive remediation programs can improve memory function in patients with TBI. They further concluded that because the treatment group was in chronic stage of recovery, the significant recovery can be attributed to the treatment rather than spontaneous recovery. The limitations of the study do not appear to have affected the outcome. One limitation was that the groups were referred for different reasons and could therefore have differed in some way, although they were not significantly different in IQ or memory deficit at the outset. Another was that the treatment group was significantly more chronic than the control group (33- vs. 12-months postinjury).

Quemada and colleagues (2003; Level III) used a one-group pretest–posttest design to assess the effectiveness of a memory rehabilitation program on a heterogeneous sample of 12 patients with TBI. The program used Wilson's structured behavioral memory program, which includes behavioral compensation techniques and mnemonic strategies. It also included adaptations to reduce environmental demands (e.g., lines on floor, labels, painting doors different colors), external aids to help coding, storing and retrieving information (e.g., tape recorders, notebooks, diary schedules, maps), and reality orientation. Reorganization and restoration techniques also were used for 11 persons. Internal aids such as mnemonic strategies and nonverbal techniques such as visualization and association were included in this program. Additional therapies, which included social skills training and problem-solving training, were offered as needed to 10 persons. Treatment was individualized and administered daily in 50-minute sessions for 6 months, reduced to 3 times per week in the last month. After treatment, 9 patients were able to travel around their town without supervision. Six relearned how to use public transportation independently and regularly used it. Four redeveloped basic shopping and cooking skills. One patient learned to use an automatic teller machine; another to drive. In the 3 patients most severely affected, functional gain was limited to improvements in dressing, personal hygiene, and organizing their daily routines to require less supervision. However, there was no significant improvement on the Rivermead Behavioral Memory Test (RBMT), the main outcome measure of the study. None of the patients or their families felt that memory had improved after treatment.

Because the neuropsychological outcome measures did not indicate improvement, the authors concluded that research into the effectiveness of memory rehabilitation requires outcome measures that take performance in ADLs into account. They stated that tests assessing memory processes tell us little about gains obtained in rehabilitation through the use of external aids or environmental modifications. The study has a serious limitation: The lack of a control group does not allow one to rule out spontaneous recovery as an explanation of the functional improvement, because a majority of the participants were in the acute stage of recovery, or cointervention as another explanation, because the participants received various treatments that potentially affected occupational performance.

Teaching Methods

Kessels and de Haan (2003) completed a Level I meta-analysis of 11 studies (out of 27 retrieved) to investigate the effects of the teaching methods of vanishing cues and errorless learning as compared with trial-and-error learning in persons with memory impairments and amnesia. The effect size for errorless-learning compared with trial-and-error learning was 0.87 (large effect; z = 2.42, p = .008), whereas the effect size for vanishing cues compared to trial-and-error learning was 0.27 (small effect; z = .38, nonsignificant). The authors concluded that patients with severe memory impairments benefit most from an errorless-learning approach. The findings do not address the problem of generalization. They stated that the errorless-learning principle is most effective in situations where implicit learning is possible (e.g., recovery of habits of self-care).

Campbell, Wilson, McCann, Kernahan, and Rogers (2007; Level IV) reported a single-case experimental design study of errorless learning in a patient with severe memory impairment following TBI. The multiple baseline study conducted 6 years after the client's TBI used daily frequency counts of everyday memory problems (e.g., writing in a memory notebook, remembering to walk his dog) as the outcome measures. The client's caregiver (i.e., his mother) was trained to facilitate errorless learning in the home environment with client-generated cues. Although no changes were seen postintervention in assessments such as the Caregiver Strain Index, RBMT, or Dysexecutive Questionnaire from the Behavioural Assessment of Dysexecutive Syndrome, there was a significant change in notebook usage from baseline to 3-month follow-up. In addition, the client, who did not walk his dog at any time during the 44-day baseline period without prompting, showed a gradual decline in the number of verbal prompts needed to initiate walking the dog. Follow-up 18 months after the intervention showed the retention of these behavioral changes and actual continued improvement. The client now walked his dog daily without prompting and successfully used his notebook as a prospective memory aid for planning everyday activities.

Tam and Man (2004; Level II) used a five group, pretest–posttest design to compare the effectiveness of four different computer-assisted memory training strategies based on the behavioral approach. Each program included four modules that were similar across programs and that related to important daily functions: remembering people's names and faces, remembering to do something, remembering what people say, and remembering where something was put. The teaching method differed between groups: (1) self-paced practice, (2) visual presentation, (3) multisensory feedback, and (4) personalized training content. There was no significant improvement on the RBMT by any of the groups. The feedback group showed a significant gain in self-efficacy score; no other group improved significantly.

The authors concluded that using computers in patients' cognitive rehabilitation is effective, although the results do not support this conclusion. They further concluded that because the feedback group showed the greatest percentage of improvement of self-efficacy, feedback is a crucial factor to improve self-efficacy. However, the analysis was on the pretest to posttest of each group separately, not across groups to determine whether any one of the treatments is significantly better than another. Further limitations were that repeated *t* tests were used without corrections, and although participants were randomly assigned to the four experimental groups, the control group was not assigned.

Egan, Worrall, and Oxenham (2005; Level III) used a one-group, pretest–posttest design to determine whether people with acquired cognitive–linguistic impairments following TBI could learn to use the Internet using specialized training materials, which had been successfully trialed with people with aphasia. The materials were cast in a simplified format and used in conjunction with a volunteer, nonprofessional tutor. The 4 modules were taught over 6 lessons, with the option of additional lessons. The modules incorporated 12 Internet tasks such as "turn on the computer," "save a site in favorites," and so on. The outcome was the ability of the participant to do each of the 12 tasks, each scored on a 5-point scale from *total independence* to *not-at-all independent*. For 6 out of 7 participants, Wilcoxon signed ranks test showed significant gains in independence ($z = -2.201$, $p = .028$, $r = .78$). Participants achieved higher levels of independence in more-concrete tasks that had fewer steps and required less abstract reasoning.

The authors concluded that it is possible for people with TBI to reach moderate-to-high levels of independence in using the Internet with assistance of structured training materials. The materials designed for patients with aphasia did not need modification for use with persons with TBI. Severe cognitive–linguistic impairment, as seen in 1 participant, prevented participation in such a training program. In addition to lack of a control group, no information was given whether there was contamination of the independent variable by the participant or tutor outside of the research.

Parente and Stapleton (1999; Level III) used a two-group design in which the data for the baseline group were obtained from retrospective records. The two groups were unbalanced: The number in the experimental group was 13 out of a possible 33, whereas in the baseline group there were 64 out of a possible 568 who had been chosen to be comparable to the experimental group in age and education. The researchers investigated the effectiveness of a Group Cognitive Skills Training Model (CSG) as a precursor to vocational placement and reentry into the workplace. The thinking skills training took place once a week for 2 months to 1 year (mean = 4 months). Ten out of 13 clients in the CSG group became employed full-time (rehabilitation rate of 76%). The rehabilitation rate for the baseline group was 58%. All employed CSG group clients were employed more than 60 days; no data were presented for the baseline group. Grade point averages for those in the CSG group who went to school ranged from 2.5 to 3.5.

The authors concluded that the best interpretation of the difference in rehabilitation rate (76% vs. 58%) is that the CSG experience facilitated a level of vocational rehabilitation that was unmatched by any other combination of available therapy services. Details of the methodology are lacking, so discerning the study limitations is not possible.

Bergman (2000; level uncategorized) did an observational posttest-only comparison of the effects of a cognitive orthotic (CO) and the ease with which a heterogeneous group of individuals with TBI demonstrated mastery when given the opportunity to try the CO. The orthoses made use of errorless-learning principles and incorporated a very simple on-screen interface. Forty-one people more than 4 years postinjury participated. Thirty-six (88%) achieved mastery of 4 or more activity modules (e.g. Journal, Telephone Log, Directory, Savings Deposit/Withdrawal, Check Writing, Appointment Scheduling) and therefore were considered successful users of the device.

The author concluded that the multifunction CO, with consistent, highly structured organization with integrated on-screen cues and feedback (error-free learning) promoted rapid, unassisted, reliable performance of targeted tasks and facilitated transfer of training across other activity tasks for most participants. The author stated that all learning occurred through active, self-directed use of the system rather than through directed instruction and repetition. The report lacks many details to allow judgment concerning the validity of the study; however, because there was no control group or condition and no pretest or pretreatment baseline, we can conclude that the evidence is weak.

Computerized Memory Orthoses

Wright and colleagues (2001; Level II) used a one-group repeated-measures, counterbalanced design to test whether a computer interface could be designed for memory aids on pocket computers, including an appointment diary and notebook that easily could be mastered by people with memory problems. The participants used two different hand-held computer interfaces for 1 month each, with a 1-month washout period between usages. The researchers measured attitude toward use of the computers and amount of usage of the two different computers. All participants could use the computers, and 83% reported them helpful. Amount of use varied widely. The only statistically reliable difference between the pocket computers was the greater use of alarms for diary entries when using the Hewlett-Packard ($t_{(11)}$ = 2.38, p < .04, r = .58).

The authors concluded that people with memory impairments resulting from brain injury can use purpose-designed computer-based memory aids, comprising an appointment diary, notebooks, and links between them. They further concluded that the data strongly suggest that different pocket computers suit different participants.

Wright, Rogers, Hall, Wilson, Evans, and Emslie (2001; Level II) also used a one-group repeated-measures, counterbalanced design to examine the hypothesis that encouraging people to use a pocket computer more often for other activities, such as games, will increase the use of the memory aids. They used the same interventions as in the first study but added

a memory aid to-do list and three games chosen to encourage planning and remembering. The first computer had Pairs, Hangman, and Mosaic games, and the second computer had Crosswords, Solitaire, and Chess. Again, the researchers measured attitude toward use and amount of usage. All participants could use the computers and 83% (10/12) found them useful. The use of games did not correlate with computer usage as memory aid (r = .11).

The authors concluded that people experiencing memory loss after brain injury can master purpose-designed electronic memory aids and find such aids of great personal benefit. Games were enjoyed by many participants, but they did not increase the use of the memory aids.

Both studies lack detail concerning possible threats to validity, including information regarding blinded evaluation, contamination, or co-intervention. No standardized outcome measures with established reliability were used.

Wilson, Emslie, Quirk, and Evans (2001; Level I) conducted an RCT with crossover design to determine whether a paging system enabled people with prospective memory and planning problems after brain injury to carry out everyday tasks as compared with people not using a pager. Although only 44% of the participants had brain injury due to trauma, this study was included in this review because occupational therapists use paging systems as an intervention for persons with TBI. Approximately 8 messages were sent on the pager to remind each person to do some agreed-upon task at a given time. Group 1 used the pager in the home and community for 7 weeks, while Group 2 did not (wait list), then Group 2 used the pager for the next 7 weeks while the first group did not. The outcome measure was individualized to participant and consisted of 4 to 7 questions to determine whether the person had remembered to do the targeted tasks. There was a significant difference in the number of targets achieved between those using the pager (~75%) and those not using it (~48% for those who had not used the pager at all and 62% for those who had used the pager in the previous 7 weeks). A total of 84.6% of participants were significantly more successful with the pager than at baseline. Seventy-three percent of those in Group 1 were still significantly better than baseline after the pager treatment was discontinued.

The authors concluded that this particular paging system significantly reduces everyday failures of prospective memory and planning and enables people with brain injury to carry out more everyday tasks at relatively low cost. This conclusion is tempered by the fact that the outcome measure was a self-report and left to the patient to fill out daily, which could be a problem for persons with memory disorders. There was no compliance or reliability information provided.

Hart, Hawkey, and Whyte (2002; Level I) used a one-group repeated-measures design with randomization to condition to test whether use of an electronic device (a voice organizer; PDA) could help clients with TBI to remember and articulate therapy goals (retrospective memory). Ten persons with moderate to severe TBI were randomly assigned to either a sequence of use of a PDA followed by no device or vice versa. In the experimental condition, the person was to listen to the list of goals on the device when it beeped (3 times per day); in the control condition, the participant was instructed to remember three goals of equal importance. The recorded goals were recalled significantly better than the unrecorded goals, and a cued recall situation was significantly better than free recall for both conditions.

The authors concluded that using a voice organizer to listen to recorded goals at multiple, consistent times each day was effective in enhancing recall of goals at the verbal level, with and without the addition of brief reminder cues. However, future research needs to evaluate whether this intervention affects actual goal-related behaviors.

Burke and colleagues (2001; Level II) used a two-condition, nonrandomized repeated-measures design to test a tracking system for patients with TBI that couples an indoor, fluorescent-light-fixture–based location system ("Talking Lights") with hand-held computer technology (called PLAM—patient locator and minder) to provide greater independence for patients in their adherence to therapy schedules without staff prompting. The PLAM provided verbal cues that an appointment was coming up, directed the patient to start moving toward the correct room, and provided feedback on the accuracy of travel to the therapy destination. The control condition was human prompting ordinarily used. The outcome measure was the number of human prompts needed and the on-time arrival at therapy destinations. Five persons with brain damage (60% TBI) used the PLAM. With the PLAM system, the average number of human prompts dropped more than 50%. The number of sessions requiring no prompting significantly increased, from 7% to 44%. The on-time arrival increased significantly with the PLAM.

The authors, noting fewer (human) commands and greater punctuality, concluded that the results imply that the constant reinforcement of external commands (whether human or mechanical) does facilitate learning and improve function. This conclusion overstates the data, however; they did not measure learning. They stated that overall this new technology has the potential to improve the lives of many individuals and move them toward greater independence. Limitations of this study include a difference in duration of the two conditions (experimental group lasted 3 days; control group lasted 1 week) and insufficient information about the methodology, including sampling procedure, outcome measurement, and statistical outcome.

Boman, Tham, Granqvist, Bartfai, and Hemmingsson (2007; Level III) used a pretest–posttest design with 8 individuals with TBI to evaluate the effectiveness of electronic aids to daily living (EADL) on functional performance. The participants, who were independent or required minimal assistance for self-care, had poor to moderate memory impairment and no additional cognitive impairments. Participants stayed in two apartments equipped with a set of basic and advanced EADL (i.e., remote or voice-controlled devices used to access, operate, and control electrical appliances designed for comfort, communication, and personal security) for 4 to 6 months during an intervention time of 2 years. Errorless learning was included in the instruction method. Outcome measures included the COPM, Sickness Impact Profile (SIP), structured observations, self-rating of EADL, and Quality of Life Visual Analogue Scale.

Results showed a significant improvement in the participants' self-perceived abilities to perform the most important activities and self-perceived quality of life between pre- and postintervention. There also was a significant improvement on the body care and psychosocial function subsets of the SIP. Occupational performance was improved, as measured by the COPM. Caution is suggested in interpreting the results, as the sample size was small and the study design did not include a control group. In addition, several participants had difficulty completing certain outcome measures, which calls into question the validity of the data.

Gentry, Wallace, Kvarfordt, and Lynch (2008; Level III) trained a group of 23 individuals living in the community who were a minimum of 1 year after a severe TBI to use PDAs as cognitive aids. Occupational performance (i.e., COPM scores) and participation in everyday life tasks (i.e., scores of the Craig Handicap Assessment and Rating Technique–Revised [CHART]) were scored pre-training and 8 weeks posttraining. Self-ratings on both outcome measures showed statistically significant improvements.

Stapleton, Adams, and Atterton (2007; Level IV) used a series of 5 single-case studies using an ABAB reversal design to evaluate the effectiveness of a "reminders" function on a mobile phone as a compensatory memory aid for persons with TBI. Participants recruited from a rehabilitation center were at least 1 year postinjury, reported to have everyday memory problems, and lived with a caregiver. Participants were provided with mobile phones that were programmed with individualized reminder messages using the reminders function. Outcomes included the speed and capacity of language processing, performance on the RBMT and Tower Test (executive functioning), the map test from the Test of Everyday Attention, and a measure of everyday memory success in achieving target behaviors.

An increase in target behaviors was noted for two participants and did not return to baseline when the phone was removed. Those who did not benefit scored within the severe impairment range on the RBMT, were significantly impaired on the Tower Test, and required 24-hour care. This study was limited by its small sample size, lack of measurement of caregiver responses, and no follow-up to determine whether improvements were maintained.

Noncomputerized Memory Orthoses

Watanabe, Black, Zafonte, Millis, and Mann (1998; Level I) used an RCT to examine the relationship among age, injury severity, and use of calendar on emergence from posttraumatic amnesia (PTA). Of the 32 participants with PTA, only 50% were post-TBI, but these were distributed equally between groups. This study was included in this evidence-based literature review because it researched an intervention commonly used by occupational therapists with person with TBI.

In the rooms of the persons in the experimental group, a 8½-x-11 inch boldly printed calendar was visible to the patient and was brought to the patient's attention once a day if the patient answered incorrectly when quizzed about time orientation. There was no calendar in the rooms of the control patients. Treatment was discontinued when the patient was accurate for 2 consecutive days on the Temporal Orientation Test or was discharged. The difference between groups was not tested. Instead, the association between calendar use and emergence from PTA was tested and found to be $R = 0.03$, accounting for only 0.09% of the variance of emergence from PTA.

The authors concluded that calendars may not be helpful in promoting reorientation despite their frequent espousal. However, this conclusion is subject to further research because this study was severely flawed; the most problematic threat to validity was possible contamination of the control group, who probably received orientation information from other staff or visitors. In addition, measurement reliability and validity were not controlled. Further, too few participants emerged from PTA to allow the planned statistical analysis to be carried out.

The primary limitations of the above studies are lack of control group or condition or comparison group for Level III studies, which limits the strength of evidence that the intervention caused the outcome; lack of detail concerning methodology to allow judgment of threats to internal validity of the study; lack of information concerning the validity and reliability of measurement; and small sample size. Although not a limitation to the internal validity of the studies, a practical limitation is the poor choice of outcome measures, for example, those that require patients with memory problems to recall behavior and those that measure the cognitive components of functional skills rather than ability to accomplish functional skills.

Schwartz (1995; Level V), an occupational therapist, reported the outcome of 3 cases in which the author applied decision-making and dynamic assessment models of occupational therapy practice. One case did not involve a patient with TBI. In the other 2 cases, the goals were to increase initiation or independence in basic ADLs. After 3 months, Case 1 became independent in tooth-brushing and shaving daily. Two years after initiation of the tape-recorded messages, Case 2 followed his morning routine with only a checklist in the bathroom. He was unable to transfer these skills to a different context. The author concluded that occupational therapy provided external compensations that facilitated the learning of specific behavior routines for these patients with severe memory impairment and other cognitive deficits. The author further stated that in the long run, this could help reduce nursing or attendant care hours and thus health care costs.

However, this report offers no trustworthy evidence that the interventions described caused the outcomes reported and the outcome was very modest in light of the extent of therapy involved, therefore negating the statement concerning cost-effectiveness. Common limitations of extremely small sample size and lack of controls for ensuring internal validity of the study prohibit the establishment of a causal relationship between the intervention and outcome.

Executive Function

Executive functions include higher-level cognitive skills of planning, judgment, decision making, organization, problem solving, self-monitoring, and cognitive flexibility that enable individuals to engage in self-directed behavior. Impairments in executive functions significantly influence functional and vocational outcomes and social participation (Cicerone, 2007; Goverover, 2004). The relative structure of daily routines during inpatient rehabilitation may not reveal the limiting nature of executive impairments. Discharge home to the community with unstructured time and unpredictable events may unmask the true extent of executive dysfunction (Toglia et al., 2008). Occupational therapy intervention addressing executive functions may occur in both individual and group sessions using a variety of unstructured tasks that required planning, organization, and flexibility. For example, clients can plan a group meal, including deciding on food to prepare that takes into account preferences and the available budget, shopping for all needed items, sequencing the items to be prepared, and assigning cooking tasks. Detailed checklists may be used to help the clients initiate the activities and self-monitoring cues to encourage self-regulation of behaviors.

Research Evidence on Executive Function Intervention

Levine and colleagues (2000; Level I) used an RCT to examine the effects of goal management training (GMT) versus a motor skills training (MST) program (control) on everyday paper-and-pencil tasks for persons with TBI to the frontal lobes. GMT included orienting to relevant goals, selecting goals, portioning goals into subgoals, encoding and retaining goals and subgoals, and monitoring outcome of action compared with goal state. The researchers found a significant difference in accuracy between groups on a proofreading task, but the difference was due to more errors by controls rather than improvement by experimental participants. The GMT group performed significantly ($p < .05$) better on the grouping task than did the

MST group, with a moderately strong effect ($r = .41$). There was no significant difference in groups on the room layout task, as both groups improved.

The authors concluded that GMT was associated with improved performance on paper-and-pencil tasks that correspond to everyday situations known to be problematic for persons with TBI. However, there was only one finding of differential improvement (grouping task), and that may have been because the tasks used to measure outcome were similar to those used in GMT (task-specific training). This study had several other flaws in addition to compromise of the independent variable, including failure to report information concerning the validity and reliability of the outcome measures or whether the evaluator was blind to group assignment.

Manly, Hawkins, Evans, Woldt, and Robertson (2002; Level I) used a one-group repeated-measures crossover design with random assignment to condition to examine whether auditory stimuli that interrupted current activity would cause the patients to pause, evaluate, plan, and change track, thereby improving performance of a complex (multistep) task. The control condition required the same tasks of the participants, but without an alerting beep. Intervention was applied in one 15-minute period in a laboratory. There was a significant ($p < .05$) improvement in the number of tasks started in the alerting condition compared with the control condition, with a strong effect ($r = .61$). Under the alerted condition, the participants performed time allocation to each task significantly ($p < .01$) better than under the control condition ($r = .79$). There was no significant difference between conditions in time spent in each activity, nor in time-specific responses, nor in use of the clock. The alert did not prompt a switch in tasks ($p = .51$, $r = .22$).

The authors concluded that the performance was significantly improved when exposed to periodic, nonpredictive tones. Although flawed in that the validity and reliability of outcome measurement were not reported, the study was fairly strong and suggests one possibly useful compensatory intervention for persons with impaired executive function post-TBI—

use of alerting beeps to catch the patient's attention and switch focus of performance. However, one study of 10 patients undergoing one 15-minute experimental treatment cannot establish this intervention as predictably effective.

Intervention Addressing Areas of Occupation

As the client emerges from the period of agitation, occupational therapy intervention can begin to focus on the client's performance of more client-centered areas of occupation, including ADLs (e.g., feeding, dressing, grooming, toileting, bathing, transfers) and IADLs (e.g., meal preparation, shopping, financial and home management, child rearing, caring for pets). The occupational therapist may delay focusing on some areas of occupation (e.g., work, education, leisure) until the client is transitioning back to his or her community.

Occupational therapists use information obtained from the occupational profile and an analysis of the client's roles (e.g., student, parent, worker, friend, volunteer) to engage in client-centered identification of priority areas of occupation to address within therapy sessions. Limitations in many performance skills (e.g., motor, cognitive, sensory and perceptual, emotional and behavioral, communication skills) can contribute to observed difficulty in ADLs and IADLs. The therapist combines knowledge of the person's assets and limitations in performance skills with an in-depth understanding of the activity demands of the occupations and supports or barriers contributed by the environment and context in which the client engages in the occupations to design an intervention plan that enables the client to engage in meaningful occupations that he or she wants or needs to do.

The occupational therapist determines where to focus intervention (i.e., the client, the activity, or the environment) based upon consideration of several questions: "Are the client's impairments expected to change?" "What activity demands or environmental conditions match the client's current capabilities?" "Can the client learn and generalize information?" "Is the client responsive to cues?" and "Is the client aware of his or her limitations?" If the client with TBI has severely limited awareness of his or her difficulties, or displays significantly limited ability to benefit from cues and potential for change, the therapist uses an approach that changes the environment or activity rather than a treatment approach that targets change in strategy use within the person (Toglia et al., 2008). Occupational therapists using an approach focused on modification of the activity complete an in-depth analysis of the task for points of breakdown in performance, then identify adaptations that support the client's performance of the task (e.g., placing an entire outfit for the next day in the top drawer of the bureau with a checklist outlining the sequence for donning so the client can dress independently in the morning). Similarly, the occupational therapist may analyze the environment for supports or barriers to independent performance of areas of occupation and structure the environment to enable more independence (e.g., placing cue signs in visible key locations to remind the individual to perform a task and minimize executive function skills).

Intervention approaches using adaptations to the task or environment require repetitive practice of the task and caregiver support and education on how to structure tasks and the environment for optimal performance. Although some adaptations to the environment may be fixed (e.g., a door alarm to prevent wandering or color-coded labels on the inside or outside of drawers and closets to reduce memory demands), other modifications depend upon the consistency and reliability of another person (e.g., filling and programming an alarmed pill box to aid the client in following a medication schedule). Throughout intervention focused on modifying and adapting tasks and the environment, the occupational therapist is acutely aware that acceptance of these interventions requires the client to accept a new vision of himself or herself and a willingness to accept change to the pattern or conditions of how he or she performs activities (Klinger, 2005).

If the individual with TBI demonstrates potential for improvement in underlying cognitive and motor impairments, shows awareness of current limitations, and shows the ability to alter performance when pro-vided cues and feedback, the occupational therapist may choose to focus intervention on restoring underlying cognitive and motor impairments that contribute to difficulties in the performance of functional tasks. Addressing executive-planning skills such as organization by developing cognitive strategies (e.g., checklists, self-monitoring strategies), occupational therapists may focus intervention on addressing underlying impairments to restore ability to enable more consistent, independent occupational performance. Application of cognitive strategies will be practiced in performance of a variety of ADLs and IADLs and individual and group intervention sessions to encourage generalization of the strategy to multiple areas of occupation. Occupational therapists working with clients during both the acute rehabilitation and community phases of recovery should incorporate functional, occupation-based activities into the intervention plan that require flexible adaptation of behavior in "What if?" situations and planning and organizing activities in time (e.g., organizing a day's activities or errands; planning a menu, lunch, picnic, vacation, or social gathering; role-playing phone calls to schedule several appointments; charting dates to pay bills on a wall calendar).

A comprehensive occupational therapy intervention program addressing ADLs and IADLs considers multiple parameters that contribute to successful performance, including familiarity of the environment and the items used; the client's typical performance patterns (i.e., habits and routines); safety risks resulting from motor and cognitive–behavioral impairments; possible adaptive devices and compensatory techniques to improve performance; team and family support for implementation of the selected approaches; and the client's ability to monitor and correct performance (McNeny, 2007). Occupational therapists working in acute rehabilitation settings engage the client in tasks such as showering, grooming his or her hair and nails, folding laundry, making a bed, vacuuming, planning and cooking a meal, sending an e-mail, dialing a cell phone, and so on. It is common to see occupational therapists modifying the clinical environment to simulate the client's home or using real-world environments like the hospital gift shop, cafeteria, or library as settings to practice performance skills. Community outings to grocery stores, banks, restaurants, and shopping centers all provide opportunities for clients with TBI to practice areas of occupational performance prior to transitioning back into their communities.

Related Evidence Focused on Occupational Performance

Occupational therapy to increase participation in occupational areas of ADLs, IADLs, work, leisure, social integration, and education involves interventions that not only reduce impairment-related disability but also reduce handicap through use of compensatory strategies and adaptation of environments. Therefore, occupational therapists are interested in knowing what evidence exists that these treatments increase participation in areas of occupation.

Recent evidence on interventions to enable persons with TBI to participate in areas of occupation (ADL, IADL, work, leisure, social participation, and education) has focused on self-selection of goals by the patient or carer in collaboration with the therapists and valuing of the goals to be worked on by the patient (meaningful occupation); compensatory strategies; environmental adaptation; and extensive, intensive practice of targeted behaviors and tasks. Limitations of the studies reviewed require occupational therapists to rely on their own clinical judgment and experience when deciding the combination of interventions that may enable their clients with TBI to engage more fully in their ADLs and IADLs. Further research is needed.

Summary of Levels I–III Evidence

Of the seven studies of evidence Levels I–III that examined the effectiveness of therapy to reduce handicap and improve participation in areas of occupation, six examined multidisciplinary treatment that included occupational therapy and one examined occupational therapy directly (Powell, Heslin, & Greenwood, 2002 [Level I; see also Hillier, 2003]; Vanderploeg et al., 2008 [Level I]; Zhu, Poon, Chan, & Chan, 2001 [Level I]; Goranson, Graves, Allison, & LaFreniere, 2003 [Level II]; Hayden, Moreault, LeBlanc,

& Plenger, 2000 [Level III]; Malec, 2001 [Level III]; Trombly, Radomski, Trexel, & Burnett-Smith, 2002 [Level III]).

Vanderploeg and colleagues (2008) randomized 360 adult veterans or active-duty military service personnel from 4 Veterans Administration Medical Centers with nonpenetrating, severe TBI to 1 of 2 groups to determine the efficacy of cognitive–didactic versus functional–experiential approaches to treatment. All participants received 1.5 to 2.5 hours of the assigned treatment protocol in addition to 2 to 2.5 hours of daily occupational and physical therapy over 20 to 60 days, depending upon client needs and progress. The cognitive–didactic treatment approach was based upon the Attention Process Training of Sohlberg and Mateer (2001) and targeted attention, memory, executive functions, and pragmatic communication using one-to-one therapy sessions incorporating paper-and-pencil or computerized tasks. Self-awareness questioning was used throughout the treatment sessions in this approach. The functional–experiential treatment was a modified version of the neurofunctional approach of Giles (an occupational therapist) and Clark-Wilson (Giles, 2005). This approach involved performance of everyday tasks in group and natural environments to mimic real-life situations and emphasized errorless-learning strategies and instructional cues. Both groups improved, but there were no significant differences between the two treatment approaches.

At 1 year follow-up, subgroup analysis found that younger participants (<30) and those with less education who participated in the cognitive–didactic approach had better work-related outcomes than participants in the functional–experiential group. However, older participants (>30) and those with more education who participated in the functional–experiential approach had better outcomes in terms of independent living. The outcomes suggest that older patients with independent living goals might benefit more from functional–experiential rather than cognitive–didactic rehabilitation treatment.

Powell and colleagues (2002), in a Level I study randomized 94 participants to 1 of 2 groups to determine whether or not outreach treatment increased the relative probability and magnitude of improvements in community integration after TBI. Individualized goals valued by the participant and carer, and considered amenable to treatment, were worked toward using a series of written contracts that specified short-term and interim goals to be achieved over a 6- to 12-week period. Treatment was carried out in patients' homes, day centers, and workplaces for 2 to 6 hours per week for a mean of 28 weeks. The program was carried out by a team of rehabilitation professionals, two of whom were occupational therapists. Outreach participants were significantly more likely to show gains on the Barthel Index and the total self-care and self-organization and psychological well-being subscales of the Brain Injury Community Rehabilitation Outcome–39 (BICRO–39) than the control group, who received a booklet listing resources and one visit by a team therapist.

Zhu and colleagues (2001), in a Level I study randomly assigned 36 persons with moderate to severe brain injury to 1 of 2 groups to evaluate the effects of intensive rehabilitation, which included occupational therapy, on functional outcome. Experimental therapy included physical and sensorimotor training, functional retraining, and psychosocial retraining for 4 hours per day (2 hours occupational therapy, 2 hours physical therapy), plus 2 hours per week of speech therapy, for up to 6 months versus the same therapy at reduced (half) intensity. There was a trend for more patients in the intensive therapy to achieve full independence FIM scores and good GOS scores at 2 and 3 months. Intensity of therapy allowed patients with TBI to resume participation sooner than the conventional intensity of therapy. Although this advantage did not prevail beyond the first 3 months, one would expect that earlier achievement of tasks of valued roles would contribute to a patient's psychological well-being and continued motivation (this assumption needs to be tested) and therefore justify increased intensity in the early period following injury. The researchers concluded that the effect of therapy is in potentiating the recovery rather than changing the final outcome.

Goranson and colleagues (2003) used a retrospective nonrandomized, two-group, pretest–posttest, matched-groups design to determine the extent to which participation in a multidisciplinary rehabilitation program and patient characteristics predicted improvement in community integration following mild to moderate TBI. The rehabilitation program, which included occupational therapy, included remediation of cognitive impairments; compensatory strategies for cognitive, physical, or emotional sequelae of TBI; mutual goal setting; and individual and group therapy. The treatment group improved significantly more than the no-treatment group on the CIQ in-home independence (14% effect size) but not in social or productive use of time.

Hayden and colleagues (2000) tested 61 persons with TBI in a Level III pretest–posttest design to determine whether manipulation of environments (graduated increase of distractions and decrease of structure) while the person was engaged in individually chosen ADL and IADL tasks that challenged each person's identified deficits would result in significant decreases in handicap. Treatment was provided 5 to 6 hours per day for an average of 35 days (for mildly injured patients admitted from home within a year postinjury) to 62 days (for acute patients who were admitted directly from inpatient care). All participants demonstrated significant gains in independence. Forty-six out of the 61 participants were independent at discharge and 92% of those remained so at the 6-month follow-up.

Malec (2001) used a Level III pretest–posttest design to study 96 participants to determine whether the Mayo Brain Injury Outpatient program, a comprehensive day treatment program, would result in positive changes in outcome measures equal to those reported for other programs. Occupational therapy participated in a "transdiciplinary" way, but the role was murky. Physical therapy and recreational therapy taught the life skills group, not the occupational therapist. Eighty-one percent of the 552 goals were met at expected or higher levels. At 1-year follow-up, 72% were living independently, and 39% were working independently. On the other hand, 24% were more depressed, and 29% were more irritable as they began to confront and realize their limitations.

Trombly and colleagues (2002), in a Level III study, used a repeated-measures design to test the effect of goal-specific outpatient occupational therapy on achievement of self-identified ADL and IADL goals, patients' ratings of their performance and satisfaction with performance of targeted activities, and level of participation in nontargeted activities. Thirty-one persons with mild to moderate brain injury from three different clinics participated. All participants received treatment focused on training of compensatory strategies and environmental adaptation to achieve the goals. Each patient received 30-minute treatments ranging in number from a mean of 24 to 63 treatments depending upon their rehabilitation site. Changes that occurred during the treatment phase were contrasted to changes during a follow-up no-treatment period ranging from 5.8 weeks to 19.6 weeks. Goal Attainment Scaling (GAS) indicated that 81% of the 149 goals identified were achieved. The effect of occupational therapy on goal achievement was strong ($r = .94$). Fifteen participants achieved 100% of their goals, 11 achieved 80%, and 2 achieved 60%. Patients were significantly more satisfied with performance and rated their performance significantly higher on the COPM after treatment than during the no-treatment phase. No change occurred during the no-treatment phase. Improvement was maintained during the no-treatment period, but no further improvement was seen. The effect sizes were strong ($r = .71$ and $.76$, respectively). There was no significant difference in scores of nontargeted activities as measured by the CIQ between the treatment and no-treatment phases.

The researchers concluded that occupational therapy directed at specific goals valued by the client and using compensatory strategies and environmental adaptation as intervention to achieve those goals is likely to be successful for persons with mild to moderate TBI. The specific interventions used at the three sites were different, but all were compensatory in nature and aimed at targeted goals identified by the client in collaboration with the occupational therapist.

The common aspects of these intervention programs offered at the different sites included

- Self-selection of goals by patient or carer in collaboration with the therapists; valuing of goals to be worked on,
- Compensatory strategies,
- Environmental adaptation, and
- Guided practice of targeted behaviors and tasks.

These studies had the following limitations: The evaluators were not blind to treatment status (Hayden et al., 2000; Trombly et al., 2002); two studies lacked control groups or conditions (Hayden et al., 2000; Malec, 2001); researchers failed to report sampling method or inclusion/exclusion criteria (Hayden et al., 2000); there were possible differences in personnel and procedures for a study whose data collection lasted 10 years (Malec, 2001); one study failed to report a statistical analysis of the data (Malec, 2001); ceiling and floor effects of the measuring instruments (Powell et al., 2002); dropouts due to researcher error (Powell et al., 2002); possible co-intervention bias (Powell et al., 2002); and experimental and control groups drawn from different populations (Goranson et al., 2003).

Summary of Levels IV–V Evidence

Three Level V case studies examined the effects of particular occupational therapy interventions on one or a few patients. We cannot say from these uncontrolled studies that the intervention was the cause of the changes reported; however, they suggest interventions that can be experimented with for other similar patients. Each paper described the treatments in detail. Careful observation of changes seen in the patient will guide continuation or discontinuation of the experimental treatment.

Gutman (2000; Level V), an occupational therapist, adapted a computer for use by a patient with hemiparesis in addition to TBI and other concurrent diagnoses. She taught the patient to use word processing and how to e-mail, and she guided him to use the computer to reestablish social roles and engage in meaningful productive activity, which he accomplished.

Walker (2002; Level V) tested a program that combined remediative and restorative interventions to enable improved participation in a man who was unable to accomplish IADL because of cognitive deficits of poor concentration, poor time management skills, and poor organizational skills. The program included task analysis, matching occupations to the patient's current abilities, grading the complexity of the occupations, developing compensatory strategies, and helping the patient to apply the strategies in actual situations. After 4 months, the patient consistently used his strategies to independently complete IADLs that were problematic before the therapy.

Kowalske, Plenger, Lusby, and Hayden (2000; Level V) described a program that focused on patient–environment interactions to improve participation in work. Treatment of three patients at different levels of severity was described. Treatment involved grading the environment (distraction/structure) from simulated environments in the clinic to actual work environments, teaching compensatory strategies, using adapted devices such as memory books, and overlearning skills until they became rote. Each of the three patients achieved return to work, commensurate with their cognitive abilities.

These Level V reports failed to control for intervening variables that could account for the outcome, and the outcomes were specific to particular persons, so the evidence they provide is weak. Because of the weak research design, causality cannot be assumed for the interventions.

Intervention During the Community Recovery Phase

"Disability is not inherent in the individual; it can only be understood in relation to the interaction between an individual and his/her environment" (Kneipp & Rubin, 2007, p. 1086). Some insurers question why community reentry services are necessary, often for long periods of time, because early rehabilitation for TBI is effective. Discharge from the relative structure and security of the acute inpatient rehabilitation setting to the unpredictable and often demanding natural environment of the person's home

and community can reveal the true challenge of reengaging in life roles and activities with residual physical, cognitive, and emotional impairments.

The National Institutes of Health Consensus Statement (Rehabilitation of Persons With Traumatic Brain Injury, 1998) recognized that cognitive and behavioral issues following brain injury can impede participation in major life roles and activities related to school, work, and family life, and that community-based programs designed to match the needs of the individual with TBI are needed to optimize recovery and outcome. At present, there is limited evidence that multidisciplinary community-based rehabilitation programs can improve activity limitations (i.e., functional performance) of individuals with TBI when targeted toward specific goals, but the beneficial effects of these community-based programs on carer issues has not been demonstrated (McCabe et al., 2007; Turner-Stokes et al., 2005). The Traumatic Brain Injury Act of 1996, amended in 2000 and reauthorized in 2008 (S. 793, 110th Congress, 1st Session, 2007–2008), mandates continued exploration of interventions that facilitate reintegration into community roles and activities.

Individuals with TBI often experience difficulty participating in areas of occupation (ADL, IADL, work, leisure, social participation, and education) after they return to their communities. Complaints of mental or cognitive fatigue can impede clients with TBI who live in the community from being able to sustain their cognitive skill performance for lengthy periods, thus influencing their participation (Cantor et al., 2008).

A total of 454 respondents with TBI living in the community participated in a Canadian post-census survey (Dawson & Chipman, 1995). The survey identified three postinjury handicaps: 66% reported the need for assistance with ADLs or IADLs, 75% reported that they were not working, and 90% reported being limited or dissatisfied with their social integration. Time postinjury was not associated with severity of handicap. The authors reported that the proportions found in this study are comparable to that reported elsewhere. Although some of the variance in this study was explained by physical and social environments, as well as by age, gender, and educational level, little of the variance was explained by disability, indicating that community reintegration does not depend simply on remediating disability.

Community-based services for individuals with TBI are provided by an array of rehabilitation professionals, including occupational therapy practitioners in both residential and nonresidential programs with varying degrees of supervision and intensity. Many of the intervention approaches detailed in literature are not specific to a particular profession and are within the scope of occupational therapy practice. Regardless of the location of service provision, the overarching goal of occupational therapy intervention at the community level is to support the client's engagement in meaningful occupations and activities that allow desired or needed participation in home, school, workplace, and community life (AOTA, 2008b).

Intervention Addressing Social and Coping Skills

Shortened lengths of inpatient hospitalizations have resulted in less time for clients and family members to prepare for the transition home to the community. Adjustment to the variety of physical, cognitive, and neurobehavioral impairments resulting from TBI require functional coping skills from both the client and family. When linked with possible preinjury impaired family functioning, individuals discharged home after TBI with neurobehavioral symptoms showed more signs of distress and depression (Testa, Malec, Moessner, & Brown, 2006). Community-based programs run using a clubhouse model may effectively meet the emotional, social, and cognitive needs of individuals with TBI and their families (Fraas et al., 2007).

Brain injury support groups, such as those run by the state affiliates of the Brain Injury Association of America (BIAA), are vital links to education, life planning, and emotional support for clients and families. These community groups offer information on life planning and real-world problem solving (Rodgers et al., 2007). They also may offer leisure and social networking opportunities in groups where the client's neurobehavioral problems are more easily understood

and accepted. Occupational therapists encourage clients and their families to connect to local brain injury support groups and may work with the groups to provide educational information sessions or develop programming to address leisure and social needs of the members.

The ability to maintain existing friendships and develop new friendships is challenged when a person experiences a TBI. Impairments in cognitive and social skills, as well as limitations in the ability to engage in shared occupations, can result in the distancing of friends from the individual who sustained the injury. Callaway, Sloan, and Winkler (2005) suggested that friends be included in educational programs and treatment sessions offered throughout inpatient rehabilitation to support and strengthen existing community-based friendships. Occupational therapy practitioners may educate friends in practical skills, such as moving a wheelchair or transferring the client into and out of a car, or more complex issues, such as managing disinhibited behaviors. Clients with TBI may engage in therapeutic activities that involve friends, such as communicating via e-mail, using photos and videos to reminisce, or sharing previous leisure activities such as TV or computer-based video gaming programs. Individuals with TBI who sustain meaningful relationships report better quality of life (Dijkers, 2004), as do those individuals who are satisfied with their level of social integration and participation within their communities (Burleigh, Farber, & Gillard, 1998; Pierce & Hanks, 2006).

Occupational therapy practitioners begin addressing social skills during inpatient rehabilitation, but often these impairments in social skills become more evident when the individual with TBI is discharged home to the community and reassumes social roles. In the community setting, the occupational therapy practitioners may conduct social skills training groups to address cognitive components of social interaction, the pragmatics of social conversation, and tasks involved in developing and maintaining friendships and relationships (Ylvisaker & Feeney, 2001). Techniques such as goal setting, individualized written contracts, role playing and rehearsal, peer mentoring and role modeling, and videotaping social interactions with self-reflection and supportive feedback may be used in individual and group sessions.

TBI is a life-changing event, and individuals who sustain brain injuries may have difficulty adjusting to the injury and its consequences. An individual's ability to cope with and adapt to physical and cognitive impairments in postinjury social situations can influence whether the individual perceives these impairments as disabling and restricting to community participation (MacLachlan et al., 2007). Individuals with TBI and impaired coping skills can show signs of depression and poorer outcomes. When impaired coping skills are coupled with neurobehavioral symptoms such as impulsivity, the person with TBI may be at greater risk for alcohol and drug abuse. Depression is, however, often amenable to treatment with a combination of psychological and pharmacological therapies.

Family-focused intervention may help the family unit manage the cognitive and neurobehavioral symptoms of their member with TBI upon return home to the community. Beliefs about caregiving, coupled with caregiver strain and inefficient problem solving, can lead to caregiver burnout, depression, and anxiety, affecting the family's well-being and perceived burden of care.

Research Evidence on Family Intervention

Research using various interventional approaches have found mixed results on the effectiveness of family-focused intervention on relieving caregiver identified issues. Boschen, Gargaro, Gan, Gerber, and Brandys (2007; Level I systematic review) reviewed four RCTs that evaluated the efficacy of various types of family-focused intervention for individuals with TBI. These interventions included education, telerehabilitation, case management, therapy (e.g., family counseling and/or cognitive behavioral), peer/support group, and multi-component programs. They found no strong evidence supporting any specific intervention method for support of family caregivers of individuals with TBI. Limitations of the studies included in the review were small sample sizes, a lack of standardized outcome measures, and a lack of consensus regarding variables to study.

Research Evidence on Interventions to Address Psychosocial, Behavioral, and Social Functions

Some persons who sustained moderate to severe TBI fail to achieve social participation without therapeutic intervention, whereas some others exhibit nonsocial or at-risk behavior that prevents participation in community life. Various treatment approaches have been developed to improve participation raising the question "What is the evidence for the effect of interventions to address psychosocial, behavioral, and social functions on the occupational performance for persons with TBI?"

Summary of Levels I–III Evidence

Ownsworth, Fleming, Shum, Kuipers, and Strong (2008; Level I RCT) compared the effectiveness of individual, group, and combined intervention formats for improving psychosocial function and goal attainment in individuals with a mean of 5.29 years since their TBI. Thirty-five participants were randomly placed into 6 groups of either immediate intervention or a wait-list control condition. The three intervention formats were all 3 hours per week for 8 weeks and included group-based support, individual occupation-based support, and a combined group and individual support intervention. Outcomes were assessed using self- and relative ratings on the COPM, Patient Competency Rating Scale (PCRS), and the BICRO–39 at pre-, post-, and 3-month follow-up.

The group-based support format targeted meta-cognitive skills through psycho-education, peer and facilitator feedback, and goal setting through group discussions and activities and homework exercises. The individualized occupation-based support intervention was based on client-centered goals (identified on the COPM) and meaningful occupation-based activities in a natural setting. The client received training in metacognitive skills focused on self-awareness and self-regulation strategies, along with family education. The combined intervention format reduced the group and individualized sessions to half the time to equalize the intervention intensity, keeping the intervention activities the same.

The results showed that individualized, occupation-based intervention led to improvements in performance in goal-specific areas (self and relative COPM ratings of satisfaction and performance for participants) and that the combined intervention format led to gains in performance and satisfaction that were maintained at the 3-month follow-up. Improvements in behavioral competency (measured by the PCRS) and psychological well-being (measured by the BICRO–39) were found more frequently in the individual and group interventions than the combined format. There were inconsistencies in the patterns of improvements between pre- and post-assessments and pre- and follow-up assessments.

Several methodological limitations were identified by the authors. Only 21 of the participants had a TBI, while the remaining 14 participants had a diagnosis of stroke ($n = 12$) and brain tumor or abscess ($n = 2$). In addition, there was heterogeneity in the time since injury, ranging from 2 to 18 years. No statistical data were provided on whether the time since injury was significantly different for the three intervention format groups. Small sample sizes in each group (5–6) reduced power in the analyses and instability in self-ratings on the COPM in the wait-list control condition participants may indicate that one of the primary outcome measures was potentially influenced by factors external to the research design (e.g., mood state, treatment expectations, acceptance of disability).

Wheeler, Lane, and McMahon (2007; Level II) used a nonrandomized controlled trial to evaluate the effect of an intensive, community-based life skills training on community integration and life satisfaction among individuals with TBI. Thirty-six individuals were separated into either the intensive treatment group ($n = 18$) or a matched comparison group ($n = 18$) of individuals living in the community, including individuals on a waiting list for the program. Treatment consisted of an intensive, community-based residential life skills training that included one-on-one sessions with a life skills trainer and involvement with an interdisciplinary team that included occupational therapy 1 to 3 hours per week. At the 90-day follow-up evaluation, there was a statistically significant improvement on overall CIQ scores for the treatment group but not for the comparison group. This also was seen on the home integration and productivity subsets of the CIQ but not for social integration. No differences were observed on the Satisfaction with Life Scale between the groups.

This study was limited in that data were collected retrospectively rather than prospectively. The lack of randomization to the groups and baseline differences limited between-group comparisons (i.e., the comparison group showed a trend toward being more educated with less time since injury and demonstrated significantly more productive engagement in community work, school, or volunteer activities, as measured by the CIQ).

Bornhofen and McDonald (2008; Level I, RCT) evaluated whether a cognitive intervention incorporating errorless learning, self-instruction training, and rehearsal could improve emotion perception, including emotional expression and nonverbal cues such as specific patterns of changes in facial features, voice tone, body posture, and movement. Twelve outpatient volunteers with severe, chronic TBI were randomized to treatment ($n = 6$) and wait-list control ($n = 6$). Although there was no statistically significant improvement on psychosocial functioning, participants in the treatment group significantly improved their accuracy in judging dynamic cues related to basic emotions such as happiness or surprise as compared to the wait-list control group. Those in the treatment group also improved in being able to draw inferences on the basis of emotional cues to determine whether a speaker was being sarcastic, sincere, or deceptive. Participants in the treatment group did not demonstrate improvement in judging static emotional cues in the form of photographed facial expressions. Several methodological limitations were identified by the authors, which limits the strength of the evidence. There was a small sample size, and a lack of comparison of postintervention performance to preintervention performance on cognitive measures to eliminate the possibility that improvements could be attributed to spontaneous recovery.

One Level I RCT (Powell et al., 2002; see also Dawson, 2002) tested the effect of a multidisciplinary, community-based outreach program using individual-ized written contracts to achieve short-term or interim goals leading to a client-valued long-term goal on 110 participants with moderate to severe TBI of 1.3 to 1.4 years' duration. The experimental treatment was administered by a team 2 to 6 hours per week in the person's home or other community setting. The team included two occupational therapists and 3.5 other professionals. The control group received limited assis-tance with pursuing referrals to outpatient services. Measuring the results on the BICRO–39 and the Barthel Index, the experimental group showed signifi-cantly ($p < .05$) greater gains in ADLs and social par-ticipation compared to the control group. The authors concluded that this study presents the strongest confir-mation to date that structured multidisciplinary reha-bilitation delivered in community settings can improve social functioning after severe brain injury.

However, the Powell and colleagues (2002) study was marred by serious threats to internal validity (e.g., inequality of time post-onset between groups, inequality of cognitive ability between groups, possible cointerven-tion bias, extreme ceiling effects on some of the sub-scales of the outcome measures, and attrition). Although significantly greater gains in ADLs and social participa-tion after the experimental treatment were reported, the role the occupational therapist played in this pro-gram, and the consequent result, was not reported. The experimental treatment consisted of writing contracts to achieve short-term goals. Certainly occupational therapists can incorporate such a treatment into their programs without detriment to the patient.

Two Level III studies (McMorrow, Braunling-McMorrow, & Smith, 1998; Murrey & Starzinski, 2004; one-group before-and-after experimental design) tested outcomes on participants before and after treat-ment. Murray and Starzinski (2004) studied the effect of the specialized neurorehabilitation program offered at the Minnesota Neurorehabilitation Hospital on a group of 44 participants with TBI and severe neurobe-havioral sequelae of an average 5 years' duration. The program was comprised of 4 stages using an individual plan and timeline. An occupational therapist was included on the team, which was led by a behavioral

neurologist and included eight other disciplines. Treat-ment was administered from 7 a.m. to 9:30 p.m. every day. At 3 years postdischarge, the stability of commu-nity placement was ascertained by questionnaire. The outcome data were reported in percentages but not tested statistically. The results indicated improvement.

McMorrow and colleagues (1998) evaluated the postdischarge outcome of a proactive behavioral–resi-dential treatment program on the functional outcomes of 71 persons with severe brain injury of 9 days to 20 years' duration. These persons generally failed to benefit from previous rehabilitation efforts. The rehabilitation team consisted of one occupational therapy practitioner and members of six other disciplines, who all used the same tenets of behavioral therapy, focusing on positive interaction, consequences, and emotional–behavioral self-management. Treatment was given all day, every day, for an average of 7 months. Seven functional out-comes were measured repeatedly up to 12 months post-discharge by record review, interview, or team process. Improvement in all seven categories (residential status, level of independence, behavioral–emotional status, level of community participation with or without assistance, level of self-awareness of personal skills and difficulties, vocational or higher education or productivity status, and level of involvement in productive activity per day and per week) was noted between the preadmission and the discharge evaluations, but the data were not tested statistically. The authors concluded that a proactive behavioral–residential treatment program is effective in improving functional outcomes and that the results are strengthened when one considers that repeated pretreat-ment measures had failed to show gains despite the pass-ing of time and use of other treatment.

These two Level III studies have serious threats to internal validity: history and maturation effects that compromise the effect of the independent variable, attrition, unblinded evaluation, and reliability of mea-sures not reported, among others. Furthermore, the data were not analyzed statistically.

Summary of Levels IV–V Evidence

Because of the paucity of strong evidence regard-ing this question, these lower-level studies have been included as the best evidence available at this time. These studies indicate that poor social skills or maladaptive social behaviors of some persons with TBI can be modified or corrected with intensive, long-term therapy. The interventions studied included

- Education about ABI using a game format with monetary incentives to increase learning (Zhou et al., 1996; Level IV);
- Operant conditioning (behavioral analysis) and feedback (Schlund & Pace, 1999; Level IV);
- Social skills training (three different programs of training for different goals), all done by by occupational therapists (Gutman & Leger, 1997 [Level V]; Sladyk, 1992 [Level V]; Yuen, 1997 [Level V]);
- Nonaversive behavioral and skills training; environmental adaptation (Rothwell, LaVigna, & Willis, 1999; Level V);
- Nonconfrontational approach and use of errorless learning and the client's implicit memory (Bieman-Copeland & Dywan, 2000; Level V); and
- Humor, reframing of the situation, diversion of attention antecedent to aggression, environmental modification, and positive rewards (Fluharty & Glassman, 2001; Level V).

These lower-level studies suggest that interventions may be therapeutic, but no study provides sufficient evidence to support any particular intervention. Only three studies specify occupational therapy interventions; those are nonexperimental case reports on a total of 5 patients (Gutman & Leger, 1997; Sladyk, 1992; Yuen, 1997). The other studies included occupational therapy as part of a multidisciplinary team or described an intervention that could become part of occupational therapy practice. These single-case designs or case reports do not support a causal relationship between intervention and outcome because there are no controls against threats to validity; because they report complex, interrelated components of a treatment program so that no one component can be identified as the causal factor; and because the reports are of a single or very few select

persons. Overall, they provide a low level of evidence of the effects of interventions aimed at improving social–behavioral functions to improve occupational performance.

Intervention Addressing Occupational Performance

Although acute inpatient rehabilitation typically focuses on the performance of ADLs, individuals more than 10 years after their brain injury can show clinically significant improvements in functional skills when engaged in rehabilitation programs focused on retraining specific skills or training of new skills previously not part of the client's roles (Parish & Oddy, 2007). Using elements of procedural learning in a natural environment with no expectations for generalization or improvement in cognitive functioning, an occupational therapist may develop a program that incorporates errorless learning, practice of a specific task with fading cues, positive prompts, and praise and encouragement. Intervention may focus on meaningful tasks such as teaching a client who was injured as a preadolescent but is now a young adult to shave his face or her legs, assisting a client to learn the public transit system to commute to new job in supported employment, training a client to prepare hot snacks, or training a client to consistently perform a morning hygiene program.

Occupational therapists also may need to assist the client and family in adapting strategies taught during acute inpatient hospitalization to sustain the same level of independence within the home environment. The natural cues offered by the familiar home and community environments may support greater independence, but these environments also challenge cognitive and physical skills due to their unpredictable nature.

Intervention Addressing Education and Work Activities in Context

Returning to community living often brings the desire to return to life roles of student or worker, yet residual cognitive, motor, and behavioral impairments may require continued rehabilitation to make these goals possible. School reintegration and vocational rehabilitation are important aspects of community recovery for clients with TBI.

Clients who wish to return to academic studies need to practice strategies that will support success in the student role. Occupational therapists may create simulated classroom instructional sessions for the client to practice taking notes and processing complex information, and review study habits and test-taking strategies. Cognitive orthotics such as PDAs, portable tape recorders, alarm watches, and laptop computers with scheduling software may be explored for their ability to compensate for residual cognitive impairments. There is strong Level I evidence that external aids are effective as compensatory strategies for functional day-to-day memory problems (Rees et al., 2007).

The occupational therapist may perform a campus visit to a community college with the client or use maps and resources from the college's Web site to help the client map out the location of classes and key student services. The therapist and client may role-play situations in which the client needs to advocate for services with the office for students with disabilities. If the client plans on residing in a dormitory on campus, the occupational therapist may perform an environmental assessment and make recommendations to accommodate the space for physical or cognitive impairments using photos and videos of the environment, or refer the client to an occupational therapist residing in the region for a more in-depth environmental assessment.

Case-coordinated early intervention focused on vocational skills can reduce unemployment among clients with TBI (Malec et al., 2000; O'Brien, 2007). Occupational therapists' unique ability to analyze task demands and environmental conditions and match these to the client's capabilities makes them well qualified to address vocational issues in individuals with TBI. Occupational therapists working in community-based return-to-work programs provide job coaching, instruction, and education in safe work practices. They also may recommend modifications to job tasks, work hours, or work positions or may recommend specialized equipment or cognitive orthoses that enable

efficient and accurate job performance. A retrospective analysis of clients with ABI who had successful employment outcomes (O'Brien, 2007) found that a client-centered team approach delivered in a realistic work environment focused on teaching compensatory strategies, followed by a graduated return to work with modification of the work environment to meet the individual's cognitive abilities was most often associated with a positive vocational outcome. Linking clients back to the preinjury employer or job or a similar one allows the client to use preserved long-term memory to meet job demands and minimizes the need for learning new skills.

Walker, Marwitz, Kreutzer, Hart, and Novack (2006) led a large multicenter study of factors leading to return to work 1 year after TBI. They found that although age, gender, marital status, hospital length of stay, functional status at rehabilitation discharge (measured by the FIM), and educational level were significantly related to return to work, the type of preinjury occupation also influenced a successful return to work. Prospects were highest for those patients who previously held professional or managerial positions work. Injury severity, classified by duration of unconsciousness, did not predict return to work.

Those clients with TBI who are able to return-to-work activities may need additional coordinated interventions and support to sustain their work status. Using qualitative research methodology, Gilworth, Eyres, Carey, Bhakta, and Tennant (2008) explored 33 individuals' expectations and experiences returning to work in a variety of white-collar and blue-collar positions. Reoccurring themes reported by the participants included a perceived lack of coordination and management of return-to-work support systems, continuing symptoms affecting their work abilities, and a lack of advice and guidance on returning to work.

Intervention Addressing Community Mobility

When the client is discharged from acute inpatient rehabilitation to his or her home, issues of community mobility, and driving specifically, should be addressed with the client and family. Most states have laws requiring physicians to report a loss of consciousness, cognitive disturbance, visual–perceptual deficit, or a seizure disorder due to a TBI to the state's department of motor vehicles. Some occupational therapists specialize in driver rehabilitation and can assist the client and family in determining if and when a return to driving for community mobility is possible.

Many of the cognitive, visual, and neurobehavioral impairments common to individuals with TBI can impair safe driving. For example, individuals with impairments in dividing attention may show declines in safe driving skills when responding to a passenger's questions, changing the radio station, or searching for street signs in unfamiliar areas. Clients with impulsivity may take risks in traffic situations, overestimating their abilities and the time available to perform the vehicle maneuvers safely.

Driving assessments should investigate the client's driving skills using Michon's (1985) hierarchically interconnected levels (operational, tactical, and strategic), considering performance in clinic-based assessments, on-road evaluations, and subsequent car accident or traffic rules violation rates to determine fitness to drive (Tamietto et al., 2006). The length of time that clients are monitored upon returning to real-life driving requires additional research. Lundqvist, Alinder, and Rönnberg (2008) retrospectively compared accident rates of 38 patients with brain injury 10 years after their injury and return to driving to accident rates of a group of 49 healthy controls. Patients had more accidents reported to insurance companies than the control group. The accident rates were not related to neuropsychological test results or to on-road test outcome 10 years previous, although the study did not report what, if any, type of driving rehabilitation the patients participated in prior to resumption of driving.

Holistic, intensive, and multidisciplinary neurorehabilitation can help individuals with TBI return to safe driving (Leon-Carrion, Dominguez-Morales, Barroso, & Martin, 2005). Occupational therapists may use driving simulators both to evaluate the client's judgment, problem solving, and reaction times and

to practice responding to simulated driving events in a safe although virtual environment. Clients who perform well in clinic-based and behind-the-wheel or on-road driving assessments typically participate in a trial of driver's training to practice and reinforce safe driving behaviors in gradually more challenging situations. Periodic follow-up on driving skills may be warranted (Lundqvist et al., 2008).

Individuals with TBI who are unable to return to driving show poorer community integration than those who drive, even after accounting for injury severity, social support, negative affectivity, and use of alternative transportation (Rapport, Coleman Bryer, & Hanks, 2008). For clients unable to resume independent driving, occupational therapists can provide intervention in use of alternatives for community mobility, including pedestrian routes, community-based transportation services for people with disabilities, taxi services, and public transportation systems (Phipps, 2006). Navigating one's community as a pedestrian after a TBI may be limited by cognitive impairments. Occupational therapists work with clients to learn the skills necessary to use these alternative forms of community mobility. For example, the client and therapist may develop a phone script for scheduling a trip with paratransit services to ensure that the client provides all required information, and then role-play scheduling the trip and using a compensatory cue to remind the client to prepare to meet the bus at the appointed time. Social interactions among the client, driver, and passengers also may be practiced.

Research Evidence on Intervention Focused on Community Mobility

Sohlberg, Fickas, Hung, and Fortier (2007; Level II) evaluated the effectiveness of different types of prompts delivered via a wrist-worn electronic device for pedestrians with severe TBI living in assisted living settings, in a nonrandomized controlled design using a within-subjects comparison. Twenty community travelers navigated four equivalent routes using four different prompting modes (i.e., aerial map image, point-of-view map image, text-based instructions with no image, and audio directions with no image). Results indicated that the participants performed significantly better when using the audio-only prompts versus the aerial image or point-of-view prompts.

Intervention Review

Intervention review is a continuous process of reevaluating and reviewing the intervention plan, the effectiveness of its delivery, progress toward targeted outcomes, and the need for future occupational therapy and referrals to other agencies or professionals (AOTA, 2008b). Reevaluation may involve re-administering assessments used at the time of initial evaluation, a satisfaction questionnaire completed by the client, or questions that evaluate each goal (Berg, 1997; Minkel, 1996). Reevaluation normally substantiates progress toward goal attainment, indicates any change in functional status, and directs modification of the intervention plan, if necessary (Moyers & Dale, 2007). Because recovery from TBI involves multiple stages of client functioning and lengthy intervention, it is important for occupational therapists to periodically review the intervention plan to determine whether it reflects the client or family's current priorities, incorporates intervention approaches that meet those needs, and integrates current available evidence.

Outcome Monitoring

Occupational therapy practitioners and occupational therapy assistants document outcomes in discharge evaluations or discontinuation notes (AOTA, 2008a) within the time frames, formats, and standards established by practice settings, agencies, external accreditation programs, and payers (AOTA, 2005). A focus on outcomes is interwoven throughout the process of occupational therapy (AOTA, 2008b), and occupational therapists may contribute their patient data and perspective to comprehensive team-based outcome assessments. The Disability Rating Scale (Rappaport et al., 1982) is a common outcome assessment used throughout the recovery of individuals with TBI. The GOS (Jennett & Bond, 1975) remains the most widely used method of measuring outcome in indi-

viduals who have sustained severe TBI, and the GOS–Extended (GOS–E) 8-point scale (Wilson et al., 1998) classifies outcomes based on the WHO categories: impairment, activity limitation (i.e., disabilities), and participation restriction (i.e., handicap; WHO, 2001). Corral and colleagues (2007) studied improvements in the GOS and GOS–E 6 and 12 months after severe TBI and concluded that over one-third of individuals with higher GCS scores (i.e., scores between 6 and 8) at admission continued to show improvement on their GOS scores between 6 and 12 months postinjury.

Occupational therapists working with clients during the coma period of recovery from TBI focus on outcomes emphasizing improvement of underlying client impairments and prevention of deterioration of these client factors. The goal is to create a positive potential for improved occupational performance upon the return of alertness and awareness. Occupational therapists monitor the client's recovery by serial administration of behavior-based assessments to determine when the client might be ready for discontinuation from rehabilitative services in the acute hospital setting and transfer to a more-comprehensive inpatient rehabilitation setting. Clients who are slow to recover may be discharged to settings that can provide longer term rehabilitation and medical care, such as subacute or nursing facilities. van Baalen, Odding, and Stam (2008) found that the risk of being admitted to an institution (i.e., rehabilitation center or nursing home) was significantly higher for individuals with severe TBI and lower cognitive status.

Clients receiving occupational therapy intervention as part of a comprehensive rehabilitation program in either an inpatient or outpatient setting typically have a greater ability to engage in the development of the intervention plan and identification of the outcomes sought. The emphasis of occupational therapy services with the client with TBI in these settings is on transitioning the client to return to previous roles and occupations. The desired outcome may focus on improving or enhancing occupational performance and patterns of occupation, adapting one's cognitive or motor responses to meet environmental challenges, and obtaining satisfaction with the quality of life after the injury. Comparison of discharge to admission status in a patient's performance on the FIM (Uniform Data System for Medical Rehabilitation, 1997) is commonly used to collect data on outcomes in the inpatient rehabilitation setting; however, the FIM is not sensitive to the gradual and subtle changes expected after acute inpatient rehabilitation discharge. The Functional Assessment Measure (FAM; Hall, 1997; Hall et al., 1996), when used in conjunction with the FIM, addresses functional areas related to cognition, communication, psychosocial adjustment, and community functioning. Discharge from a comprehensive rehabilitation program should include consideration of the need for future occupational therapy and for referrals to other agencies or professionals.

Clients with TBI living in the community who are assuming new or previous life roles within their community may have similar needs and desired outcomes to those focused on during the acute rehabilitation period. In addition, clients living in the community may benefit from training in self-advocacy skills (e.g., requesting and receiving reasonable accommodations in a work setting). An emphasis on improved health and wellness and quality of life may be lifelong goals of individuals with TBI as they seek to engage in meaningful occupations and participate in their communities. The concept of participation as described in the *ICF* is involvement in one's life situation, encompassing the lived experience in the actual context. Community participation is a dynamic interaction among the individual's residual impairments and contextual factors of the activity and the environment. Assessment of community participation is difficult to make by observation of performance alone because it does not capture the unique lived experience of the individual (Häggström & Lund, 2008). Assessments such as the Mayo–Portland Adaptability Inventory (MPAI–4; Malec, 2005), CHART (Whiteneck et al., 1992), CIQ, and BICRO–39 scales (Powell et al., 1998) may provide more global data on the client's outcome within the community setting. A "good" outcome from TBI may be described differently by the members of the health care team, client, and family, and a single outcome assessment may not be

capable of capturing these perspectives or measuring the quantitative and qualitative changes throughout each recovery phase from TBI (Golisz, 2006).

In addition to monitoring outcomes of individuals with TBI, aggregate data from outcome assessments are used by occupational therapists to evaluate the effectiveness of specific interventions and programs. Together with other members of the rehabilitation team, collection of standardized outcomes data contributes to program development and the establishment of a research foundation for evidence-based practice.

Discontinuation, Discharge Planning, and Follow-Up

The existing health care reimbursement system in the United States bases eligibility for medical rehabilitation, length of stay, and discharge from services on motor impairments limiting function more than the cognitive behavioral impairments limiting resumption of life roles and independent living (Katz et al., 2007). When clients with TBI are discharged from structured inpatient rehabilitation programs to their homes and communities, the true extent of their limitations may be revealed, often at a time when their financial and supportive resources are depleted. Occupational therapists' strength in analyzing and adapting functional tasks can be of great assistance in helping clients with TBI living in the community in resuming meaningful roles and occupations.

The course of recovery from TBI may last over a longer period of the lifespan than other ABI and neurological disorders that tend to evolve more quickly or affect persons at later stages of life (Corrigan, Smith-Knapp, & Granger, 1998; Hammond, Hart, Bushnik, Corrigan, & Sasser, 2004; Katz et al., 2007; Millis et al., 2001; Olver, Ponsford, & Curran, 1996). Over two-thirds of persons who sustain a TBI prior to age 30 live an additional 30 to 40 years (Brown et al., 2004; Harrison-Felix, Whiteneck, DeVivo, Hammond, & Jha, 2004). The effects of aging following TBI may require continued rehabilitation as new clinical issues arise, with existing impairments becoming more pronounced with age (Colantonio, Ratcliff, Chase, & Vernich, 2004), and community supports (e.g., family relationships) changing.

Clients with TBI may flow in and out of the various service provision settings on the basis of their needs, being periodically discharged from occupational therapy services as they reach goals typically addressed within one rehabilitation setting and transitioned to another setting. New referrals for continued rehabilitation may be made when the client with TBI, discharged from active rehabilitation, experiences a change in medical status (e.g., surgical release of a contracted muscle, revision of a joint contracted with heterotopic bone), needs to adjust to a change in life roles or living arrangements (e.g., adolescent with TBI preparing for college), or adopts a maladaptive coping style (e.g., alcohol abuse). During discharge planning, occupational therapists should assist the client in exhausting all options and resources for continued services and transitioning to the new settings and available services.

The Traumatic Brain Injury Model Systems (TBIMS) program is working with 16 centers nationwide in collecting and analyzing longitudinal data from persons with TBI in their communities to improve comprehensive systems of care for individuals with TBI (Rehabilitation of Persons With Traumatic Brain Injury, 1998). This program recommends that rehabilitation services should be interdisciplinary and comprehensive matching the current needs, strengths, and capacities of the client and that "persons with TBI should have access to rehabilitation services through the entire course of recovery, which may last for many years after the injury" (Rehabilitation of Persons With Traumatic Brain Injury, 1998).

Occupational Therapy Services to Organizations and Populations

Occupational therapists may work with organizations such as businesses, industries, or agencies that serve individuals with TBI in a variety of ways by

- Providing consultation or educational information to community groups;

- Developing programs or grant proposals for funding agencies to develop community programs for individuals with TBI;
- Serving on brain injury support groups' advisory boards to establish services and programs for recovering individuals and their families;
- Consulting for community groups of individuals with TBI who are engaging in self-advocacy efforts to develop supported living and work environments that meet their capabilities and needs;
- Consulting on job tasks and environmental structures for local businesses who contracted with an agency to employ individuals with TBI;
- Consulting for the state department of health to evaluate existing occupational therapy services for individuals with TBI and recommend or assist in developing improved methods, services, and programs; or
- Consulting for universities on the effect of cognitive and behavioral impairments on the classroom performance of students with TBI and performing environmental assessments of dorm space, classroom space, and so on.

Occupational therapists who provide services to organizations rather than individuals with TBI enter the therapeutic relationship with respect for the values and beliefs of the organization. They seek to understand the collective abilities and needs of the members of the organization and how the features and structure of the organization support or inhibit the overall performance of individuals within the organization (AOTA, 2008b). The skills of an occupational therapist with experience in community-based programming, program development, and management and reimbursement can assist community organizations and agencies in dealing with the issues and needs of the TBI population. Therapists work to affect the organization's design and ability to more effectively and efficiently meet the needs of individuals with TBI and other stakeholders while empowering the members with TBI to seek satisfying lives.

Occupational therapists may facilitate occupational justice for the TBI population by assisting groups of individuals with TBI to organize to address social policies, actions, and laws that enable people to engage in meaningful occupations, and ensuring that the TBI population is considered in ongoing discussions on health care reform. They may lobby for legislation that funds community programming, prevention education, or access to appropriate housing. Occupational therapists may volunteer in community advocacy and prevention activities that enhance the health of all people by engaging in activities such as educating community groups on prevention activities to minimize the incidence of TBI, fundraising for a bicycle helmet program for local schools, advocating for safer playground equipment, or lobbying state legislature for stricter drinking and driving laws.

Implications for Research, Education, and Clinical Practice

Research

The diverse clinical presentation of TBI makes "accurate prognostication, sensitive outcome assessment, and effective conduct of clinical trials challenging issues in TBI research" (Wagner, 2007, p. 33). When investigating both the extent of injury and recovery in the TBI population, primary (i.e., focal or diffuse) injuries coupled with secondary brain injuries resulting from the biochemical cascade of neurological events must be considered along with premorbid and demographic characteristics and contextual factors that can affect both physical and cognitive functioning. Additional factors may complicate the study of individuals with TBI. For example, research participant recruitment and selection may be biased by either a focus on neurological injury parameters or behavioral presentation of impairments. In addition, identical injuries on neuroimaging may generate markedly different patterns of symptoms in different individuals, and similar neurobehavioral patterns may be attributed to very different brain injuries (National Institute of Neurological Disorders and Stroke, 2005).

The multidisciplinary nature of TBI rehabilitation of which occupational therapy is typically a compo-

nent, coupled with individualization of treatment on the basis of injury variables, client demographics, and the treatments themselves, makes it difficult to determine which specific components of the overall rehabilitation are critical to achieving a positive client outcome. Assessing the effectiveness of comprehensive multidisciplinary treatment programs is difficult because of overlap of many of the areas of intervention and practitioners providing services and an inability to separate the effects of individual interventions attributable to a specific profession. Likewise, occupational therapy rehabilitation is complex, as targeting functional performance requires simultaneous intervention focused on multiple cognitive domains combined with physical performance skills. In addition, occupational therapy treatment regimens are individualized on the basis of the needs of a given client. Other demographic variables, such as social and financial supports, discharge environments, and client comorbidities and complications, can all influence the long-term outcome in isolation of the actual brain injury confounding research results. Separating the effects of natural recovery from recovery influenced or improved by rehabilitation services is difficult to research ethically, but long-term clients many years past the anticipated natural recovery period have shown functional improvements attributed to focused rehabilitation (Parish & Oddy, 2007).

To assist in the investigation of outcomes and development of evidence to support rehabilitation with individuals with TBI, the U.S. Department of Education, Office of Special Education and Rehabilitative Services, National Institute on Disability and Rehabilitation Research (NIDRR) supports research through the 16 Traumatic Brain Injury Model System (TBIMS) centers. Using multicenter prospective, longitudinal studies (several of which engage occupational therapists on the research teams), NIDRR aims to advance rehabilitation interventions by increasing the rigor and efficiency of scientific efforts. TBIMS sites contribute to a national database that presently contains over 7,000 cases with up to 15 years of follow-up (Traumatic Brain Injury Model Systems of Care,

2008). Long-term follow-up of a clinical data set is a challenge, particularly in clients who are socioeconomically disadvantaged, have experienced an injury from a violent event, or had a history of substance abuse. This loss to follow-up diminishes the generalizability of the research findings to the TBI population at large (Wagner, 2007).

Multicenter research studies, however, are not without their challenges. Variations in the standard of care across the centers can contribute to a significant portion of the variance in study results (Wagner, 2007). Work by the American Association of Neurological Surgeons and Brain Trauma Foundation to develop national practice guidelines for early management of care of patients with TBI has had positive affects on patient outcomes (Bulger et al., 2002; Palmer et al., 2001). Due to the foundation of client-centered intervention in naturalistic environments, occupational therapy practice may more easily lend itself to single-subject research designs. Documentation of these single-subject research designs can contribute to the available evidence supporting the effectiveness of occupational therapy clinical practice with individuals with TBI and drive development of larger cohort or even RCTs to provide evidence at higher levels.

Ethical challenges exist to conducting research in a population often unable to give informed consent due to altered states of consciousness or cognitive impairments diminishing the ability to understand the risks or benefits of research participation. The potential for diminished self-awareness typically associated with TBI raises the question of the reliability of self-reported information and the need to use proxy reports for research data collection. We cannot assume high levels of agreement between proxy and client ratings, so the level of agreement between the client and proxy ratings need to be continually investigated (Cusick, Gerhart, & Mellick, 2000).

Outcome is best reflected when measures are comprehensive in nature and involve an element of client-centered goal setting and evaluation. Use of valid and reliable assessments is important to contribute to

generalizable evidence of intervention effectiveness. The WHO's *ICF* provides a framework for rehabilitation research broadening our assessment of outcome from life-altering injuries such as TBI. It is important to measure outcome across these *ICF* domains and ensure that the selected measures appropriately match the intended targets of the intervention.

For example, intervention focused on impairments may not have meaningful affect on a more global outcome such as quality of life because many factors contribute to this qualitative construct. Global measures of outcome such as the Disability Rating Scale (DRS; Rappaport et al., 1982) may be too general to capture meaningful change in a client that results from rehabilitation. Other more functionally based assessments such as the FIM focus primarily on need for physical assistance and do not take into considerations the need for verbal or environmental cues to perform functional tasks imposed by residual cognitive impairments. More recent outcome measures such as the GOS–E (Wilson, Pettigrew, et al., 1998), the Functional Status Exam (FSE; Dikmen, Machamer, Miller, Doctor, & Temkin, 2001; Hudak et al., 2005; Temkin, Machamer, & Dikmen, 2003), and the MPAI–4 (Malec, 2005) measure abilities, adjustment, and participation and offer promise for monitoring recovery and assessing functional status in clinical trials.

Despite the many challenges to conducting quality research with the TBI population, the volume of research supporting the beneficial effects of early and aggressive rehabilitative intervention on functional recovery of clients emerging from coma continues to grow (Cope & Hall, 1982; High et al., 2006; Mackay et al., 1992; Mysiw et al., 2007; Sirois et al., 2004; Zhu et al., 2007). Therapists need to document their intervention routinely in sufficient detail to permit investigation and replication of the intervention to determine efficacy of the action, intensity, and client participation. As Tickle-Degnen (2000) states, "It is a short step from monitoring data for evidence-based practice with a single client to collecting data for a research study involving one or more clients" (p. 436).

It is strongly recommended that occupational therapy researchers continue to research the effectiveness of occupational therapy–specific interventions and increase collaboration with colleagues also interested in investigating interventions that may contain components of occupational therapy interventions. Occupational therapists need to continue to research the effects of interventions used to address psychosocial, behavioral, social, and cognitive components of occupational performance for persons with TBI, as well as interventions that utilize compensatory strategies and environmental adaptation to enable occupational performance by persons recovering from TBI.

Education

The nature of a TBI with potential comorbidities that can result from the event causing the injury (particularly if of a violent or accident-related nature) can result in a client with a clinical presentation that incorporates many neurological, orthopedic, psychosocial, and functional impairments learned in the course of an occupational therapist's academic preparation for practice. The frequent presentation of a potentially overwhelming number of impairments in a single client can challenge a student therapist's ability to prioritize treatment goals and select intervention approaches. Occupational therapy curricula must contain comprehensive information on neuroscience as well as neurorehabilitative and cognitive rehabilitative approaches to prepare student therapists to meet the needs of the TBI population.

Educators presenting information on the TBI population simultaneously need to present existing evidence supporting occupational therapy interventions and integrate literature published by psychologists, neuropsychologists, and members of other disciplines who also are treating persons with TBI into lectures and lesson plans. Exposing students to existing and newly developed standardized assessments for use with the TBI population is required not only by accreditation standards but by ethical obligations to adequately prepare the next generation of occupational therapy practitioners. Student therapists must

learn to examine systematically the effect of their interventions and develop the habit of applying their research competencies in everyday practice to support or negate particular interventions with clients (Holm, 2000). Student therapists and practicing occupational therapists must examine their intervention by observing closely, interpreting observations, reflecting on goals and outcomes and intervening variables, and experimenting with variations of therapy to determine the key therapeutic processes.

Students engaging in health promotion academic assignments should consider focusing on brain injury prevention community projects using the available resources from organizations such as the ThinkFirst campaign from the National Injury Prevention Foundation (http://www.thinkfirst.org/home.asp); Preventing Traumatic Brain Injury in Older Adults (http://www.cdc.gov/braininjuryinseniors); or the Heads Up Program, focused on teens in sports (http://www.cdc.gov/ConcussionInYouthSports/default.htm), all available from the CDC.

Because intervention with the TBI population can cross the traditional separation of fieldwork into physical disabilities and mental health settings, occupational therapy educators and fieldwork coordinators need to place these terms aside and recognize that this population requires a consistent integration of physical and psychosocial factors in all phases of recovery. Exposing students to community-based practice settings that treat clients with TBI can assist student therapists in not only learning to think outside the medical model but also to address client-centered goals to "support health and participation in life through engagement in occupation" (AOTA, 2008b, p. 626).

Continued efforts to bridge the gap between research and practice can be achieved by increasing research partnerships between faculty and students from academic programs and occupational therapists in clinical settings providing services to clients with TBI. These research partnerships can lead to meaningful evidence supporting occupational therapy practice with the TBI population.

Clinical Practice

The rehabilitation of clients with severe TBI is complex, requiring the integrated efforts and skills of practitioners from many specialties. Reinforcement of the strategies and goals for the client across disciplines is encouraged for successful outcomes. A multidisciplinary team is essential to coordinate care during all phases of recovery. This multidisciplinary, and sometimes transdisciplinary, approach to rehabilitation requires occupational therapists and other professionals to be proficient in negotiation and teamwork skills to advocate for particular approaches to intervention and the contributions that they and their profession can make to the client's care.

Occupational therapists in centers treating clients with TBI need to critically review national guidelines and recent clinical research, both within their profession and in other professions providing services to the TBI population, and to integrate this information into client care. Occupational therapy administrators in clinical settings need to encourage integration of evidence-based practice into the clinical setting by providing therapists with access to resources to search for evidence, focusing in-service training sessions on evidence-based practice, and collaborating with academic-based occupational therapy faculty to design and develop research projects that can contribute to evidence supporting occupational therapy practice.

The research reviewed for this guideline offers some specific recommendations for rehabilitation of the client with TBI (see Table 5). Occupational therapy practitioners need to integrate all relevant, valid, and available research evidence when making clinical decisions and consider whether a hierarchical model of evidence organization or a heterarchical organization with a network of parallel goals provides better guidance for intervention planning (Tickle-Degnen & Bedell, 2003). Occupational therapists must constantly assess whether the available evidence is applicable to the needs of their particular client and feasible to carry out in their intervention setting. Any intervention decision must consider not only the research findings

but also the individual client's preference and therapist's expertise. More recent research by Vanderploeg and colleagues (2008) illustrates that there may be subpopulations of patients with TBI that respond differently to selected interventions.

There is a growing body of evidence supporting interventions focused on motor recovery and cognitive recovery in clients with TBI. Occupational therapists must review and extrapolate the elements that fit into the philosophy of occupational therapy practice and further investigate the effectiveness of these intervention components in enhancing occupational performance in clients with TBI.

So, what guidance does the existing research offer? Although case reports suggest that tasks that require mental manipulation of information or solving novel problems do affect brain organization, there is no direct evidence that challenging demands placed on the clients engaged in rehabilitation reorganize brain function beyond spontaneous recovery after TBI. Despite the inability to demonstrate reorganization of brain function, research with clients past the point of expected spontaneous recovery supports the potential for improved occupational performance with focused rehabilitation (Coetzer & Rushe, 2005; High et al., 2006; Parish & Oddy, 2007). Because recovery from TBI is a lengthy process, routine periodic evaluation of the individual with TBI would be beneficial to determine whether the client is demonstrating change (e.g., improvement or decline in status) that may require short-term rehabilitative services to improve or sustain his or her ability to engage in meaningful occupations. Clients long after their TBI may present with new rehabilitative needs as they assume new life roles or change their living environments. These clients, who may have sustained their initial injury during adolescence or young adulthood, may need short-term occupational therapy intervention to learn to perform new areas of occupation, adapt to their new environment, alter their cognitive strategies to include new technology or roles, or adjust their daily routines and care to their new roles. Short-term occupational therapy intervention may assist clients to improve or sustain

Table 5. Recommendations for Occupational Therapy Interventions for Clients With Traumatic Brain Injury*

Intervention	Recommendation for Inclusion of Intervention in Occupational Therapy Services		
	Recommended (supported by strong or moderate evidence)	**No Recommendation** (existing evidence is limited, insufficient, or inconclusive)	**Recommended Against** (supported by strong or moderate evidence)
Overall recovery	Early and aggressive rehabilitative intervention to reduce length of stay and improve short-term functional outcomes (B)	Continued outpatient therapy sustains early gains (C)	
	Post-acute functionally based rehabilitation (B)	Challenging therapeutic interventions requiring mental manipulation to reorganize brain function (I)	
		Family intervention (I)	
		Short-term intervention for individuals with MTBI (I)	
Interventions focused on client factors/impairments	CIMT (A)	Sensory stimulation or coma arousal programs (I)	Nocturnal hand splinting to improve ROM, pain, or function (D) is not effective
	Serial casting of ankle plantar contractures (A)	Cognitive–behavioral therapy for insomnia (I)	
	Serial casting of upper-extremity contractures (B)	CPM for HO in lower extremity (I)	
	Purposeful activities for fine motor recovery (B)	Calendars for temporal reorientation (I)	
		Telerehabilitation for cognitive impairments (I)	
Interventions focused on performance skills	Errorless learning (A)	GMT (C)	Drills and computerized practice training is not effective for improving attention or memory (D)
	Compensatory approaches to cognitive rehabilitation (A)	Behavioral approach using positive reinforcement (C)	
	Memory rehabilitation utilizing restorative (visualization, mnemonics); compensatory (internal mnemonics and external aids); and external change/adapt environment strategies for clients with mild-to-moderate impairments (A)	Attention processing therapy (C)	
		Prospective memory training (I)	
		Treating the client within environments that are graded to reduce structure and to increase distractions equal to real-life situations (I)	
	Computerized memory orthoses for prospective memory (A)	Positive talk training (I)	
	Awareness training embedded in functional task performance (A)	Organizational supports to reduce everyday memory problems (I)	
	Group-based cognitive rehabilitation (A)	Multidisciplinary cognitive rehabilitation (I)	
	Social skills training (B)	TEACH–M approach for using a simple e-mail interface (I)	
	Establishment of goals valued by the client, combined with compensatory training and environmental adaptation (B)	Self-determination model to address integrated self-awareness (I)	
		Intervention focused on perception of emotion on psychosocial functioning (I)	

Table 5. Recommendations for Occupational Therapy Interventions for Clients With Traumatic Brain Injury*
(cont.)

Intervention	Recommendation for Inclusion of Intervention in Occupational Therapy Services		
	Recommended (supported by strong or moderate evidence)	**No Recommendation** (existing evidence is limited, insufficient, or inconclusive)	**Recommended Against** (supported by strong or moderate evidence)
Interventions focused on performance skills *(cont.)*	Pager systems for memory and planning problems (B) PDA to remind client about therapy goals (B) Mobile phones as compensatory memory aids (B) Environmental cues for performance of ADLs and IADLs (B) Attention remediation programs for clients in the chronic phase of recovery (B)	Gross motor activities for attention (I) Sustained attention training for hemi-attention disorder (I) Web-based interactive assistance for performance of targeted functional activity (I) Modified memory diary with a pair of pages for each day of the week (i.e., timetable and to-do list) (I) Use of an alphanumeric pager system to increase memory notebook use (I) Computer-related activities designed to enhance participation in desired social roles (I) Game format to teach information about TBI (I) Role-playing to achieve friendships and intimate relationships (I) Cognitive groups to achieve return to employment (I)	
Interventions focused on occupational performance areas and/or participation	Functional–experiential treatment for older clients with TBI and independent living goals (B) Written contracts to achieve short-term goals (B) Life skills training to increase community participation (B) ICRP to return to work for military personnel (B)	EADLs (I) Wrist-worn electronic device for community navigation (I)	

A—Strongly recommend that occupational therapy practitioners routinely provide the intervention to eligible clients. Good evidence was found that the intervention improves important outcomes and concludes that benefits substantially outweigh harm.

B—Recommend that occupational therapy practitioners routinely provide the intervention to eligible clients. At least fair evidence was found that the intervention improves important outcomes and concludes that benefits outweigh harm.

C—No recommendation is made for or against routine provision of the intervention by occupational therapy practitioners. At least fair evidence was found that the intervention can improve outcomes, but concludes that the balance of the benefits and harm is too close to justify a general recommendation.

D—Recommend that occupational therapy practitioners do not provide the intervention to eligible clients. At least fair evidence was found that the intervention is ineffective or that harm outweighs benefits.

I—Insufficient evidence to recommend for or against routinely providing the intervention. Evidence that the intervention is effective is lacking, of poor quality, or conflicting, and the balance of benefits and harm cannot be determined.

Recommendation criteria are based on standard language from Agency for Healthcare Research and Quality (2009).

*Suggested recommendations are based on the available evidence and content experts' opinions. See Appendix E for a list of supporting evidence used to develop these recommendations.

their level of independence in their home and community. Occupational therapists need to advocate for the potential benefit of ongoing evaluation and intervention for the TBI population with insurance companies and legislators. Continued research on the benefits of occupational therapy with long-term survivors of TBI also will help provide the evidence to support access to services throughout life.

The current research on controlled sensory stimulation to arouse persons in coma or persistent vegetative state is not consistent or strong enough to support or rule out the use of this commonly used intervention. There is evidence that arousal procedures do not have detrimental effects on clients. More research is needed to verify the effectiveness of sensory stimulation to arouse patients from coma or persistent vegetative state, to verify the effectiveness of familiar and meaningful stimuli over a standard protocol of stimulation, and to relate the arousal enabled by such an adjunctive therapy to ultimate functional outcome.

Four therapeutic interventions (i.e., self-selected goals, compensatory strategies, environmental adaptation, intensive practice) were shown to enable persons with TBI to participate in areas of occupation (i.e., ADLs, IADLs, work, leisure, social participation, education), although the strength of the evidence is limited by methodological issues in the research designs. Self-selection of goals by the client or carer in collaboration with the therapist and valuing of the goals to be worked on by the client (i.e., meaningful occupation) hold promise and support occupational therapy's belief in client-centered practice. Intervention that incorporates compensatory strategies, environmental adaptation, and intensive practice of targeted behaviors and tasks has the potential to improve participation in areas of occupation for clients with TBI. Occupational therapists need to continue to research the ideal combination of interventions and the crucial elements of intervention that enable persons with TBI to engage more fully in ADLs and IADLs.

Individual written contracts; individualized therapy; and skills training with extensive guided practice addressing psychosocial, behavioral, or social functions

to improve occupational performance for persons with TBI have mixed levels of support in the research. Because these residual impairments can significantly limit the recovery client's participation in social and community activities, occupational therapists applying these interventions need to contribute to the evidence supporting or refuting their effectiveness.

Conclusions regarding the effectiveness of interventions aimed at recovery of cognitive functions to restore occupational performance are as follows:

- Memory rehabilitation is effective (Cicerone et al., 2004; Freeman et al., 1992; Loya, 1999) but, on the basis of available research, no one intervention can be considered more effective than another (Loya, 1999).
- Using a computer to play games to increase frequency of computer use does not increase the usage of the computer for memory compensation (Wright et al., 2001a; Wright et al., 2001b).
- The evidence regarding whether multidisciplinary (including occupational therapy) or unidisciplinary (e.g., neuropsychologists, psychiatric nurses) cognitive rehabilitation is more effective (Braverman et al., 1999; Cicerone et al., 2004; Salazar et al., 2000) is not definitive. However, more intensive therapy early postinjury facilitates the client's ability to engage in some occupational areas sooner (Zhu et al., 2001).
- Older patients with independent living goals might benefit more from functional–experiential intervention rather than cognitive–didactic rehabilitation treatment (Vanderploeg et al., 2008).
- Errorless learning is more effective than vanishing cues or trial-and-error methods of teaching patients with memory impairment after TBI, especially in situations in which implicit learning is possible (e.g., habit recovery; Bergman, 2000; Kessels & de Haan, 2003).
- Treatment aimed at relearning functional tasks through task-specific training or by learning compensatory strategies for memory impairment appear to be effective (Ho & Bennett, 1997; Mills et al., 1992; Parente & Stapleton, 1999; Que-

mada et al., 2003), but the evidence is weak and needs further study.

- Simplified computer interfaces and training materials facilitate mastery of computer use for persons with memory impairment (Bergman, 2000; Egan et al., 2005; Wright et al., 2001a; Wright et al., 2001b). This is important because computerized memory orthoses are effective in compensating for deficits of prospective memory (Burke et al., 2001; Wilson et al., 2001) and retrospective memory (Hart et al., 2002). Occupational therapists need to continue to explore how everyday technological devices such as PDAs, computers, and cell phones can be used to improve the occupational performance of clients with TBI.
- Although members of the rehabilitation team, including occupational therapists, typically use environmental objects and cues to try to orient confused clients to time and place, the use of a calendar with only minimal orientation was not found to be effective in orienting post-TBI amnesic patients (Watanabe et al., 1998).
- Current research shows that neuropsychological measures do not correlate with ADL ratings (Ho & Bennett, 1997; Quemada et al., 2003). Occupational therapists need to continue to contribute observational findings to team discussions, because functional performance in naturalistic settings may provide a different picture of clients' occupational performance than existing standardized neuropsychological assessments. Therapists also need to collaborate with neuropsychologists to further research the correlation of function performance to standardized assessments of cognitive impairments.
- For persons with mild TBI, a single session of patient education and discussion of concerns was as adequate as a more-intense treatment regime (Paniak et al., 1998, 2000).

Conclusions regarding the effectiveness of interventions aimed at motor impairments to restore occupational performance are as follows:

- The growing body of evidence supporting the use of CIMT and mCIT to address upper-extrem-

ity hemiparesis recommends that occupational therapists consider this intervention approach to enhance motor function in clients with TBI (Cho et al., 2005; Page & Levine, 2003; Shaw et al., 2005).
- Occupational-based functional activities may be more effective than remedial activities (e.g., pegboards, puzzles) in improving fine motor coordination (Neistadt, 1994).
- Application of nocturnal hand splinting in combination with conventional therapy does not improve ROM, function, or pain control in the spastic hand (Lannin et al., 2003), but the role of splinting in prevention of loss of ROM needs further investigation.
- Serial casting of the upper extremity for shortened periods (e.g., 1–4 days) can result in significant improvements in ROM and fewer complications as compared to the conventional casting period (e.g., 5–7 days; Pohl et al., 2002).

In Summary

In summary, recovery from TBI is a long process, and occupational therapy practitioners may encounter recovering clients in many different clinical and community settings. The lengthy natural recovery period and potential for functional improvements long after spontaneous recovery is anticipated to be complete suggests that occupational therapists retain hope for the potential effect of occupational therapy intervention with clients with TBI, regardless of the setting or phase of recovery in which they encounter the client.

The growing body of evidence supporting the overall effectiveness of rehabilitation with clients who sustained TBI encompasses many components that fit the philosophy and practice of occupational therapy. Occupational therapists need to collaborate with clients, families, and colleagues from other professions to address the needs of clients with TBI in all intervention settings and phases of the recovery process. The overarching goal of occupational therapy intervention with clients recovering from TBI is to provide client-centered, occupation-based, evidence-supported intervention with consideration of the person's residual impairments, potential for improvement, personal motivation, and contextual influences to promote health and enable client participation in meaningful occupations.

■ ■ ■

Appendix A. Preparation and Qualifications of Occupational Therapists and Occupational Therapy Assistants

Who Are Occupational Therapists?

To practice as an occupational therapist, the individual trained in the United States

- Has graduated from an occupational therapy program accredited by the Accreditation Council for Occupational Therapy Education (ACOTE®) or predecessor organizations;
- Has successfully completed a period of supervised fieldwork experience required by the recognized educational institution where the applicant met the academic requirements of an educational program for occupational therapists that is accredited by ACOTE or predecessor organizations;
- Has passed a nationally recognized entry-level examination for occupational therapists; and
- Fulfills state requirements for licensure, certification, or registration.

Educational Programs for the Occupational Therapist

These include the following:

- Biological, physical, social, and behavioral sciences
- Basic tenets of occupational therapy
- Occupational therapy theoretical perspectives
- Screening and evaluation
- Formulation and implementation of an intervention plan
- Context of service delivery
- Management of occupational therapy services (master's level)
- Leadership and management (doctoral level)
- Use of research
- Professional ethics, values, and responsibilities.

The fieldwork component of the program is designed to develop competent, entry-level, generalist occupational therapists by providing experience with a variety of clients across the life span and in a variety of settings. Fieldwork is integral to the program's curriculum design and includes an in-depth experience in delivering occupational therapy services to clients, focusing on the application of purposeful and meaningful occupation and/or research, administration, and management of occupational therapy services. The fieldwork experience is designed to promote clinical reasoning and reflective practice, to transmit the values and beliefs that enable ethical practice, and to develop professionalism and competence in career responsibilities. Doctoral-level students must also complete a doctoral experiential component designed to develop advanced skills beyond a generalist level.

Who Are Occupational Therapy Assistants?

To practice as an occupational therapy assistant, the individual trained in the United States

- Has graduated from an occupational therapy assistant program accredited by ACOTE or predecessor organizations;
- Has successfully completed a period of supervised fieldwork experience required by the recognized

educational institution where the applicant met the academic requirements of an educational program for occupational therapy assistants that is accredited by ACOTE or predecessor organizations;

- Has passed a nationally recognized entry-level examination for occupational therapy assistants; and
- Fulfills state requirements for licensure, certification, or registration.

Educational Programs for the Occupational Therapy Assistant

These include the following:
- Biological, physical, social, and behavioral sciences
- Basic tenets of occupational therapy
- Screening and assessment
- Intervention and implementation
- Context of service delivery
- Assistance in management of occupational therapy services
- Professional literature
- Professional ethics, values, and responsibilities.

The fieldwork component of the program is designed to develop competent, entry-level, generalist occupational therapy assistants by providing experience with a variety of clients across the life span and in a variety of settings. Fieldwork is integral to the program's curriculum design and includes an in-depth experience in delivering occupational therapy services to clients, focusing on the application of purposeful and meaningful occupation. The fieldwork experience is designed to promote clinical reasoning appropriate to the occupational therapy assistant role, to transmit the values and beliefs that enable ethical practice, and to develop professionalism and competence in career responsibilities.

Regulation of Occupational Therapy Practice

All occupational therapists and occupational therapy assistants must practice under federal and state law. Currently, 50 states, the District of Columbia, Puerto Rico, and Guam have enacted laws regulating the practice of occupational therapy.

Note. The majority of this information is taken from the *Accreditation Standards for a Doctoral-Degree-Level Educational Program for the Occupational Therapist* (AOTA, 2007a), *Accreditation Standards for a Master's-Degree-Level Educational Program for the Occupational Therapist* (AOTA, 2007b), and *Accreditation Standards for an Educational Program for the Occupational Therapy Assistant* (AOTA, 2007c).

Appendix B.
Selected *CPT*^{TM} Coding for Occupational Therapy Evaluations and Interventions

The following chart is a guide to assist in making clinically appropriate decisions in selecting the most relevant *CPT* code to describe occupation therapy evaluation and intervention. Occupational therapy practitioners should use the most appropriate code from the current *CPT* based on specific services provided, individual patient goals, payer policy, and common usage.

Examples of Occupational Therapy Evaluation and Intervention	Suggested *CPT*^{TM} Code(s)
• Provide instruction and training in compensatory techniques for performing daily self-care activities • Assist patient to incorporate cognitive strategies to facilitate participation in instrumental activities of daily living (IADLs) • Provide training in use of environmental controls and adaptive equipment to assure safe, independent living within the home environment	97535—Self-care/home management training (e.g., activities of daily living [ADL] and compensatory training, meal preparation, safety procedures, instructions in use of assistive technology devices/adaptive equipment), direct (one-on-one) contact by the provider, each 15 minutes
• Assess patient requirements for specialized mobility equipment, such as powered wheelchairs, to enable community and work participation • Provide recommendations for wheelchair modifications to ensure optimal sitting posture in order to maintain skin integrity, prevent pressure sores, and facilitate performance in ADLs and IADLs	97542—Wheelchair management (e.g., assessment, fitting, training), each 15 minutes

• Evaluate/assess changes in such areas as
  – neuromusculoskeletal and movement-related functions, presence of movement dysfunction (e.g., tremor, spasticity, flaccidity, rigidity, bradykinesia, ataxia, dyskinesia, athetosis)
  – sensory functions and pain
  – mental functions, depression, denial, anxiety about the progressive nature of the disease
	97003—Occupational therapy evaluation
	97004—Occupational therapy reevaluation
	97750—Physical performance test or measurement (e.g., musculoskeletal, functional capacity), with written report, each 15 minutes

• Evaluate changes in neurocognitive function including memory (short-term, long-term, and organizational), reasoning, sensory processing, visual, perceptual status, orientation, social pragmatics, and elements of decision making and executive function	96125—Standardized cognitive performance testing (e.g., Rivermead Behavioral Memory Test) per hour of a qualified health care professional's time, both face-to-face time administering tests to the patient and time interpreting these test results and preparing the report

(continued)

Examples of Occupational Therapy Evaluation and Intervention	Suggested *CPT*™ Code(s)
• Train in use of a cognitive orthoses to enhance the ability to remember telephone numbers, e-mail addresses, and appointment/events while at home or work • Develop strategies to ensure completion of morning routine, such as medication management, safely preparing breakfast and school lunches, and organizing daily schedule for completion of household activities • Teach client to use a memory notebook to compensate for memory impairments (e.g., schedule daily activities such as appointments, to do lists, child's play dates, shopping lists) • Develop self-cueing strategies with client to check and correct work	97532—Development of cognitive skills to improve attention, memory, problem solving (includes compensatory training), direct (one-on-one) patient contact by the provider, each 15 minutes
• Provide occupation-based activities to increase ability to perform avocational or work tasks such as reaching into cabinets to grasp items for functional cooking task or balancing and bending to transfer laundry items from washer to dryer	97530—Therapeutic activities, direct (one-on-one) patient contact by the provider (use of dynamic activities to improve functional performance), each 15 minutes
• Have client gather information on possible leisure/social activities (e.g., phone calls, search newspaper, Internet sites for local businesses/cultural exhibits) and plan/carry out a community outing considering time and financial needs and hypothetical problem solving of emergency situations • Analyze client routines and train in modifying/changing daily routines, roles, and habits to reintegrate client into independent shopping, work, or volunteer activities	92537—Community/work reintegration training (e.g., shopping, transportation, money management, avocational activities and/or work environment/modification analysis, work task analysis, use of assistive technology device/adaptive equipment), direct one-on-one contact by the provider, each 15 minutes
• Provide functional exercises to increase self range of motion, strength, and mobility to enable increased participation in daily activities • Engage client in pool-based activities to improve strength and endurance	97110—Therapeutic procedure, one or more areas, each 15 minutes; therapeutic exercises to develop strength and endurance, range of motion, and flexibility 97113—Aquatic therapy with therapeutic exercises
• Design graded tasks to increase coordination and balance • Provide training in proper use of adaptive equipment to assist with balance and facilitate community mobility	97112—Therapeutic procedure, one or more areas, each 15 minutes; neuromuscular reeducation of movement, balance, coordination, kinesthetic sense, posture, and/or proprioception for sitting and/or standing activities
• Prevent loss of range of motion by fabricating dynamic hand for radial nerve injury [Refer to Medicare National Level II HCPCS Codes for billing actual orthosis]	97760—Orthotic(s) management and training (including assessment and fitting when not otherwise reported), upper extremity(s), lower extremity(s) and/or trunk, each 15 minutes 97762—Checkout for orthotic/prosthetic use, established patient, each 15 minutes
• Assess and fabricate a serial cast to stretch a contracted elbow to enable proper hygiene and functional use of the limb in daily activities such as dressing and feeding	29065—Application, cast; shoulder to hand (long arm) 29075—Application, cast; elbow to finger (short arm) 29085—Application, cast; hand and lower forearm (gauntlet) 29086—Application, cast; finger (e.g., contracture)
• Provide joint mobilization to the wrist and fingers to maintain joint play and joint integrity in order to grasp utensils and other items such as pens and toothbrush	97140—Manual therapy techniques (e.g. mobilization/manipulation, manual lymphatic drainage, manual traction), one or more regions, each 15 minutes
• Assess body structure and body functions that influence feeding and eating, environmental influence, positioning, physical and cognitive problems that affect feeding, eating, and swallowing	92610–92612—Clinical evaluation of swallowing function (see CPT for precise descriptions of possible tests)
• Train in the use of compensatory strategies, appropriate positioning, adaptive equipment, and food textures to maximize oral intake and nutritional status	92526—Treatment of swallowing dysfunction and/or oral function for feeding
• Meet with the rehabilitation team and the patient and his/her family to discuss and plan transition to the home environment • Meet with the rehabilitation team without the family/patient to develop behavior management program to deal with patient's agitation and inappropriate social behaviors	99366—Medical team conference with interdisciplinary team of healthcare professionals, face to face with patient and/or family; 30 minutes or more, participation by nonphysician qualified health care professional. 99368—Medical team conference with interdisciplinary team of health care professionals, patient, and/or family not present; 30 minutes or more; participation by nonphysician qualified health care professional

Note. The *CPT 2009* codes referenced in this document do not represent all of the possible codes that may be used in occupational therapy evaluation and intervention. Not all payers will reimburse for all codes. Refer to *CPT 2009* for the complete list of available codes. *CPT*™ is a trademark of the American Medical Association (AMA). *CPT* five-digit codes, nomenclature, and other data are copyright 2008 by the American Medical Association. All Rights Reserved. No fee schedules, basic units, relative values, or related listings are included in *CPT.* The AMA assumes no liability for the data contained herein. Codes shown refer to *CPT 2009. CPT* codes are updated annually. New and revised codes become effective January 1. Always refer to annual updated *CPT* publication for most current codes.

Appendix C.
Evidence-Based Practice

Why Evidence-Based Practice?

One of the greatest challenges facing health care systems, service providers, public education, and policymakers is to ensure that scarce resources are used efficiently. The growing interest in outcomes research and evidence-based medicine over the past 30 years, and the more recent interest in evidence-based education, can in part be explained by these system-level challenges in the United States and internationally.

In response to demands of the cost-oriented health care system in which occupational therapy practice is often embedded, occupational therapists and occupational therapy assistants routinely are asked to justify the value of the services they provide on the basis of the scientific evidence. The scientific literature provides an important source of legitimacy and authority for demonstrating the value of health care and education services. Thus, occupational therapists, other health care practitioners, and educators increasingly are called on to use the literature to demonstrate the value of the interventions and instruction they provide to clients and students.

What Is an Evidence-Based Practice Perspective?

According to Law and Baum (1998), *evidence-based occupational therapy practice* "uses research evidence together with clinical knowledge and reasoning to make decisions about interventions that are effective for a specific client" (p. 131). An evidence-based perspective is based on the assumptions that scientific evidence of the effectiveness of occupational therapy intervention can be judged to be more or less strong and valid according to a hierarchy of research designs and an assessment of the quality of the research. AOTA uses standards of evidence modeled from standards developed in evidence-based medicine. This model standardizes and ranks the value of scientific evidence for biomedical practice using the grading system in Table 6. In this system, the highest levels of evidence include those studies that are systematic reviews of the literature, meta-analyses, and randomized controlled trials. In randomized controlled trials, the outcomes of an intervention are compared to the outcomes of a control group, and participation in either group is determined randomly. This design provides strength to the conclusion that the effect (dependent variable) was caused by the treatment (independent variable).

The evidence-based literature review presented within this document includes primarily evidence Levels I–III. *Level I* evidence consists of meta-analyses, critical reviews, and randomized controlled trials. *Level II* evidence consists of studies in which assignment to a treatment or a control group is not randomized (cohort study). *Level III* evidence consists of studies that do not use a control group. In this review, if Levels I, II, and III evidence for occupa-

Table 6. Levels of Evidence for Occupational Therapy Outcomes Research

Levels of Evidence	Definitions
Level I	Systematic reviews, meta-analyses, randomized controlled trials
Level II	Two groups, nonrandomized studies (e.g., cohort, case-control)
Level III	One group, nonrandomized (e.g., before and after, pretest and posttest)
Level IV	Descriptive studies that include analysis of outcomes (e.g., single-subject design, case series)
Level V	Case reports and expert opinion that include narrative literature reviews and consensus statements

Source. Adapted from "Evidence-based medicine: What it is and what it isn't" by D. L. Sackett, W. M. Rosenberg, J. A. Muir Gray, R. B. Haynes, & W. S. Richardson, 1996, *British Medical Journal, 312,* pp. 71–72. Copyright © 1996 by the British Medical Association. Adapted with permission.

tional therapy practice was adequate, then only those levels are used to answer a particular question. If, however, higher-level evidence was lacking, and the best evidence provided for occupational therapy specifically is ranked as only Levels IV and V, then those levels are included. *Level IV* studies are experimental single-case studies, with at least marginal manipulation of the independent variable. *Level V* evidence includes descriptive case reports in which therapists simply described what they did and the outcome for one or a few persons.

Best Practice of Occupational Therapy for Persons With Traumatic Brain Injury: An Evidence-Based Literature Review

Four focused questions and one subquestion were developed for the evidence-based literature review on rehabilitation of adults after TBI. The questions were generated to provide needed information to update the previously published guidelines for the practice of occupational therapy with persons after TBI (Radomski, 2001). The questions reviewed were

1. What is the evidence that **challenging demands** to the brain, such as therapy, activity, or sensory stimulation, **reorganizes brain function** beyond spontaneous recovery after traumatic brain injury?
   1a. What is the evidence for the **effect of sensory stimulation on the arousal level** of persons in coma or persistent vegetative state after traumatic brain injury?

2. What is the evidence for the **effect of interventions** (published between 2000 and 2006) to enable persons with TBI **to participate in areas of occupation** (activities of daily living, instrumental activities of daily living, work, leisure, social participation, and education)?
3. What is the evidence for the **effect of interventions** to address **psychosocial, behavioral, and social functions** on the occupational performance of persons with TBI?
4. What is the evidence for the **effect of interventions** to address **cognitive/perceptual functions** (attention, memory, executive functions) on the occupational performance of persons with TBI?

The results of the evidence-based review are interwoven in the above guidelines for the practice of occupational therapy with persons after TBI.

Literature Review Methodology

Search items for the review were developed by the reviewer. Search terms used for all questions included the following: *brain injury* AND *rehabilitation, brain injury* AND *rehabilitation* AND *community, brain injury* AND *rehabilitation* AND *critical reviews, brain injury* AND *rehabilitation* AND *meta-analysis, brain injury* AND *effects* AND *social* AND *therapy, brain injury* AND *effects* AND *behavioral, brain injury* AND *effects* AND *memory therapy, brain injury* AND *effects* AND *attention therapy, brain injury* AND *effects* AND *problem solving, brain injury* AND *RCT* AND *rehabilitation, brain injury* AND *effects* AND *cognitive therapy, brain injury* AND *task-specific train-ing, brain injury* AND *school* NOT *children, brain injury* AND *participation, brain injury* AND *motor tasks, brain injury* AND *activities of daily living* AND *effects, brain injury* AND *sensory stimulation, brain injury* AND *enriched environment, brain injury* AND *use-dependent plasticity, brain injury* AND *leisure, brain injury* AND *plasticity* (1985–2006), *brain injury* AND *occupational therapy, brain injury* AND *education* NOT *children, brain injury* AND *return to work, Prigitano, Ben-Yishay.*

The search consisted of peer-reviewed literature published between 1990 and April 2006, with the following exceptions. For question 1, the plasticity literature was searched from 1985, when studies of human brain plasticity first appeared. For question 3, the search consisted of peer-reviewed literature published from 2000 to April 2006, because the previous guidelines included literature through 1999. The databases searched included PubMed (Medline of the National Library of Medicine; nlm.gov); PsycINFO; Web of Science, which includes the Science Citation Index and the Social Science Citation Index; and CINAHL. Consolidated information sources searched included OTSeeker.com; OTCATS.com; DARE (Database of Abstracts of Reviews of Effects) at http://www.crd.york.ac.uk/crdweb/; and the Cochrane Collaboration (www.cochrane.org), which maintains a database of systematic reviews. These databases provide peer-reviewed summaries of research journal articles with commentary on the overall strength of the evidence. Reference lists of retrieved articles were examined for potential additional articles.

The inclusion criteria for primary research included
1. Participants were diagnosed with acquired brain injury, but not stroke.
2. Participants were adults (≥18 years of age).
3. The research studied the effects of occupational therapy intervention or interventions claimed and researched by other disciplines but also used by occupational therapists. The intervention had to represent current occupational therapy practice or theoretically could be occupational therapy practice. Studies of the effects of multidisciplinary

rehabilitation that included occupational therapy were included.
4. Outcome was measured in terms of occupational performance. In cases in which outcome was reported via multiple assessments, only those pertaining to occupational performance were examined for this review.
5. Research was written in English.
6. Meta-analyses or critical reviews, which are judged to be strong Level I evidence, were included if available.

The following types of studies were excluded
1. Prediction studies
2. Correlational studies
3. Measurement studies
4. Multidisciplinary intervention without occupational therapy mentioned
5. Observational studies of the course of outcome post–traumatic brain injury.

The review author reviewed the articles that met criteria for their quality (i.e., scientific rigor, lack of bias) and levels of evidence. Guidelines for reviewing quantitative studies were based on those developed by Law (2002) and colleagues to ensure that the evidence is ranked according to uniform definitions of research design elements.

- *Level I* studies included systematic reviews, meta-analyses, and randomized controlled trials.
- *Level II* studies included two-group nonrandomized studies, such as cohort and case control studies.
- *Level III* studies were one-group nonrandomized studies, such as before-and-after and pretest–post-test designs.
- *Level IV* studies were single-case experimental designs.
- *Level V* material included descriptive studies, case reports, case series, expert opinion, book chapters, and conference proceedings. Only descriptive studies and case reports were considered for the review.

A total of 2,297 titles were retrieved. After duplicates were discarded, 1,832 abstracts were reviewed. A total of 278 articles were retrieved from Boston University's Mugar Library, the Boston University Library of Science and Engineering, the Boston University Medical Library, the Boston University e-journal subscription, and the Wilma L. West Library of the American Occupational Therapy Foundation. After review, 38 articles of Levels I through III were included for critical review (Level I = 18; Level II = 9; Level III = 11). In addition, one uncategorizable (posttreatment observation) article was included. Twenty-seven articles ranked as Levels IV and V were critically reviewed; some are included in this guideline. The decision to include or not include was made on the basis of whether studies ranked Levels I–III provided strong evidence for a particular question or not. If not, then studies ranked Levels IV and V were included because they presented the best evidence of effectiveness of the interventions available at this time. All studies included in the review, as well as those not specifically described in this review, are summarized and cited in full in the evidence tables in Appendix D. Readers are encouraged to read the full articles for more details.

In May 2008, a review was completed to update the information from the initial review. The search included evidence-based information published between May 2006 and May 2008 and some earlier seminal articles and followed the original search terms, inclusion and exclusion criteria, and databases. Articles selected from this review were included in the appropriate evidence tables. This review resulted in a total of 99 articles (Level I, 32; Level II, 10; Level III, 16; Level IV, 20; Level V, 20; uncategorized, 1). In addition, the decision was made to incorporate evidence from the systematic review on constraint-induced movement therapy (CIMT) completed for the *Occupational Therapy Practice Guideline for Adults With Stroke* (Sabari, 2008). Readers should refer to the CIMT table for studies included in this review that address CIMT for persons with hemiparesis.

All studies included in the review, as well as those not specifically described in the evidence-based literature review section of the practice guideline, are summarized, critically appraised, and cited in full in the evidence tables in Appendix D. The evidence tables also include implications for occupational therapy practice. Readers are encouraged to read the full articles for more details. In addition, recommendations for occupational therapy practice can be found in Table 6. The recommendations are based upon the strength of the evidence for a given topic in combination with the expert opinion of review authors and the advisory group reviewing this practice guideline. The strength of the evidence is determined by the number of articles included in a given topic, the study design, and the limitations of those articles. Recommendation criteria are based on standard language developed by the U.S. Preventive Services Task Force of the Agency for Health Care Quality and Research (2009).

■ ■ ■

Appendix D.
Evidence Tables

EVIDENCE TABLE. CONSTRAINT-INDUCED MOVEMENT THERAPY

Author/Year	Study Objectives	Level/Design/ Participants	Intervention and Outcome Measures	Results	Study Limitations	Implications for Occupational Therapy
Lin et al. (2007)	Assess outcomes of modified constraint-induced movement therapy (mCIMT) on motor control characteristics during performance of functional reach-to-grasp task (as measured by motion analysis technology) and functional performance	I—Pre–post randomized controlled trial. *N* = 32 patients with stroke who meet motor criteria for participation in CIMT	Participants were randomly assigned to mCIMT or control groups. Participants in both groups received individualized, 2-hour occupational therapy sessions, 5 times per week, for 3 weeks Therapy for mCIMT participants consisted of shaping and adaptive, repetitive task practice techniques, with 15 minutes of therapy time spent on reducing abnormal muscle tone, when needed. In addition, they wore mitts on the less affected hand every weekday for 6 hours during a time of frequent arm use. TR group members received traditional rehabilitation at the same dosage. *Outcome measures:* ■ Kinematic analysis of spatial and temporal movement efficiency and type of movement control when reaching forward to grasp a beverage can ■ MAL ■ FIM. Outcomes were assessed immediately after the 3-week intervention.	Analysis of covariance revealed significantly greater improvements for the mCIMT group in temporal, spatial, and preplanning measures generated by kinematic analysis, but more so when performing the bilateral task. The mCIMT improvements on MAL and FIM were also significantly greater than the control group.	No follow-up assessments were made to assess long-term effects. Study did not include objects of different sizes to detect treatment efficacy on grasping.	This study provides additional support for the efficacy of mCIMT during rehabilitation of stroke survivors who meet the motor criteria for CIMT participation

Lin, K.-C., Wu, C. Y., Wei, T. H., Lee, C. Y., & Liu, J. S. (2007). Effects of modified constraint-induced movement therapy on reach-to-grasp movements and functional performance after chronic stroke: A randomized controlled study. *Clinical Rehabilitation, 21,* 1075–1086.

Page et al. (2008)	Assess the effectiveness of a reimbursable program, mCIMT on motor function in chronic stroke survivors as compared with traditional rehabilitation (proprioceptive neuromuscular facilitation; PNF) and no treatment	I—Randomized controlled trial, comparing three groups of chronic stroke survivors: treatment group, no treatment control, and traditional rehabilitation control. N = 35 subjects, all more than 12 months poststroke, and meeting standard criteria for CIMT programs (n = 13 mCIMT, n = 12 traditional rehabilitation, n = 10 no treatment)	For a 10-week period, mCIMT participants wore a constraining mitt on the less-affected hand for 5 hours per day, 5 days per week and participated in half-hour one-on-one shaping sessions 3 times per week. Traditional rehabilitation participants received the same dose of arm therapy, focusing on PNF. Control group members received no therapy. *Outcome measures*: On completion of 10-week period ■ Action Research Arm Test (ARAT) ■ FMA ■ MAL.	The mCIMT group demonstrated significantly greater improvements on the MAL, FMA, and ARAT as compared with the other two groups.	No follow-up assessments were made to assess long-term effects. The authors speculate that the use of a behavioral contract, only for the mCIMT group, might have unfairly strengthened these subjects' commitment to the therapy.	This study provides additional support for mCIMT in chronic stroke survivors and, indirectly, for the efficacy of task-specific repetitive training to improve motor function in the paretic arm after stroke.

Page, S. J., Levine, P., Leonard, A., Szaflarski, J. P., & Kissela, B. M. (2008). Modified constraint-induced therapy in chronic stroke: Results of a single-blinded randomized controlled trial. *Physical Therapy, 88*, 1–8.

Ro et al. (2006)	Determine feasibility of using TMS to assess functional motor reorganization after CIMT in patients in subacute phase of stroke; determine feasibility, safety, and effectiveness of using constraint-induced movement therapy with patients in subacute phase of stroke; and determine	I—Randomized controlled trial N = 8 participants (5 men, 3 women), all within 2 weeks after stroke; 4 in group receiving CIMT and 4 in control group Average age: 61.4 years	Participants were randomly assigned to group receiving CIMT or control group. CIMT includes constraint to unaffected hand (by wearing a mitt) during 90% of waking hours and intensive task-based practice sessions using shaping.	At 3-month follow-up, CIMT group showed significantly larger representations for movement than control group showed. At end of treatment and 3-month follow-up, CIMT group was significantly faster in motor performance on Grooved Pegboard Test (GPT) than con-	Small sample size	TMS can safely and effectively assess brain function in patients in subacute state of stroke. CIMT may enhance motor reorganization and accelerate motor recovery when started within 2 weeks following stroke.

(continued)

EVICENCE TABLE. CONSTRAINT-INDUCED MOVEMENT THERAPY (cont.)

Author/Year	Study Objectives	Level/Design/ Participants	Intervention and Outcome Measures	Results	Study Limitations	Implications for Occupational Therapy
Ro et al. (2006) (cont.)	whether brain reorganization of movement control correlates with improved motor function		Control group received traditional therapy, focused on increasing function with use of both hands. Therapy, delivered by 1 occupational therapist and 1 physical therapist in laboratory, occurred 3 hours per day 6 days per week for 14 consecutive days. *Outcome measures:* ■ Location and extent of motor representation of hand movement (TMS) ■ Motor performance (GPT; FMA) ■ Amount of use and quality of movement (MAL).	trol group and scored significantly higher on FMA. At 3-month follow-up, performance on GPT and FMA was significantly and highly correlated with motor representation of impaired hand. There were no differences in performance on the MAL between groups at any stage of the study.		
Sterr et al. (2002)	Compare the effectiveness of 3-hour versus 6-hour daily training sessions in CIMT	I—Randomized controlled trial, comparing 2 groups of CIMT participants. 15 adults with chronic hemiparesis (13 poststroke; *n* = 8 [3-hour group], *n* = 7 [6-hour group]). Repeated measures were administered on two occasions before treatment, immediately following the standard 2-week CIMT intervention, and on 2 occasions weekly following CIMT.	Participants in a CIMT program were randomly assigned to shaping sessions whose duration was either 3 hours per day or 6 hours per day (6 hours is standard in CIMT protocols). *Outcome measures:* ■ MAL ■ Wolf Motor Function Test (WMFT).	MAL scores improved significantly posttreatment for both groups and remained well above baseline level during follow-up. WMFT scores improved significantly, using a two-tailed test, for the group receiving 6-hour daily shaping sessions. For the group receiving 3-hour daily shaping sessions, WMFT scores improved significantly, using a one-tailed test.	Small sample size.	Shaping sessions of 3 hours per day in a CIMT protocol may be effective in improving motor function in patients with chronic hemiparesis, but the standard protocol of 6 hours per day of directed task practice is more effective in improving motor function.

Ro, T., Noser, E., Boake, C., Johnson, R., Gaber, M., Speroni, A., et al. (2006). Functional reorganization and recovery after constraint-induced movement therapy in subacute stroke: Case reports. *Neurocase, 12,* 50–60.

Sterr, A., Elbert, T., Berthold, I., Kolbel, S., Rockstroh, B., & Taub, E. (2002). Longer versus shorter daily constraint-induced movement therapy of chronic hemiparesis: An exploratory study. *Archives of Physical Medicine, 83,* 1374–1377.

Author/Year	Study Objectives	Level/Design/Participants	Intervention and Outcome Measures	Results	Study Limitations	Implications for Practice
Underwood et al. (2006)	Explore relationship between intensity of CIMT and fatigue and pain	I—Randomized controlled trial *N* = 32 (22 men, 10 women); 18 in subacute group, 14 in chronic group Average age: 61.6 years	Participants were randomly assigned to a group that would receive therapy during subacute phase of stroke or a group that would receive therapy during chronic phase of stroke, using a process designed to ensure balance between groups in functional capability, sex, hemiplegic side, and hand dominance. The subacute group received CIMT 3–9 months after stroke; the chronic therapy group received therapy 1 year after enrollment in study. Both groups received therapy 6 hours per day for 10 days. Therapy relied on shaping and repetitive practice. *Outcome measures:* ■ Upper-extremity motor function (WMFT) ■ Upper-extremity joint pain (FMA) ■ Intensity of therapy (minutes actually spent in task practice) ■ Fatigue and pain during training (single-item rating scales of 1–10).	Both groups showed significant improvement in motor function from before therapy to after therapy. Both groups achieved same intensity of therapy. For both groups, there was no change in morning or afternoon pain and fatigue during treatment period.	Small sample size.	CIMT can improve motor function in patients in subacute or chronic phase of stroke with minimal to moderate impairment. With careful screening, neither pain nor fatigue should be of concern in using CIMT with these patients.

Underwood, J., Clark, P. C., Blanton, S., Aycock, D. M., & Wolf, S. L. (2006). Pain, fatigue, and intensity of practice in people with stroke who are receiving constraint-induced movement therapy. *Physical Therapy, 86,* 1241–1250.

(continued)

EVIDENCE TABLE. CONSTRAINT-INDUCED MOVEMENT THERAPY (cont.)

Author/Year	Study Objectives	Level/Design/ Participants	Intervention and Outcome Measures	Results	Study Limitations	Implications for Occupational Therapy
Wittenberg et al. (2003)	Compare effects of CIMT and less-intensive intervention on motor function and brain physiology in stroke patients 1 year or more after stroke	I—Randomized controlled trial

$N = 16$ (13 men, 3 women); 9 in experimental group, 7 in control group

Average age: 64 years | Participants were randomly assigned to receive CIMT or control therapy. CIMT involved restraint of unaffected upper extremity during waking hours and task-oriented therapy with affected upper extremity. Control therapy involved task performance on unaffected side.

CIMT, delivered in clinical center, occurred 6 hours per day for 8 days, 4 hours per day for 2 days (1 weekend). Control therapy, also delivered in clinical center, occurred 3 hours per day for 8 days. Participants rested on weekend.

Outcome measures:
- Motor function (WMFT)
- Function during daily activities (MAL)
- ADL (Assessment of Motor and Process Skills [AMPS])
- Changes in motor cortex (transcranial magnetic stimulation) | Experimental group performed significantly better than control group on MAL but not on AMPS and WMFT.

TMS-center of gravity of map of unaffected side shifted significantly in both groups, in medial direction. Difference between groups was not significant.

TMS-map volume ratio (map volume of affected side divided by map volume of unaffected side) increased more in experimental group than in control group, and difference approached significance.

Paired-pulse facilitation on unaffected side increased significantly more in experimental group than in control group.

Motor cortical activation on affected side decreased (improved) more in experimental group than in control group. | Study is of good quality. | Measurable physiological changes may accompany rehabilitation interventions emphasizing practice. |

- Changes in motor task–related activation (positron emission tomography).

Wittenberg, G. F., Chen, R., Ishii, K., Bushara, K. O., Eckloff, S., Croarkin, E., et al. (2003). Constraint-induced therapy in stroke: Magnetic-stimulation motor maps and cerebral activation. *Neurorehabilitation and Neural Repair, 17*, 48–57.

| Wolf et al. (2008) | To evaluate the effectiveness of constraint-induced movement therapy (CIMT) 24 months after the intervention. | I—Randomized controlled trial—single blind crossover trial—control group received treatment after one year

N = 222 participants with mild to moderate poststroke impairments *n* = 106 CIMT, *n* = 116 usual care

Analysis of data was done only for group receiving CIMT immediately after randomization | *Intervention* – Constraint-induced movement therapy – Participants wore a padded protective mitt on less impaired wrist and hand for 90% of waking hours during 2-week treatment period. Participants did adapted task practice and repetitive task practice (e.g., grooming or eating) using more impaired wrist and hand.

Outcomes measure: Impaired upper limb function
■ Wolf motor function test (WMFT)
■ Motor Activity Log (MAL) health-related quality of life—Stroke Impact Scale (SIS). | Improvements were maintained 24 months after CIMT for time to complete the WMFT, weight lifted on the WMFT, grip strength on the WMFT, amount of use in the MAL, and how well the limb was used in the MAL. In addition, improvements observed at 12 months were maintained on the SIS domains of strength, memory, activities of daily living, instrumental activities of daily living, social participation and the physical domain. | Study is of good quality | This study provides support for the long-term impact of CIMT on improving hand motor function in stroke survivors who meet criteria for participation |

Wolf, S. L., Winstein, C. J., Miller, J. P., Thompson, P. A., Taub, E., Uswatte, G., et al. (2008). Retention of upper limb function in stroke survivors who have received constraint-induced movement therapy: The EXCITE randomized trial. *Lancet Neurology, 7*(1), 33–40.

(continued)

Author/Year	Study Objectives	Level/Design/ Participants	Intervention and Outcome Measures	Results	Study Limitations	Implications for Occupational Therapy
Wolf et al. (2006)	Compare effects of 2-week multisite program of CIMT and usual and customary care for patients in subacute phase of stroke (3–9 months since occurrence)	I—Randomized controlled trial

$N = 222$ (142 men, 80 women); 106 in experimental group, 116 in control group

Average age: 62.2 years | Participants were randomly assigned to a group receiving CIMT (experimental group) or a group receiving usual and customary care (control group). Experimental group received therapy 6 hours per day for 10 weekdays and were encouraged to wear a mitt on the unaffected hand for a target of 90% of waking hours on those 10 days and related weekends. Therapy involved both shaping and repetitive-task training.

Control group received care ranging from no treatment to use of orthotics to various occupational and physical therapy approaches.

Outcome measures:
- Quality and speed of arm movement (WMFT)
- Quality and amount of real-world arm use (MAL). | Immediately following treatment, experimental group showed significantly larger improvements than control group in quality and speed of arm movement, except on 2 motor-function strength items, and in quality and amount of real-world arm use.

At 4-, 8-, and 12-month follow-ups, experimental group showed significantly greater improvements on speed of arm movement and in quality and amount of real-world arm use. | Possible bias from difference between groups in intensity of treatment. | CIMT produces improvements in patients in subacute phase of stroke. These improvements persist for at least 1 year. |

Wolf, S. L., Winstein, C. J., Miller, J. P., Taub, E., Uswatte, G., Morris, D., et al. (2006). Effect of constraint-induced movement therapy on upper extremity function 3 to 9 months after stroke: The EXCITE randomized clinical trial. *JAMA, 296,* 2095–2104.

| Wu, Chen, et al. (2007) | Assess the benefits of mCIMT on motor function, daily function, and health-related quality of life (HRQL) in elderly stroke survivors. | I—Randomized controlled trial

26 elderly patients with stroke (mean = 72 years) who met motor criteria for participation (n = 13 mCIMT, n = 13 traditional rehabilitation) | Participants were randomly assigned to mCIMT or control groups. Participants in both groups received individualized, 2-hour occupational therapy sessions, 5 times per week for 3 weeks.

For mCIMT participants, therapy consisted of shaping and adaptive, repetitive task practice techniques, with 15 minutes of therapy time spent on reducing abnormal muscle tone when needed. In addition, participants wore mitts on the less-affected hand every weekday for 6 hours during a time of frequent arm use.

For control group participants, therapy consisted of approximately 75% traditional rehabilitation focused on neurodevelopmental technique and 25% training in compensatory techniques using the unaffected limb to perform functional tasks.

Outcome measures:
■ FMA
■ FIM
■ MAL
■ SIS. | Compared with controls, the mCIMT group showed significantly greater gains on FMA, FIM, MAL, and SIS scores when assessed immediately posttreatment. | No follow-up assessments were made to assess long-term effects. | Elderly stroke survivors, who may tolerate the demands of mCIMT better than standard CIMT, benefit from a modified CIMT program during inpatient rehabilitation. |

Wu, C. Y., Chen, C. L., Tsai, W. C., Lin, K. C., & Chou, S. H. (2007). A randomized controlled trial of modified constraint-induced movement therapy for elderly stroke survivors: Changes in motor impairment, daily functioning, and quality of life. *Archives of Physical Medicine and Rehabilitation, 88,* 273–278.

(continued)

EVIDENCE TABLE. CONSTRAINT-INDUCED MOVEMENT THERAPY *(cont.)*

Author/Year	Study Objectives	Level/Design/ Participants	Intervention and Outcome Measures	Results	Study Limitations	Implications for Occupational Therapy
Wu, Lin, et al. (2007)	Use motion analysis technology to compare motor control during functional reach in patients who participated in mCIMT with patients who participated in traditional rehabilitation	I—Randomized controlled trial 30 patients with stroke who meet motor criteria for participation in mCIMT (*n* = 15 mCIMT, *n* = 15 traditional rehabilitation [TR])	Participants were randomly assigned to mCIMT or control group. Participants in both groups received individualized, 2-hour occupational therapy sessions, 5 times per week for 3 weeks. For mCIMT participants, therapy consisted of shaping and adaptive, repetitive task practice techniques, with 15 minutes of therapy time spent on reducing abnormal muscle tone when needed. In addition, participants wore mitts on the less-affected hand every weekday for 6 hours during a time of frequent arm use. TR group members received neurodevelopmental treatments at the same dosage. *Outcome measures:* ■ Kinematic analysis of spatial and temporal movement efficiency and type of movement control during unilateral (reaching forward to depress a bell) and bilateral (opening a drawer and reaching	Analysis of covariance revealed significantly greater improvements for the mCIMT group in temporal, spatial, and preplanning measures generated by kinematic analysis, but more so when performing the bilateral task. The mCIMT improvements on MAL and FIM were also significantly greater than the control group.	No follow-up assessments were made to assess long-term effects.	In addition to its impact on functional outcomes, mCIMT also results in improved quality of movement during arm reach, as measured with motion analysis technology.

inside to retrieve an eyeglass case) tasks
- MAL
- FIM.

Outcomes were assessed immediately after the 3-week intervention.

Wu, C. Y., Lin, K. C., Chen, H. C., Chen, I. H., & Hong, W. H. (2007). Effects of modified constraint-induced movement therapy on movement kinematics and daily function in patients with stroke: A kinematic study of motor control mechanisms. *Neurorehabilitation and Neural Repair, 21,* 460–466.

Author/Year	Purpose	Level/Design	Sample	Intervention & Outcome Measures	Results	Limitations	Conclusions
Taub et al. (2006)	Conduct placebo-controlled trial of CIMT with patients in chronic phase of stroke	II—Nonrandomized controlled trial N = 41 (27 men, 14 women); 21 in CIMT group, 20 in control group Average age: 52.7 years	Participants were assigned in blocks to CIMT group or control group, on basis of scores on WMFT (to match groups on initial motor deficit). CIMT includes constraint to unaffected hand (by wearing a mitt) during 90% of waking hours and intensive task-based practice sessions using shaping. Control group participated in fitness program (exercises and games). Treatment occurred 6 hours per day, 5 days per week, for 2 weeks. *Outcome measures:* • Quality of movement (QOM scale of MAL) • Actual amount of use (upper-extremity actual-amount-of-use test)	CIMT group showed significantly greater improvement in quality of movement (on MAL), actual amount of use, and speed. At 4-week follow-up, CIMT group had retained gains on MAL. At 2-year follow-up, CIMT group showed only 23% decrease from MAL levels immediately following treatment.	Lack of randomization.	CIMT is effective in rehabilitating upper-extremity motor function in chronic stroke survivors.

(continued)

Author/Year	Study Objectives	Level/Design/ Participants	Intervention and Outcome Measures	Results	Study Limitations	Implications for Occupational Therapy
Taub et al. (2006) *(cont.)*			▪ Motor ability (speed and quality; performance-time and functional-ability scales of WMFT).			

Taub, E., Uswatte, G., King, D. K., Morris, D., Crago, J. E., & Chatterjee, A. (2006). A placebo-controlled trial of constraint-induced movement therapy for upper extremity after stroke. *Stroke, 37,* 1045–1049.

Author/Year	Study Objectives	Level/Design/ Participants	Intervention and Outcome Measures	Results	Study Limitations	Implications for Occupational Therapy
Uswatte et al. (2006)	Evaluate effect of type of training provided to affected arm and type of restraint used on unaffected arm in CIMT with patients in chronic phase of stroke	II—Nonrandomized control trial *N* = 17 (10 men, 7 women); 4 in sling-and-task-practice group, 4 in sling-and-shaping group, 5 in half-glove-and-shaping group, and 4 in shaping-only group Average age: 63.8 years	Participants were consecutively assigned to sling-and-task-practice group, sling-and-shaping group, half-glove-and-shaping group, and shaping-only group. Sling-and-task-practice group engaged in repetitive practice of functional tasks (eating lunch, throwing ball, etc.) 6 hours per day for 10 consecutive weekdays. Sling-and-shaping group received shaping of affected-arm use on same schedule. In both groups, movement of unaffected arm was restricted by splint/ sling combination worn for target of 90% of waking hours. Half-glove-and-shaping group received same treatment as sling-and-shaping group but wore half-glove rather than splint/sling combination. Shaping-only group received shaping of affected arm on same schedule as other groups but wore no restraint.	Immediately following treatment, all four groups combined showed significant improvement in real-world arm use from before treatment to after treatment. All four combined also showed significant improvement in motor ability. Further, there were no significant differences among groups. One month after treatment, all four groups combined continued to show significant gains in real-world arm use from before treatment to after treatment. There were no significant differences among groups. Two years after treatment, three groups combined (shaping-only excluded because of missing data) still showed significant gains in real-world arm use from before treatment to after treatment.	Possible bias from difference in training intensity; possible confounding from similarity of task practice to shaping; possible confounding from failure to monitor compliance with wearing of restraint; small sample size; lack of no-treatment group.	In terms of immediate outcomes, shaping and task practice may be equivalent methods for training affected arm. Physical restraint of unaffected arm may not be necessary to promote use of affected arm. Other components of therapy (training of affected arm, contract with patient, etc.) may suffice

Therapy was delivered in laboratory by therapists (type not reported).

Outcome measures:
- Real-world arm use (Quality of Movement Scale of MAL)
- Motor ability (WMFT).

Uswatte, G., Taub, E., Morris, D., Barman, J., & Crago, J. (2006). Contribution of the shaping and restraint components of constraint-induced movement therapy to treatment outcome. *NeuroRehabilitation, 21,* 147–156.

Brogardh & Sjölund (2006)	Investigate effectiveness of 6 hours of constraint-induced group therapy wearing mitt on unaffected hand and investigate added benefits of use of mitt beyond therapy	III and I—Combined case control and randomized controlled trial, respectively *N* = 16 (9 men, 7 women); 9 in active-treatment group, 7 in control group Average age: 56.7 years	All participants had had a stroke at least 6 months earlier. They agreed to use a mitt on the less affected hand 90% of waking hours for 12 consecutive days. They received constraint-induced movement therapy in small groups of 2–3 people 6 hours per day 5 times per week for 2 weeks. Therapy was delivered by occupational therapists, physical therapists, and nurses.	During constraint-induced group therapy, 11 of 16 participants significantly improved quality and speed of movement, and 12 of 16 improved the ability to grasp. Changes in self-reported quality and amount of use (MAL) also were significant. After 3 months of extended use of the mitt, the active treatment group showed no further significant improvement. The control group also showed no further significant improvement. Participants then were assigned randomly to receive active treatment or no further treatment (control). The active-treatment group used the mitt at home 90% of waking hours every other day for 2 weeks during	The first phase of study lacked a control group; small sample size; possible bias from the failure of some members of the active treatment group to comply fully with extended wearing of the mitt. Conducting constraint-induced movement therapy in small groups (2–3 patients per therapist) may be a realistic alternative to one-on-one treatment of stroke patients.

(continued)

Author/Year	Study Objectives	Level/Design/ Participants	Intervention and Outcome Measures	Results	Study Limitations	Implications for Occupational Therapy
Brogardh & Sjölund (2006) (cont.)			3 months—a total of 21 days. The control group stopped use of the mitt after group therapy but was encouraged to use affected hand in real-life situations. *Outcome measures:* ▪ Quality of movement and speed of performance (modified Motor Assessment Scale) ▪ Ability to grasp different objects (Sollerman Hand Function Test) ▪ Sensory discrimination (Two-Point Discrimination Test) ▪ Quality and amount of movement (Motor Activity Log [MAL]).			

Brogardh, C., & Sjölund, B. H. (2006). Constraint-induced movement therapy in patients with stroke: A pilot study on effects of small group training and of extended mitt use. *Clinical Rehabilitation, 20,* 218–227.

Author/Year	Study Objectives	Level/Design/ Participants	Intervention and Outcome Measures	Results	Study Limitations	Implications for Occupational Therapy
Flinn et al. (2005)	Investigate the outcome of constraint-induced movement therapy (CIMT) on arm use, coordination, and perceptions of participation in meaningful activities	III—Before-and-after design *N* = 11 participants at least 6 months poststroke (7 males, 4 females) Average age: 61.4 years	Participants took part in a constraint-induced movement therapy program for 8 hours per day for 8 days, receiving therapy for 3½ hours per day. The therapy included participation in activities with the affected hand and arm. Logs were kept during therapy and at home and included records of how long participants wore mitts on their unaffected arm.	Following treatment, participants significantly increased the use of their affected arm in daily activities as measured by the MAL. Coordination of the affected arm did not change as measured by the WMFT. While there was no change in satisfaction immediately following treatment, there was significant improvement in satisfaction with performance	Small sample size, lack of a control group. The authors report that the social component of the program may have contributed to the positive improvements in performance	CIMT is effective in increasing the use of the affected arm in daily activities and may increase satisfaction in the performance of occupations that require the use of the hand.

			Outcome measures:		
			■ MAL ■ Wolf Motor Function Test (WMFT) ■ COMP.	of activities at 4–6 months posttreatment, as measured by the COPM. Participants did not identify improvements in occupational performance or satisfaction as an outcome of CIMT.	

Flinn, N. A., Schamburg, S., Fetrow, J. M. & Flanigan, J. (2005). The effect of constraint-induced movement treatment on occupational performance and satisfaction in stroke survivors. *OTJR: Occupation, Participation and Health, 25,* 119–127.

| Fritz et al. (2006) | Investigate 6 potential predictors of outcomes of CIMT | III—Before-and-after design

N = 55 (33 men, 22 women)

Average age: 62.1 years | Participants received CIMT involving task practice with the affected hand and arm. They wore a mitt on the unaffected hand for goal of 90% of waking hours. Therapy occurred 6 hours per day 5 days per week for 2 weeks.

Potential predictors were side of stroke, time since stroke, hand dominance, age, sex, and ambulatory status.

Outcome measures:
■ Movement capability (performance–time scale of WMFT)
■ Amount of perceived use. | Age was the only significant predictor of outcome at 4–6 months, and only for amount of perceived use. | Lack of randomization and possible bias from withdrawals | Age may be a significant predictor of favorable outcome from constraint-induced movement therapy. Side of stroke, time since stroke, hand dominance, sex, and ambulatory status were not predictors and therefore should not be considered as inclusion criteria in CIMT programs. |

Fritz, S. L., Light, K. E., Clifford, S. N., Patterson, T. S., Behrman, A. L., & Davis, S. B. (2006). Descriptive characteristics as potential predictors of outcomes following constraint-induced movement therapy for people after stroke. *Physical Therapy, 86,* 825–832.

(continued)

EVIDENCE TABLE. CONSTRAINT-INDUCED MOVEMENT THERAPY *(cont.)*

Author/Year	Study Objectives	Level/Design/ Participants	Intervention and Outcome Measures	Results	Study Limitations	Implications for Occupational Therapy
Liepert (2006)	Investigate excitability of motor cortex in stroke patients before and after CIMT	III—Before-and-after design *N* = 12 (7 men, 5 women) Average age: 59.5 years	Researchers used transcranial magnetic stimulation (TMS) and peripheral electrical stimulation to assess excitability of motor cortex in participants. Participants then received constraint-induced movement therapy 6 hours per day for 12 days. Afterward, researchers reassessed excitability of motor cortex. *Outcome measures:* ■ Motor thresholds (MTs) ■ Motor evoked potential (MEP) latency and central motor conduction time ■ Duration of silent period obtained by TMS with stimulus intensity 50% above MT ■ Intracortical inhibition (ICI) ■ Intracortical facilitation ■ Amount and quality of use ■ Motor function (WMFT) ■ Spasticity (MAS).	MEP amplitudes were significantly different after therapy. MEP size was significantly and inversely correlated with MT. Before therapy, participants had significantly less ICI in the affected hemisphere than in the unaffected hemisphere. After therapy, mean ICI value remained almost identical in both hemispheres, but a significant difference in amount of ICI changes was evident. ICI changes were stronger in the affected hemisphere. Participants significantly improved motor function following therapy, and significantly reduced spasticity.	Lack of control group and randomization.	CIMT enhances motor function in patients in the chronic phase of stroke and also produces evidence of recordable motor cortex excitability.

Liepert, J. (2006). Motor cortex excitability in stroke before and after constraint-induced movement therapy. *Cognitive and Behavioral Neurology, 19,* 41–47.

Liepert et al. (2000)	Use CIMT as a model to assess therapy-induced plasticity in stroke patients	III—Before-and-after design $N = 13$ (10 men, 3 women) Average age: 56.7 years	Participants received CIMT for 12 days. They wore a splint on the nonparetic arm all 12 days for 90% of waking hours and were trained in use of paretic arm 6 hours per day for 8 days. Intervention was delivered in laboratory. *Outcome measures:* ■ Arm use in 20 ADL (MAL) ■ Changes in cortical output area (TMS).	Participants significantly improved arm use. Size of muscle output area in affected hemisphere was significantly enlarged (nearly double in size).	Lack of control group and randomization	CIMT may induce alteration in brain function and improvement in motor function.

Liepert, J., Bauder, H., Wolfgang, H. R., Miltner, W. H., Taub, E., & Weiller, C. (2000). Treatment-induced cortical reorganization after stroke in humans. *Stroke, 31*, 1210–1216.

Page & Levine (2006)	Determine efficacy of combining electromyography-triggered neuromuscular stimulation (ETMS) and mCIMT in treatment of patients in chronic phase of stroke	III—Before-and-after design $N = 6$ (2 men, 4 women) Average age: 62.8 years	Participants used ETMS device at home in 35-minute sessions 2 times per day, 5 days per week for 8 weeks. After 1-week interval, they received mCIMT in 30-minute sessions 3 days per week for 10 weeks. They also wore slings and mitts 5 hours per day 5 days per week, to restrain unaffected arm and hand. *Outcome measures:* ■ Motor recovery (upper-extremity motor component of Fugl-Meyer Assessment [FMA]) ■ Grasp, grip, pinch, and gross movement (Action Research Arm Test) ■ Active wrist extension (goniometry).	Before ETMS, participants could minimally activate affected extensors but could not functionally use wrists and fingers. After ETMS, although there were no functional changes, participants had adequate active wrist extension and requisite movement in affected hand to qualify for mCIMT. After mCIMT, participants had improved ability to perform FMA wrist items and new ability to perform FMA hand items. They also had improved grasp and grip and new ability to pinch small objects.	Small sample size and lack of control group.	ETMS may be useful in preparing some stroke patients for participation in CIMT.

Page, S. J., & Levine, P. (2006). Back from the brink: Electromyography-triggered stimulation combined with modified constraint-induced movement therapy in chronic stroke. *Archives of Physical Medicine and Rehabilitation, 87*, 27–31.

(continued)

EVIDENCE TABLE. CONSTRAINT-INDUCED MOVEMENT THERAPY (cont.)

Author/Year	Study Objectives	Level/Design/ Participants	Intervention and Outcome Measures	Results	Study Limitations	Implications for Occupational Therapy
Szaflarski et al. (2006)	Determine whether cortical changes occur in patients in chronic phase of stroke following mCIMT	III—Before-and-after design N = 14 (7 men, 7 women); 4 with stroke, 10 without disability Average age: 59.3 years	Stroke patients received mCIMT 30 minutes per day, 3 times per week, for 10 weeks. Therapy was delivered by an occupational therapist. Patients wore mitt on unaffected hand 5 hours per day for same 10 weeks. Participants without disability acted as control group for data on typical activation patterns in finger-tapping tasks. *Outcome measures:* ■ Cortical reorganization (functional magnetic resonance imaging [fMRI]) ■ Motor function (FMA) ■ Impairment (ARAT) ■ Amount and quality of use (MAL).	Three of 4 stroke patients showed cortical reorganization on fMRI. Same 3 showed increases in motor function, reductions in impairment, and increases in amount and quality of use.	Small sample size, lack of randomization, and lack of true control group.	mCIMT appears to induce cortical reorganization. In patients who responded to therapy, cortical reorganization was positively related to degree of increase in use of affected arm and in ability.

Szaflarski, J. P., Page, S. P., Kissela, B. M., Lee, J-H., Levine, P., & Strakowski, S. M. (2006). Cortical reorganization following modified constraint-induced movement therapy: A study of 4 patients with chronic stroke. *Archives of Physical Medicine and Rehabilitation, 87*, 1052–1058.

Citation	Study objective	Design/Participants	Methods/Outcome measures	Results	Limitations	Conclusion
Liepert et al. (2004)	Study impact of lesion in central somatosensory system, lesion in cerebellum, and CIMT on excitability of motor cortex	IV—Single-subject design Part 1: $N = 3$ Part 2: $N = 6$ Part 3, study A: $N = 15$; study B: $N = 8$ (Gender not reported for any part) Average age: Not reported	Researchers studied participants in part 1 for interaction between central somatosensory lesions and excitability of motor cortex; participants in part 2 for interaction between cerebellar lesions and excitability of motor cortex; and participants in part 3, studies A and B, for effects of constraint-induced movement therapy on excitability of motor cortex. Latter intervention occurred 6 hours per day 5 days per week for 2 weeks. *Outcome measures:* ■ Interaction between central somatosensory lesion and motor excitability (TMS) ■ Interaction between cerebellar lesion and motor excitability ■ Motor function (MAL) ■ Changes in cortical motor output area (TMS and functional magnetic resonance imaging [fMRI]).	Participants in part 1 showed loss of intracortical inhibition on the affected side. Participants in part 2 showed loss of intracortical facilitation in the primary motor cortex. Participants in part 3, study A, showed significant improvement in motor function and enlarged motor output area for the paretic hand following therapy. Participants in part 3, study B, showed less intracortical inhibition after therapy, and 4 showed more. Difference in values of intracortical inhibition before and after therapy was significantly stronger in the affected hemisphere than in the nonaffected hemisphere. Also, motor thresholds were reduced after therapy.	Small sample size and a lack of control group and randomization	CIMT may induce changes in neural excitability, mainly in affected hemisphere.

Liepert, J., Hamzei, F., & Weiller, C. (2004). Lesion-induced and training-induced brain reorganization. *Restorative Neurology and Neuroscience, 22,* 269–277.

EVIDENCE TABLE. FOCUSED QUESTION 1.

What is the evidence that challenging demands to the brain, such as therapy, activity, or sensory stimulation, reorganizes brain function beyond spontaneous recovery after traumatic brain injury?

Author/Year	Study Objectives	Level/Design/ Participants	Intervention and Outcome Measures	Results	Study Limitations	Implications for Occupational Therapy
Marshall et al. (2007)	Evaluate the efficacy of interventions used to manage motor impairments following acquired brain injury (ABI)	I—Systematic review Searched CINAHL, Medline, EMBASE, PsycINFO for articles from 1980 to 2006. All published literature related to acquired brain injury was included (study participants with ABI were at least 50% of the population). Bibliographies of selected articles also were reviewed. Review included experimental (randomized trials, prospective and retrospective controlled trials, single group interventions) and nonexperimental designs (retrospective and case studies).	*Interventions in the review included:* Constraint-induced movement therapy functional fine motor retraining, hand splinting, electrical stimulation, vestibular rehabilitation, and aerobic exercise *Outcome measures:* ■ Activities of daily living ■ Test of motor and hand function ■ Range of motion ■ Balance scales ■ Pain scales.	36 studies were included in the review. There is moderate evidence that functional fine motor retraining activities improve fine motor coordination and functional performance, and that aerobic activity increases aerobic capacity in ABI. There is moderate evidence that nocturnal splinting is not effective in improving range of motion or function. There is limited evidence that reach training with occupational-embedded intervention is more effective in reducing upper extremity spasticity than a traditional reaching program. The evidence also is limited for balance and vestibular rehabilitation programs, visual feedback grip force training, serial casting, and electrical stimulation.	Small sample sizes, low quality of study designs, and heterogeneity of study populations and study interventions.	Modified constraint-induced therapy may be an effective intervention for upper extremity movement improvement. Shorter duration between serial casts can lead to fewer complications and no difference in range of motion outcome when compared to more traditional casting time frames. Nocturnal hand splinting does not improve range, function, or pain in patients with TBI. Functional fine motor activities may be more effective in improving fine motor coordination than tabletop activities.

Marshall, S., Teasell, R., Bayona, N., Lippert, C., Chundamala, J., Villamere, J., et al. (2007). Motor impairment rehabilitation post acquired brain injury. *Brain Injury, 21,* 133–160.

| Cho et al., 2005 | Investigate the effect of CIMT on fine motor ability in clients with upper limb hemiparesis after traumatic brain injury (TBI)

Functional plasticity in motor cortex accompanies recovery associated with CIT (Nudo, 2003). | III—One group pretest–posttest design

N = 9 individuals with chronic hemiparesis; 6 had sustained a stroke and 3 had TBI; mean age = 42.1 years (range 29–62 years)

Participants were at least 12 weeks post–brain injury onset; showed no abnormal movement pattern due to spasticity, compensation, or tremor; demonstrated Medical Research Council (MRC) grade above 4; able to complete basic activities of daily living (ADLs) with only affected hand; and displayed no serious cognitive problems (aphasia, attention deficits, visual neglect, disorders of reasoning and memory)

Participants were included in the study after they showed 3 consecutive weeks of no further recovery of fine motor ability by Purdue Pegboard (PP) test and motor function by the MRC grade. | *Intervention:* The affected hand was restricted with an opposition restriction orthosis worn during all waking hours except during showering, defecation, urination, or driving. Participants continued training with the same physical and occupational therapy programs.

Outcome measures: Weekly scores from the PP test were taken and the constraint-induced movement therapy (CIMT) was stopped when the participant obtained the same PP score for 3 consecutive weeks. The mean restriction period was 3.6 weeks (range 2–5 weeks). | PP score increased in all participants. The mean posttreatment PP score was significantly increased over the pre-treatment mean score. | Small sample size with mixed diagnoses and lack of control group; lack of description of time since injury may have resulted in inclusion of TBI participants who still were in the spontaneous recovery period; no description of the interventions included in the standard physical and occupational therapy programs—it is possible some therapists focused more on fine motor practice tasks; no follow-up assessments were made to assess long-term effects. | Constraint-induced movement therapy may enhance motor function in patients with TBI. |

Cho, Y. W., Jang, S. H., Lee, Z. I., Song, J. C., Lee, H. K., & Lee, H. Y. (2005). Effect and appropriate restriction period of constraint-induced movement therapy in hemiparetic patients with brain injury: A brief report. *NeuroRehabilitation, 20,* 71–74.

(continued)

Author/Year	Study Objectives	Level/Design/ Participants	Intervention and Outcome Measures	Results	Study Limitations	Implications for Occupational Therapy
Shaw et al., 2005	Determine the effectiveness of a 2-week program of constraint-induced movement therapy (CIMT) for clients with chronic traumatic brain injury (TBI)	Level III One group pretest–posttest design. 22 participants with chronic TBI (onset >1 year) with moderate disability in the more-affected upper limb	CIMT was provided for a 2-week period; treatments included massed practice, shaping, behavioral contracts, and other behavioral techniques for affecting transfer to a real-world setting. *Outcome measures:* ■ Wolf Motor Function Test ■ Fugl-Meyer Motor Performance Assessment ■ Motor Activity Log.	All outcome measures improved significantly. More-adherent participants had more improvement compared with less-adherent participants.	The study lacked a control group.	These preliminary results suggest that CIMT may be effective for improving motor function in the upper limbs following TBI.

Shaw, S. E., Morris, D. M., Uswatte, G., McKay, S., Meythaler, J. M., & Taub, E. (2005). Constraint-induced movement therapy for recovery of upper-limb function following traumatic brain injury. *Journal of Rehabilitation Research and Development, 42,* 769–778.

Author/Year	Study Objectives	Level/Design/ Participants	Intervention and Outcome Measures	Results	Study Limitations	Implications for Occupational Therapy
Sterr & Freivogel (2003)	Examine the benefits of a modified regimen designed to be applicable in clinical environment	Level III—One group pretest–posttest design N = 13 participants aged 17 to 21 years with chronic upper limb hemiparesis after severe TBI (n = 11; chronicity, 38 ± 39 months [range, 24 to 150 months]) or stroke (n = 2; chronicity, 12 months).	During the baseline phase of the study, participants received 90 minutes of occupational therapy per day. During the 3-week intervention phase, participants were trained individually for 90 minutes per day to perform specific movements of progressive difficulty using the learning principle of shaping. Constraint was not used to the other limb. *Outcome measures:* The Motor Activity Log, Wolf Motor Function Test, and Frenchay Arm Test were administered four times by teams	Statistically significant improvements were found in the amount of use and quality of movement for each participant on the MAL between the pre-intervention to post-intervention period but not during the baseline to pre-intervention post-intervention to follow-up periods. Improvements in the Frenchay Arm Test and the quality of movement component of the Wolf Motor Function Test were found for pre- to post-treatment but not for baseline to follow-up periods. No significant results were	Small sample size, lack of a control group, and limited follow-up period.	Increased use of the affected limb in everyday situations can be achieved for low-functioning patients well beyond spontaneous recovery.

			obtained for the speed component in the Wolf Motor Function Test.	of two blinded control physiotherapists: at the beginning of the baseline period, the week after the baseline interval (pre), after the intervention (post), and 1 month after intervention (follow-up).	

Sterr, A., & Freivogel, S. (2003). Motor improvement following intensive training in low-functioning chronic hemiparesis. *Neurology, 61,* 842–844.

| Page & Levine (2003) | Determine the efficacy of mCIT in improving upper limb use and function in patients with traumatic brain injury (TBI)

Functional plasticity in motor cortex accompanies recovery associated with CIT (Nudo, 2003). | IV—Multiple-baseline, pre–post, case series

N = 3 patients greater than 1 year after TBI who exhibited stable upper limb hemiparesis and learned non-use | Patients participated in 10 sessions of 30-minute, structured physical and occupational therapy, emphasizing use of the affected limb in valued, functional activities combined with 3 times/week for 10 weeks shaping techniques and constraint of their less affected upper limbs 5 days/week during 5 hours identified as times of frequent use.

Outcome measures:
■ The Action Research Arm Test (ARA)
■ Wolf Motor Function Test (WMFT)
■ Motor Activity Log (MAL). | Following intervention, subjects exhibited improvements >2.0 in their amount and quality of more affected limb use, as measured by the MAL. Subjects 1, 2, and 3 also displayed functional improvements on the ARA (14.0, 5.5, and 6.0, respectively), improvements in ratings of WMFT task performance (1.15, 1.7, and 1.35, respectively) and diminished time needed to perform all WMFT tasks.

Conclusion: mCIT is a promising approach by which improved more affected limb use and function can be realized following TBI. Repeated affected limb ADL practice is believed to be the critical variable of the program. | Limited sample size; use of a qualitative measure such as the MAL may be subject to rater bias.

The reliability and validity of the MAL and the WMFT tests were not reported. The MAL required recall of use of the extremity during the past week. No information about compliance with restraint at home was given. | mCIT participation can overcome learned non-use syndrome and elicit functional improvements in clients with TBI and hemiparesis. |

Page, S., & Levine, P. (2003). Forced use after TBI: Promoting plasticity and function through practice. *Brain Injury, 17,* 675–684.

(continued)

EVIDENCE TABLE. FOCUSED QUESTION 1 *(cont.)*

Author/Year	Study Objectives	Level/Design/ Participants	Intervention and Outcome Measures	Results	Study Limitations	Implications for Occupational Therapy
Laatsch et al. (1997)	Determine whether brain reorganization occurred during cognitive rehabilitation therapy (CRT) as determined by serial relative cerebral blood flow (rCBF) examination during the course of recovery	V—Longitudinal, repeated measure case series. $N = 3$ participants with mild, moderate, and severe TBI 2 participants were in the acute phase of recovery and one was in chronic stage (20 mos. postinjury). Mean age = 30 years; above average education and employment level	Individualized, developmental CRT program with a clinical psychologist present. Training was structured so that the use of residual, intact cognitive mechanisms was maximized to increase cognitive efficiency in areas where there were neuropsychological impairments. Number of weekly sessions varied. *Outcome measures:* ■ Wechsler Adult Intelligence Test–Revised (WAIS–R) ■ Test of Non-Verbal Intelligence ■ Single Photon Emission Computed Tomography.	Case 1 (mild) became especially efficient in the use of memory strategies; his stimulating posttreatment employment (office manager) continued his cognitive improvement. Case 2 (moderate) was able to demonstrate improvements in problem solving and verbal memory, which she sustained over a 23-month period, probably also due to challenging job (computer programmer). Case 3 (severe) showed slow but consistent improvement in memory abilities; processing speed remained unchanged. Problem solving improved during the nontreatment period, probably due to her job (dentist). There was enhanced rCBF during the period of cognitive rehabilitation, especially near the area of injury. These changes continued postdischarge when the patient returned to work.	Sample size was small and participants were older, more educated, and more professionally employed than many persons with TBI. Age and preinjury brain functioning are believed to affect recovery from brain injury. No statistical analysis.	Developmentally structured cognitive rehabilitation therapy was shown, in these 3 highly selected persons with various severity of traumatic brain injury, to be effective in reorganizing brain function and improving cognitive functioning.

Laatsch, L., Jobe, T., Sychra, J., Lin, Q., & Blend, M. (1997). Impact of cognitive rehabilitation therapy on neuropsychological impairments as measured by brain perfusion SPECT: A longitudinal study. *Brain Injury, 11,* 851–863.

Conclusion: The specific changes in rCBF appear to be related to the location of the patient's brain injury and strategies particular to cognitive rehabilitation therapy.

Study	Purpose	Design/Subjects	Intervention/Outcome measures	Results	Conclusion
Laatsch et al. (2004)	Demonstrate, through functional magnetic resonance imaging (fMRI), brain plasticity in response to cognitive rehabilitation therapy (CRT) following mild traumatic brain injury.	V—Pretest–posttest case series *N* = 5 (mean age = 33 years) referred by physicians; 3 in acute phase of recovery and 2 in chronic phase No psychiatric symptoms	Intervention: Outpatient computerized and noncomputerized cognitive rehabilitation that concentrated on visual scanning and expressive language processing. Hours of CRT varied from 12–24, 30 min. sessions per week for 4–13 mos., and weekly homework. *Outcome measures:* ■ Neuropsychological tests of visual attention and scanning (WAIS-III, Trails A & B, and Digit Vigilance Test) ■ Expressive language processing subtests of the WAIS-III and the FAS Verbal Fluency Test ■ fMRI.	All subjects experienced improvement >1 standard deviation (SD) on at least one of the 5 neuropsychological tests. A total of 32 pre–post comparisons; 10/32 scores demonstrated improvement at 1 SD and 6/32 at 2 SD or greater. Qualitatively, all subjects experienced improvements in their everyday abilities and jobs or school. Post-CRT fMRI showed changes in the distribution of activated voxels (a measure of brain sections using fMRI) during CRT. *Conclusion:* In this preliminary study, five subjects with a history of mild TBI demonstrated re-distribution of cognitive workload across existing large-scale neurocognitive networks during a period of treatment involving CRT.	Small, diverse sample; possible spontaneous recovery in some subjects. This was a longitudinal study that has the confounding of changes that occur over time outside of the treatment being studied (no control group). Testing effects. These case studies indicate that in some people with mild TBI, a structured, developmental, individualized cognitive rehabilitation therapy program results in improved visual scanning and expressive language abilities and that the brain reorganizes during the period of CRT. Patients with a history of other brain injuries or other neurological diagnoses do not benefit as much as do those without such a history.

Laatsch, L., Thulborn, K. R., Krisky, C. M., Shobat, D. M., & Sweeney, J. A. (2004). Investigating the neurobiological basis of cognitive rehabilitation therapy with fMRI. *Brain Injury, 18,* 957–974.

(continued)

EVIDENCE TABLE. FOCUSED QUESTION 1 (cont.)

Author/Year	Study Objectives	Level/Design/ Participants	Intervention and Outcome Measures	Results	Study Limitations	Implications for Occupational Therapy
Scheibel et al. (2003), Scheibel et al. (2004)	Test the hypothesis that disruption of a patient's frontal circuitry would result in recruitment of more extensive frontal and associated cortical regions to perform working memory and inhibition tasks than neurologically intact adults; working memory and inhibition are used in problem solving and response selection; more extensive recruitment than normal would suggest remodeling of the neural networks subserving these executive functions	V—Case comparison study $N = 1$ 46-year-old man with severe diffuse TBI, 1 year postinjury; 1 44-year-old man and 3 women (ages 20–26 years) for control comparison	*Visual Working Memory Task:* 10 black-and-white photographs of faces of adult men and women were presented for 24 sec. each; the subject signaled (0-back) every time a man's face was presented; (1-back) every time a face presented matched the previous face presented; (2-back) every time the face presented was identical to the face presented immediately before the previous face. The entire task lasted 4 min., repeated 4 times. *Inhibition Task:* In the congruous (noninhibition) condition, participants saw blue arrows that pointed either left or right, and were told to hit the response key ipsilateral to the direction the arrow was pointing. In the incongruous (inhibition) condition, the arrows were red and participants were instructed to press the response key contralateral to the direction the arrow was pointing, thus inhibiting	The scores for the patient and one female control subject were: 0 omission errors on the 0-back condition for both; 4 errors versus 1 error for the 1-back condition; and 14 errors versus 8 errors for the 2-back condition. The male control subject scored 100% correctly on noninhibition trials and 99.25% on inhibition trials, while the patient scored 85.5% on noninhibition trials and 63.5% on inhibition trials. In all subjects, frontal activation increased when the subject was asked to remember (working memory) pictures presented 2-back from present as compared to when asked to remember pictures 1-back from present. The activation was greater in the person with TBI. Frontal activation increased similarly in the inhibition task, with the person with TBI having greater activation. *Conclusion:* Severe diffuse TBI results in recruitment of additional	This was a laboratory experiment rather than therapy, per se. Only one patient was tested. Three of the control subjects were female and younger than the patient.	The authors extrapolated their findings to suggest that nonroutine activities that involve solving novel problems, manipulating information held in short-term memory, inhibiting a prepotent response, reallocating attention, and selecting responses also would necessitate recruitment of more extensive frontal and associated cortical regions to support cognitive performance. This study provides tentative evidence to support the use of such activities in the treatment of persons with diffuse TBI.

response in the direction of the pointing arrow.

Outcome measures:
Accuracy of responses: Number of correct responses, commission errors, omission errors, and multiple presses; brain scans using MRI scanner.

neural resources for cognitive control.

Scheibel, R. S., Pearson, D. A., Faria, L. P., Kotrla, K. J., Aylward, E., Bachevalier, J., et al. (2003). An fMRI study of executive functioning after severe diffuse TBI. *Brain Injury, 17,* 919–930.

Scheibel, R. S., Pearson, D. A., Faria, L. P., Kotrla, K. J., Aylward, E., Bachevalier, J., et al. (2004). Erratum: An fMRI study of executive functioning after severe diffuse TBI. *Brain Injury, 18,* 219–220.

Reference
Nudo, R. J. (2003). Adaptive plasticity in motor cortex: Implications for rehabilitation after brain injury. *Journal of Rehabilitation Medicine, 41*(Suppl.), 7–10.

EVIDENCE TABLE. FOCUSED QUESTION 1A.

What is the evidence for the effect of sensory stimulation on the arousal level of persons in a coma or persistent vegetative state after traumatic brain injury?

Author/Year	Study Objectives	Level/Design/ Participants	Intervention and Outcome Measures	Results	Study Limitations	Implications for Occupational Therapy
Johnson et al. (1993)	Investigate the efficacy of a program of multisensory stimulation to patients with severe diffuse traumatic brain injury (TBI) while they are in the intensive care unit (ICU); measure outcome in terms of physiological and biochemical changes as well as observation of response	I—Randomized controlled trial $N = 14$ males with severe brain injury (Glasgow Coma Scale [GCS] ≤ 8) People with neurological psychiatric disorders, alcohol or drug abuse, or previous head injuries were excluded. Experimental group = 7 (mean age 27.7 years, mean GCS 4.8) Control group = 7 (mean age 31.4 years, mean GCS 4.8)	*Experimental group:* Stimulation, in random order, of 5 senses for 20 min. per day while in ICU (median stay 8.1 days). *Control group:* Usual care without stimulation (median stay 3.7 days). *Outcome measures:* ■ GCS ■ State of ventilation ■ Spontaneous eye movements ■ Oculocephalic response assessed daily. Physiological and biochemical measures taken 20 min. before and 20 min. after stimulation.	GCS—not reported. Only 3-methoxy, 4-hydroxyphenylglycol showed a significant difference in stimulation effect between the 2 groups ($F = 8.54$, $p < 0.006$). It rose in the treated group and declined in the control group, but the authors could not explain the meaning. There was no significant difference between groups for heart rate ($F = .70$, $p = .499$) or skin conductance ($F = 2.51$, $p = .092$). The results give no unequivocal support for the effectiveness of multisensory stimulation in the acute stage of recovery after severe diffuse TBI. Unable to confirm that early multisensory stimulation is of any benefit to the patient.	Method of randomization not reported; observation time was less for the control group (not tested statistically); more of the control group died; attrition rate for total sample > 50%; assessor not blind to assignment.	The outcome measures gave no indication of functional recovery and therefore were not clinically relevant to occupational therapy. This study does not provide guidance to occupational therapy practice.

Johnson, D. A., Roethig-Johnson, K., & Richards, D. (1993). Biochemical and physiological parameters of recovery in acute severe head injury: Responses to multisensory stimulation. *Brain Injury, 7,* 491–499.

| Lombardi et al. (2002) | Review the literature to assess the effectiveness of sensory stimulation programs compared to standard rehabilitation for patients in a coma or vegetative state | I—Systematic review of randomized controlled trials (RCT) and controlled clinical trials (CCT) of people in a coma or vegetative state | *Intervention:* Any type of stimulation program compared to standard rehabilitation. | Results: 25 studies that addressed the topic were located. 22 were excluded because participants underwent concomitant interventions, historical control groups were used, or the studies were case series without control group or individual case reports. Three studies (1 RCT and 2 CCTs) with 68 patients with traumatic brain injury in total met inclusion criteria. Overall methodological quality of these studies was poor. Quantitative meta-analysis was not possible because of diversity of reporting of outcome measures among the studies. | None | There is no reliable evidence to support or rule out multisensory stimulation as an intervention to arouse patients with traumatic brain injury from a coma or vegetative state. Larger and better-controlled research studies that measure disability outcomes are needed. |
| | | Sources of studies:
■ The Injuries Group specialized register
■ Cochrane Controlled Trial register
■ EMBASE
■ Medline
■ CINAHL
■ PsychLit, 1966–January 2002
■ Reference lists and contact of experts.

Three reviewers independently identified relevant studies, extracted data, and assessed study quality. Disagreements were resolved by consensus. | *Outcome measures:*
■ Duration of unconsciousness (time between trauma and ability to respond to verbal commands)
■ Level of consciousness (Glasgow Coma Scale [GCS])
■ Level of cognitive functioning
■ Functional outcomes (Glasgow Outcome Scale or Disability Rating Scale)
■ Negative effects. | *Conclusion:*
There is no reliable evidence to support the effectiveness of multisensory stimulation programs in patients in coma or in vegetative state | | |

Lombardi, F., Taricco, M., De Tanti, A., Telaro, E., & Liberati, A. (2002). Sensory stimulation of brain-injured individuals in coma or vegetative state: Results of a Cochrane systematic review. *Clinical Rehabilitation, 16,* 464–472.

(continued)

EVIDENCE TABLE. FOCUSED QUESTION 1A. *(cont.)*

Author/Year	Study Objectives	Level/Design/ Participants	Intervention and Outcome Measures	Results	Study Limitations	Implications for Occupational Therapy
Davis & Gimenez (2003)	Measure, using behavioral assessments, whether an auditory stimulation program increased arousal of patients who had intact auditory pathways and who were in a coma secondary to traumatic brain injury (TBI); determine whether the auditory sensory stimulation program had detrimental physiologic effects	II—Two-group, repeated measures pretest–posttest *N* = 12 males with TBI; mean postinjury day at admission to study 9 for experimental group and 6.3 for control group; mean Glasgow Coma Scale (GCS) score of 5.5 for experimental group and 6.0 for control group; medically stable; intact auditory pathways; mean age = 30 years; at Levels I to III of the Rancho Los Amigos Cognitive Functioning Scale	*Intervention:* Routine nursing care with routine rehabilitation services and a unimodal (auditory) sensory stimulation program: various tone frequencies (bells, blocks, and claps); music (favorite or researcher selected); familiar (taped) and unfamiliar (TV or radio) voice patterns; spoken messages requiring simple to complex interpretive processes. Sequence varied; randomly distributed throughout the day. *Control:* Routine nursing care with routine rehabilitation services and hourly GCS and Rancho Los Amigos Cognitive Scale (RLA) administration. *Outcome measures:* ■ Change in arousal measured by GCS ■ Sensory Stimulation Assessment Measure (SSAM) ■ RLA ■ Disability Rating Scale (DRS) ■ Physiological changes in central nervous system and cardiac pressures and function.	Intervention group improved more than control group: DRS (*p* = .0005; effects size, *r* = .95); SSAM (*p* = .015; *r* = .63); GCS (*p* = .14; *r* = .31); RLA (*p* = .278; *r* = .17). No statistically or clinically significant changes in the physiologic measures (heart rate, mean arterial pressure, intracranial pressure, cerebral perfusion pressure).	No random assignment to group; all control participants recruited after treatment participants; unknown whether treatment site or who treated was kept constant; unknown whether the assessor was blind to assignment; too few subjects; lacked power to detect significant difference on 2 of the 4 outcome measures.	The results suggest that a program of controlled auditory stimulation may be effective in improving functional level and response to sensory stimulation in acute, comatose patients following TBI. The study was not powerful enough to determine whether the program was effective in improving the level of coma or cognition. The auditory stimulation program was not detrimental to vital functions. These findings suggest that using such a program in occupational therapy may be of some benefit for similarly affected patients.

Davis, A. E., & Gimenez, A. (2003). Cognitive–behavioral recovery in comatose patients following auditory sensory stimulation. *Journal of Neuroscience Nursing, 35,* 202–209, 214.

Mitchell et al. (1990)	Evaluate the efficacy of a Coma Arousal Procedure (CAP) to expedite recovery from coma of patients with severe head injury	II—Two group matched pairs (age, sex, type, and location of head injury; surgical intervention; and Glasgow Coma Scale [GCS] on admission to hospital) N = 24 persons with traumatic brain injury Treatment group: 10 male and 2 female, aged 17–40 years (mean = 22.3), GCS range 4–6 Control group: 10 male and 2 female, aged 17–42 years (mean = 22.75), GCS range 4–6	Treatment group: Cyclical visual, auditory, olfactory, tactile, gustatory, kinesthetic, and vestibular stimulation 1 hour, once or twice a day for 6 days per week for 4 weeks maximum, starting when clinically stable (about 1 week postinjury). Control group: No arousal procedure. Outcomes: Total duration of coma in days as measured by the GCS's measure of responsiveness.	Treatment group in coma for significantly fewer days—22 days (±9.7) versus 26.9 days (±6.6) for the control group (p < 0.05). Conclusion: "The findings of the present study support the efficacy of the CAP" (p. 278).	Criterion for decision regarding the intensity of the treatment is not stated; the assessor was not blind to assignment because the treatment and evaluation were done by the patient's relatives; it was not reported who evaluated the control group; the extent of training of the relatives was not reported.	The arousal procedure reduced the time in coma by almost 5 days. However, the clinical relevance of this without any functional indicator is questionable.

Mitchell, S., Bradley, V. A., Welch, J. L., & Britton, P. G. (1990). Coma arousal procedure: A therapeutic intervention in the treatment of head injury. *Brain Injury, 4*, 273–279.

Wilson, Brock, et al. (1996)	Describe how arousal profiles (frequency of eyes open and frequency of spontaneous movements) are produced; discuss the potential use of this technique for monitoring patients diagnosed as being in a vegetative state using case studies	IV—Single case study; ABA design: 5-day baseline, 15-day treatment phase, 5-day baseline All participants confirmed to be in vegetative state. P1: 35-year-old male, 18 months postinjury P2: 16-year-old female, 6 months postinjury P3: 39-year-old male, 61 months postinjury	Baseline phase: 10-min. time sample taken every morning and every afternoon. Treatment phase: Treatment given in morning and afternoon. Time sample taken immediately before and immediately after each treatment. Random allocation of type of sensory stimulation if two or more forms of sensory stimulation were being used. Multimodal stimulation: Each of	P1: No significant behavior changes were noted in response to either unimodal or multimodal treatment. P2: No significant treatment effects on frequency of eyes open for either unimodal or multimodal stimulation. In fifth treatment block, mother's and therapist's communication resulted in significant (p < 0.05, p < 0.025) improvement in time of eyes open.	Participants were receiving other therapy interspersed with rest periods; did not control for spontaneous recovery; other threats to internal validity were not controlled for (e.g., deteriorating health for P1)	Neither unimodal nor multimodal stimulation were supported or ruled out by this study. The procedure of time sampling behavior for 10 min. immediately before and after treatment seems useful in documenting effects of sensory stimulation or treatment of patients who cannot respond to verbal commands.

(continued)

EVIDENCE TABLE. FOCUSED QUESTION 1A. (cont.)

Author/Year	Study Objectives	Level/Design/ Participants	Intervention and Outcome Measures	Results	Study Limitations	Implications for Occupational Therapy
Wilson, Brock, et al. (1996) (cont.)			the senses was stimulated in turn, using everyday or individually familiar stimuli, to the highest level at which a response could be achieved. Unimodal stimulation: One sense, selected randomly, was treated using everyday or individually familiar stimuli. Stimuli were presented in a graded and structured manner. Rest periods of 20 min. preceded each session.

Outcome measures: Arousal profile from time sampling of behavior. 7 behaviors involving eyes open or closed and movement were sampled every 10 sec.; the beginning of the sampling period was prompted by a sound in the rater's ear piece. | *P3:* In three treatment blocks, no significant effects were found. Toward the end of the third treatment block, the patient was no longer in vegetative state and treatment was stopped.

Conclusion: Arousal profiles are useful source of information of how the patient is responding to treatment | | |

Wilson, S. L., Brock, D., Powell, G. E., Thwaites, H., & Elliott, K. (1996). Constructing arousal profiles for vegetative state patients—A preliminary study. *Brain Injury, 10,* 105–113.

Author/Year	Study Objectives	Level/Design/ Participants	Intervention and Outcome Measures	Results	Study Limitations	Implications for Occupational Therapy
Wilson, Powell, et al. (1996)	Evaluate the immediate effects of sensory stimulation treatment on patients in a vegetative state following traumatic brain injury; determine the relative effectiveness of different treatment protocols; determine the	IV—ABA single case studies: 5-day baseline, 15-day treatment phase, 5-day baseline.

For first 11 cases, treatment blocks with data collection were carried out 3 months after first block. The | Same as in Wilson, Brock, Powell, Thwaites, and Elliott (1996). All patients received multimodal stimulation; 23 received unimodal stimulation and 8 received familiar as well as everyday stimuli. | Pretreatment and post-treatment mean scores for each behavioral category in the time sampling schedule were calculated for each participant in each treatment block. The data from the multiple cases were | Participants were receiving other therapy interspersed with rest periods; the study did not control for spontaneous recovery; it is unclear, but possible, that these participants are the same as reported on | The use of familiar sensory stimuli offered to many senses in a graded, organized way in order to arouse a person from a persistent vegetative state seemed somewhat beneficial, within the *serious limitations* |

effects of age, gender, and time since injury on the magnitude of behavior change; test for a correlation between response to treatment and emergence from vegetative state

number of treatment blocks given to each patient varied from 1 to 8; participants stayed in the study until no longer vegetative ($n = 12$) or discharged.

$N = 24$ (all in the vegetative state in a neuro-disability hospital, secondary to injury of the brain; age 12–50 years [mean = 28.75 years])

Time since injury: 2–61 months (mean = 16.2 months)

Outcome measures: Arousal profile from time sampling of behavior as in Wilson, Brock, et al. (1996).

treated as a group (though not using meta-analytic analysis to group them) and the data were analyzed using 24 1-tailed *t* tests for related samples without adjusting the alpha level for multiple testing.

Multimodal stimulation using everyday stimuli resulted in significant changes in poststimulation behavior as compared to prestimulation behavior ($p < 0.001$), although only total instances of eyes open reached adjusted (by this author) alpha level (.002).

Unimodal stimulation with everyday stimuli did not result in significant change in post-treatment behavior.

Conclusion:
Multimodal familiar stimulation resulted in 3 out of 4 of significant (although not at the adjusted alpha level) behavioral changes after treatment. Graphic representation shows that the multimodal familiar type of stimulation had the greatest effect in terms of percent of total time spent in the aroused behavior.

in other articles by this group; participants were collected over a period of 5 years, during which concomitant treatments and personnel could have changed; some significant findings could have occurred by chance because of multiple t-tests used in the analysis; the study did not control for other threats to validity; each participant received different amounts of treatment and some participants also received treatment between the treatment blocks in which the responses were documented.

of this study, but definitive research is required. Although not explicitly stated, it appears that the professional carrying out the treatment was an occupational therapist.

(continued)

EVIDENCE TABLE. FOCUSED QUESTION 1A. (cont.)

Author/Year	Study Objectives	Level/Design/ Participants	Intervention and Outcome Measures	Results	Study Limitations	Implications for Occupational Therapy
Wilson, Powell, et al. (1996) (cont.)				Age at injury positively correlated with increase in eyes opening (r = .61). Females responded significantly better than males. No correlation between time since injury and behavioral changes. The 12 patients who were known to emerge from the vegetative state were not significantly different from those who had not emerged in terms of age, gender, and time since onset; 7 showed a response during at least 1 treatment block. 9 of those not known to have emerged also showed a response in at least 1 treatment block. Sensory stimulation produced statistically significant increases in arousal as compared to no treatment. Multimodal stimulation produced greater behavioral changes than unimodal stimulation. Personally salient multimodal stimulation produced greatest changes. Age and gender affected outcome: older and female people responded better. Time since injury showed		

Wilson, S. L., Powell, G. E., Brock, D., & Thwaites, H. (1996). Vegetative state and responses to sensory stimulation: An analysis of 24 cases. *Brain Injury, 10,* 807–818.

			no effect. There was no correlation between response to stimuli and emergence from vegetative state	
Watson & Horn (1991)	Illustrate that people with severe brain injury can show promising signs late following brain injury when stimuli of personal relevance are used to evoke responsiveness	V—Anecdotal case reports N = 2 P1: 36-year-old male, 103 days postinjury, severe brain injury (unconscious 10 days) P2: 35-year-old male, 190 days postinjury	P1: The therapist offered the patient a 10 pound note and asked whether he would like it. He immediately reached out and took it. Then the therapist said it was only a test and he'd have to give it back. He did so with a grin. P2: A motor car magazine was held within view. Within seconds, the patient turned his head in the direction of the magazine and seemed to be focusing on it and scanning the photos. *Outcome measures:* Observation of behavior.	P1: Since the incident with the 10 pound note, the patient makes more meaningful responses, can indicate yes or no, indicates a need for the bathroom, and feeds himself. P2: The patient continued to show interest in the magazine, then started focusing on people in his room and sustained attention for 3+ min. on a video showing car racing. At 344 days postinjury, he began to feed himself. *Conclusion:* These two cases demonstrate that unusual, imaginative, or innovatory "tests," including those of personal relevance, may sometimes elicit responses in the patient with severe brain injury who has previously demonstrated a limited repertoire of behavior.	No causal relationship can be established between treatment and outcome because there were no controls used against threats to validity. These anecdotes suggest that personally salient (meaningful) stimuli may have an effect when other stimuli do not. Definitive studies are required before this treatment can be supported.

Watson, M., & Horn, S. (1991). "The ten pound note test": Suggestions for eliciting improved responses in the severely brain-injured patient. *Brain Injury, 5,* 421–424.

What is the evidence for the effect of interventions to enable persons with traumatic brain injury to participate in areas of occupation (activities of daily living, instrumental activities of daily living, work, leisure, social participation, and education)?

Author/Year	Study Objectives	Level/Design/ Participants	Intervention and Outcome Measures	Results	Study Limitations	Implications for Occupational Therapy
Cullen, Bayley, et al. (2007)	Evaluate the effectiveness of interventional strategies for heterotopic ossifications (HO) and venous thromboembolism following TBI	I—Meta-analysis *N* = 19 studies with 10 studies focused on HO and 1 Level V study focused on a non-invasive, non-medical intervention approach (continuous passive motion)	One case study looked at continuous passive motion for 4 weeks to reduce development of HO in a patient's knees. *Outcome measure:* Range of motion (ROM) of the joint.	Case study participant showed significant improvements in both knees that were sustained 2 years postintervention.	Case report cannot establish the intervention as the cause of change observed because there are no controls for threats to internal validity. In addition, pharmacotherapy may have contributed to the outcome.	Heterotopic ossifications can result in significant limitations to joint mobility, which in turn can limit independence and participation in many areas of occupation. Continued ROM of the joint with HO may be beneficial for the maintenance of ROM, thus enhancing opportunities to engage in meaningful areas of occupation.

Cullen, N., Bayley, M., Bayona, N., Hilditch, M., & Aubut, J. (2007). Management of heterotopic ossification and venous thromboembolism following acquired brain injury. *Brain Injury, 21,* 215–230.

Cullen, Chundamala, et al. (2007)	Evaluate the efficacy of rehabilitation interventions for acquired brain injury	I—Systematic review Searched CINAHL, Medline, EMBASE, PsycINFO for 1980–2005. All published literature related to acquired brain injury was included. Bibliographies of selected articles also were reviewed. Review included experimental (randomized trials, prospective and retrospective controlled trials, single-group interventions) and non-experimental designs (retrospective and case studies)	Interventions include: Inpatient rehabilitation, timing and intensity of rehabilitation, community rehabilitation, vocational rehabilitation, supported employment, and support groups. *Outcome measures:* ■ Activities of daily living ■ Glasgow Coma Scale ■ Length of stay ■ Cognitive levels at discharge ■ Likelihood of discharge to home ■ Independence and need for care	There is moderate evidence that inpatient rehabilitation results in successful return to work and successful return to duty for military service members. In addition, there is moderate evidence that increasing the intensity of rehabilitation (studies ranged from low intensity of 2 hours per day 5 days per week to high intensity of 4–8 hours per day 7 days per week) reduces length of stay and improves short-term functional outcomes for motor	Limited number of randomized controlled trials (4). Wide range of outcome measures in each intervention explored with no standardization of timing of measurement limits comparison between studies.	Occupational therapists should engage clients in goal setting and, as members of a multidisciplinary team, provide intensive inpatient rehabilitation early in the recovery process. Transfer of clients to transitional living settings during the last weeks of inpatient rehabilitation may result in greater independence. There is limited evidence that community-based programs lead to more independence and social participation, and less need for caregiver support.

Author/Year	Purpose	Design/Level	Interventions/Outcome measures	Results	Limitations
			▪ Social activity level ▪ Return to work ▪ Psychosocial functioning.	and functional recovery. There is moderate evidence that client involvement in goal setting yields significant improvement to reaching and maintaining rehabilitation goals. There is limited evidence for the efficacy of the remaining interventions.	

Cullen, N., Chundamala, J., Bayley, M., & Jutai, J. (2007). The efficacy of acquired brain injury rehabilitation. *Brain Injury, 21*, 113–132.

Author/Year	Purpose	Design/Level	Interventions/Outcome measures	Results	Limitations
McCabe et al. (2007)	Evaluate interventions and strategies used for transition from acute care or rehabilitation to the community after brain injury	I—Systematic review Searched multiple databases for 1980–2005. Review included experimental (randomized trials, prospective and retrospective controlled trials, single-group interventions) and non-experimental designs (retrospective and case studies).	Interventions: Aspects of community reintegration measured were independence in ADL, IADL, and social integration, caregiver burden, satisfaction with quality of life, productivity, and return to driving. *Outcome measures:* ▪ Activities of daily living ▪ Level of supervision ▪ Caregiver stress ▪ Quality of life ▪ Return to work ▪ Return to driving.	There is limited evidence, due to the absence of randomized controlled trials, that interventions related to increasing self care independence and social integration, quality of life, productivity, and driving were effective. There is moderate evidence, as noted by one randomized controlled trial, that behavioral management in conjunction with caregiver education did not improve caregiver burden.	Only one randomized controlled trial was included in the review; wide range of outcome measures used in a given area There is only limited reliable evidence to support the major aspects of community integration following brain injury. There is moderate evidence that behavioral management and education do not improve caregiver perceived burden. Larger and better controlled research studies that measure disability outcomes are needed.

McCabe, P., Lippert, C., Weiser, M., Hilditch, M., Hartridge, C., & Villamere, J. (2007). Community reintegration following acquired brain injury. *Brain Injury, 21*, 231–257.

(continued)

EVIDENCE TABLE. FOCUSED QUESTION 2 (cont.)

Author/Year	Study Objectives	Level/Design/Participants	Intervention and Outcome Measures	Results	Study Limitations	Implications for Occupational Therapy
Powell et al. (2002)	Evaluate multidisciplinary community-based outreach rehabilitation after severe traumatic brain injury (TBI); determine whether or not outreach treatment increased the relative probability and magnitude of improvements	I—Randomized controlled trial N = 94 (75.5% male) with moderate to severe TBI aged 16 to 65 years, in acute to chronic stages of recovery	*Experimental*—Outreach treatment: Long-term goals valued by the participants and caregivers and considered amenable to intervention by the staff were worked toward via a series of written contracts which specified interim and short-term goals to be achieved over a 6- to 12-week period. Carried out in patients' homes, day centers, and workplace (2–6 hr per week, mean of 28 weeks). *Control*—A collated booklet listed alternative resources. Patient seen on one visit by a team therapist. *Outcome measures:* ■ Barthel Index (BI) ■ Brain Injury Community Rehabilitation Outcome–39 (BICRO–39).	Outreach participants were significantly more likely to show gains on the BI ($p < .05$), and on the total score ($p < .05$) and self-organization ($p < .05$) and psychological well-being ($p < .05$) subscales of the BICRO–39. The maximum gain index was significantly better for the outreach group than the control group ($p < .05$). *Conclusion:* Community rehabilitation after severe TBI can yield benefits that outlive the active treatment period, even if offered years postinjury.	The ceiling effects of the BI and the floor effects of the BICRO–39 limited the amount of achievement that could be measured. There was a 15% dropout rate due to lack of information at baseline on the BICRO–39. There was a possible co-intervention bias—the information group received "limited treatment and support from the outreach team" (p. 194) over the month immediately following discharge from inpatient rehabilitation. These limitations did not offer alternative explanations for the outcome.	This outreach program was carried out by a team of rehabilitation professionals, two of whom were occupational therapists. Their role was not described. However, since the goal of the intervention was independence in activities of daily living, it can be extrapolated that community-based occupational therapy will produce significant improvement in self-care and self-organization for persons with moderate to severe TBI over that expected from an informational home program alone. Further research is needed to determine the specific effectiveness of occupational therapy community-based treatment for TBI patients.

Powell, J., Heslin, J., & Greenwood, R. (2002). Community-based rehabilitation after severe traumatic brain injury: A randomized controlled trial. *Journal of Neurology, Neurosurgery, and Psychiatry, 72,* 193–202.

| Turner-Stokes et al. (2005) | Assess the effectiveness of multidisciplinary rehabilitation (including occupational therapy) for adults with acquired brain injury (ABI) | I—Systematic review

This Cochrane review searched Medline (1966–2004), EMBASE (1988–2004), CINAHL (1983–2004), AMED (2004), ISI Science Citation Index (1981–2004), and Cochrane Central Register of Controlled Trials | Review included all randomized controlled trials (RCTs) comparing multi-disciplinary rehabilitation either with routinely available local services or lower levels of intervention, or trials comparing interventions in different settings or different levels of intensity. Quasi-randomized and quasi-experimental design studies were included if they met predefined methodological criteria.

Outcome measures:
■ Functional independence
■ Care burden and stress
■ Return to work
■ Discharge destination
■ Social integration
■ Health-related quality of life. | Ten trials of good quality and four of lower quality were included. There is strong evidence that patients with mild brain injury make a good recovery with provision of information, without additional specific intervention. There is strong evidence that those with moderate to severe ABI benefit from formal intervention. For those already in intervention, there is strong evidence that more intensive programs result in earlier functional gains. There is moderate evidence that continued outpatient therapy sustains early gains. There is limited evidence that specialist in-patient rehabilitation and specialist multi-disciplinary community rehabilitation may result in additional functional gains. | Studies included in the review may have had small sample sizes; the expanding body of evidence for the effectiveness of multidisciplinary research (e.g., stroke) make it difficult ethically and practically to randomize those with ABI to no treatment or standard care | Due to the heterogeneousness of the TBI population, the variety of intervention approaches, and the lack of RCTs, the implications for practice from this systematic review are limited to the recommendations that clients with TBI should be engaged in intensive rehabilitation and have access to follow-up outpatient or community-based programs appropriate to their needs. Recommendations are made regarding research on the cost-effectiveness and efficacy of TBI rehabilitation. |

Turner-Stokes, L., Disler, P. B., Nair, A., & Wade, D. T. (2005). Multi-disciplinary rehabilitation for acquired brain injury in adults of working age. *Cochrane Database of Systematic Reviews,* Issue 3. Art. No.: CD004170. DOI: 10.1002/14651858.CD004170.pub2.

(continued)

EVIDENCE TABLE. FOCUSED QUESTION 2 *(cont.)*

Author/Year	Study Objectives	Level/Design/ Participants	Intervention and Outcome Measures	Results	Study Limitations	Implications for Occupational Therapy
Vanderploeg et al. (2008)	Determine the efficacy of cognitive–didactic versus functional–experiential approaches to treatment for different patient subpopulations with traumatic brain injury (TBI)	I—Randomized controlled trial (RCT) *N* = 360 adult veterans or active duty military service with nonpenetrating moderate to severe TBI admitted to acute inpatient rehabilitation TBI programs at 4 Veterans Administration Medical Centers	Participants received 1.5 to 2.5 hours of protocol-specific rehabilitation therapy within an interdisciplinary (included OT) TBI program in addition to another 2 to 2.5 hours daily of occupational and physical therapy targeted to the specific protocol. Duration of protocol treatment varied from 20 to 60 days, depending on the clinical needs and progress of each participant. *Functional–Experiential treatment:* A modified version of the neurofunctional approach of Giles and Clark-Wilson (1993). It used real-life performance situations and common tasks in group settings and natural environments using errorless treatment strategies and instructional cues. *Cognitive–Didactic treatment:* A version of Attention Process Training of Sohlberg and Mateer (2001) and targeted attention, memory, executive functions, and pragmatic communication using primarily paper-and-pencil or computerized cognitive tasks in 1:1 sessions.	Though both groups showed improvements there were no significant differences between the groups at 1 year on the primary outcome measures. Subgroup analysis found that younger participants (<30) and those with less education who participated in the cognitive group had better work-related outcomes at 1 year follow-up than participants in the functional–experiential group. However, older participants (>30) and those with more education had better outcomes in terms of independent living at 1 year if they participated in the functional experiential approach.	There is some overlap between the two types of approaches, as both use compensatory techniques, though the functional–experiential approach uses more compensatory techniques. Memory notebooks were common to both approaches, though the purpose was different. The primary outcome measures of return to work and independent living are dependent upon more than cognitive and functional levels. Intervening factors may have contributed to the outcome. Additional outpatient therapy during the follow-up period was not controlled for and may have influenced outcomes. The gender composition of the sample (93% male) may limit the generalization of the findings to women.	The outcomes suggest that both cognitive–didactic and functional–experiential treatment, in addition to standard care, may have specific advantages in certain subpopulations and for achieving specific outcomes in acute rehabilitation following TBI. Specifically, older patients with independent living goals might benefit more from functional–experiential rather than cognitive–didactic rehabilitation treatment.

Self-awareness questions were used throughout this approach.

Primary outcome measures:
Functional independence in living (less than 3 hours of assistance per week), and return to work and/or school assessed by independent evaluators at 1-year follow-up via structured telephone interview

Secondary outcome measures:
- Functional Independence Measure (FIM™)
- Disability Rating Scale score
- Items from the Present State Exam, Apathy Evaluation Scale, and Neurobehavioral Rating Scale.

Vanderploeg, R. D., Schwab, K., Walker, W. C., Fraser, J. A., Sigford, B. J., Date, E. S., et al., for the Defense and Veterans Brain Injury Center Study Group. (2008). Rehabilitation of traumatic brain injury in active duty military personnel and veterans: Defense and Veterans Brain Injury Center randomized controlled trial of two rehabilitation approaches. *Archives of Physical Medicine and Rehabilitation, 89,* 2227–2238.

(continued)

EVIDENCE TABLE. FOCUSED QUESTION 2 *(cont.)*

Author/Year	Study Objectives	Level/Design/ Participants	Intervention and Outcome Measures	Results	Study Limitations	Implications for Occupational Therapy
Zhu et al. (2001)	Evaluate the effects of intensive rehabilitation (occupational therapy included) on the functional outcome of patients with traumatic brain injury (TBI; 6 month interim report)	I—Randomized controlled trial (RCT) $N = 36$ (78% male) with moderate to severe TBI	*Intensive therapy* ($N = 15$): Individual treatment, including physical and sensorimotor training, functional retraining (activities of daily living and instrumental activities of daily living), and psychosocial retraining (social skills, hearing, speech). 4 hr/day in 2 2-hr sessions (1 hr physical therapy, 1 hr occupational therapy) + 2 hr/wk speech therapy. 5 days/wk for up to 6 months. *Conventional therapy* ($N = 21$): Same therapy at reduced intensity: 2 hr/day (1 hr physical therapy, 1 hr occupational therapy) + 1 hr/ week speech therapy. 5 days/wk for up to 6 months. *Outcome measures:* ■ Glasgow Outcome Scale (GOS) ■ Functional Independence Measure (FIM™).	There was a trend of more patients in the intensive group achieving full FIM scores and good GOS scores at 2 and 3 months, but the control group was catching up at 6 months. A significant percentage of patients in the intensive group achieved "good" status at 2 months (40% vs. 10%, $p = .046$). There was no significant difference between groups on the FIM motor or cognitive subscales, but a greater percentage of persons in the intensive group achieved full independence at 3 months. The advantage diminished to nonsignificant levels at 4 months and following. *Conclusion:* Increasing the amount of rehabilitation therapy (physical therapy and occupational therapy) from the conventional 2 hr to 4 hr per day improved the functional outcome of TBI patients as measured by the GOS. The improvement was most significant in the early period (2–3 months). The effect of therapy is in potentiating the recovery, rather than changing the final outcome.	Well-controlled	More-intensive therapy early postinjury facilitates the person's ability to engage in some occupational areas sooner. However, conventional dosage of therapy results in comparable outcome as spontaneous recovery slows (after 4–6 months). Managers need to consider whether doubling the expense of therapy early is worth the cost. If hospitalization is to be brief, then intensive therapy is needed to prepare the patient for discharge. Whether the intensive therapy would result in higher levels of functional achievement in a longer hospitalization is an interesting question that this study did not answer because the FIM and the GOS do not measure higher levels of functional achievement.

Zhu, X. L., Poon, W. S., Chan, C. H., & Chan, S. H. (2001). Does intensive rehabilitation improve the functional outcome of patients with traumatic brain injury? Interim result of a random-

| Zhu et al. (2007) | Evaluate the effects of differing levels of intensity on functional outcomes of patients with traumatic brain injury (TBI) | Level I—Randomized controlled trial

$N = 68$ patients with moderate-to-severe TBI at the early post-traumatic stage (up to 6 months postinjury; $n = 36$ in intensive group; $n = 32$ in control group); age range 12–65 years | *Interventions*: Patients were randomized to either 4 or 2 hours of therapy per day. Patients in both groups received occupational therapy (OT), physical therapy, and speech therapies. OT included functional retraining and psychosocial retraining including social skills. The duration of treatment varied based on individual needs for a maximum of 6 months.

Outcome measures:
■ Functional Independence Measure (FIM™)
■ Glasgow Outcome Scale (GOS)
■ Neurobehavioral Cognitive Status Examination (NCSE)
■ Outcomes were measured at baseline, monthly until 6 months, then bimonthly from 8–12 months. | There were no differences between the levels of intensity on the FIM and NCSE. At 3 months, there were significantly more in the high (49%) than low (19%) intensity group who achieved a maximum total FIM and GOS scores. | Heterogeneity of the TBI population; outcome measures may not fully capture all impairments contributing to independence in activities of daily living and return to work | Early intensive multidisciplinary rehabilitation, including occupational therapy, can improve the functional outcome after TBI, increasing patients' potential early return to work. Final level of outcome was not different, just the rate of recovery. |

Zhu, X. L., Poon, W. S., Chan, C. C., & Chan, S. S. (2007). Does intensive rehabilitation improve the functional outcome of patients with traumatic brain injury (TBI)? A randomized controlled trial. *Brain Injury, 21*, 681–690.

(continued)

EVIDENCE TABLE. FOCUSED QUESTION 2 (cont.)

Author/Year	Study Objectives	Level/Design/ Participants	Intervention and Outcome Measures	Results	Study Limitations	Implications for Occupational Therapy
Goranson et al. (2003)	Determine the extent to which participation in a multidisciplinary rehabilitation program and patient characteristics predict improvement in community integration following mild-to-moderate traumatic brain injury (TBI)	II—Retrospective, non-randomized two-group pretest–posttest case control (matched groups) *N* = 42 persons with mild-to-moderate brain injury 2 groups, divided into the rehabilitation program and control	*Rehabilitation group:* Intensive outpatient rehabilitation, using multimodal interventions to remediate and/ or teach compensatory strategies for cognitive, physical, or emotional difficulties incurred as a result of TBI. Included mutual goal setting, attention process training, and individual and group therapy. *Control group:* No treatment. *Outcome measures:* ■ Community Integration Questionnaire (CIQ; measures home independence, social integration, and productivity).	The rehabilitation group improved significantly more than the no-treatment group ($F[1,37] = 4.193$, $p = 0.024$). Significant improvement was seen in home independence (14% effect size), but not in social integration or productive use of time. Female subjects improved more than males (21% effect of gender). *Conclusion:* Patients who participated in the multidisciplinary rehabilitation program achieved greater improvement on the CIQ than patients who did not participate. 14% of the variance associated with improvement on the Home Independence subscale was accounted for by the multidisciplinary program. As a group, TBI patients did not improve on the Community Socialization or Productivity subscales over the study interval.	Although the groups were statistically similar on age, length of posttraumatic amnesia, education, pretest scores, and legal case pending, and although the authors presented an argument against the groups being different, the people who did not qualify for rehab are different from those who did on one or more inclusion/exclusion criteria.	This study offers no specific guidance to occupational therapy practice other than to say that occupational therapy's involvement in an intensive multidisciplinary rehabilitation program may contribute to the successful outcome for patients postinjury.

Goranson, T. E., Graves, R. E., Allison, D., & LaFreniere, R. (2003). Community integration following multidisciplinary rehabilitation for traumatic brain injury. *Brain Injury, 17,* 759–774.

Author/Year	Study Objectives	Level/Design	Intervention and Outcome Measures	Results	Study Limitations	Implications/Conclusions
Wheeler et al. (2007)	Evaluate the effect of an intensive, community-based life-skills training on community integration and life satisfaction among persons with traumatic brain injury (TBI)	II—two group pre-post test design N = 36 individuals (n = 18 intensive group, mean age = 34; n = 18 control, mean age = 35)	*Intervention:* Involvement in Radical Rehab Solutions, an intensive, community-based residential life skills training that included one-on-one sessions with a life skills trainer and involvement with an interdisciplinary team that included occupational therapy 1–3 hours per week. *Control:* Individuals living in the community and not participating in Radical Rehab Solutions, including being on the waiting list for the program. *Outcome measures:* ■ Community Integration Questionnaire (CIQ) ■ Satisfaction with Life Scale (SWLS).	At follow-up, there was a statistically significant improvement on overall CIQ scores for the treatment group, but not for the control group. This was also seen on the home integration and productivity subsets of the CIQ, but not for social integration. No significant differences were observed on the SWLS within or between groups.	Data were collected retrospectively rather than prospectively; lack of randomization; baseline differences limited between-group comparisons.	Life satisfaction is a complex concept that involves more than increased community participation in individuals with TBI. Residual cognitive and physical impairments may be more evident upon return to community activities. Social integration may be most resistant to change. Occupational therapists working in community reintegration programs need to provide emotional support for clients as they struggle to increase their community participation and redefine their self-identity.

Wheeler, S. D., Lane, S. J., & McMahon, B. T. (2007). Community participation and life satisfaction following intensive, community-based rehabilitation using a life skills training approach. *OTJR: Occupation, Participation, and Health, 27,* 13–22.

Author/Year	Study Objectives	Level/Design	Intervention and Outcome Measures	Results	Study Limitations	Implications/Conclusions
Hayden et al. (2000)	Present a treatment model with a primary goal of minimizing handicap through treatment using carefully simulated environments; present an outcome measurement system that corresponds to the treatment model; determine whether a treatment milieu that gradually increases environmental distractions and reduces structure	III—Pretest–posttest of the group subdivided into 4 subgroups on the basis of time since injury and severity of injury N = 61 (75.4% male) persons with TBI of various severities and times since onset	Environmental simulation to control and gradually increase the degree of distraction tolerated and gradually decrease the degree of structure provided while the person was engaged in individually chosen activities of daily living and instrumental activities of daily living; community mobility and volunteer or vocational tasks that challenged each	All subjects demonstrated significant gains in independence (p < .01). 46 out of the 61 participants were independent at discharge and 92% of them remained so at 6-month follow-up. *Conclusion:* The majority of individuals in this study left treatment much more independent than they were at admission.	The method of sampling was not reported; inclusion/exclusion criteria for participation in the study were not reported; evaluators were not blind to treatment status; there was no control group	This program was successful. Treatment was implemented through engagement in occupational tasks (occupation-as-means) to address patients' specific deficits within environmental (distractions/structure) scaffolding based on activity analysis of their information processing abilities and executive functioning.

(continued)

Author/Year	Study Objectives	Level/Design/ Participants	Intervention and Outcome Measures	Results	Study Limitations	Implications for Occupational Therapy
Hayden et al. (2000) (cont.)	provided would result in significant decreases in handicap at discharge and at 6 months postdischarge		person's identified deficits. Participants worked for 5–6 hr per day for 35–62 days. *Outcome measures:* ■ Pate Environmentally Relevant Program Outcome System (PERPOS), which measured the amount of distraction tolerated and the amount of structure required, as well as overall functioning.	However, their increased level of independence was bought at the price of considerable energy and effort to maintain.		The treatment is occupational therapy, although the program was administered by a multidisciplinary team (including occupational therapy), and the study was designed by neuropsychologists. There is a need for occupational therapy researchers to document the effectiveness of such occupational therapy treatment.

Hayden, M. E., Moreault, A. M., LeBlanc, J., & Plenger, P. M. (2000). Reducing level of handicap in traumatic brain injury: An environmentally based model of treatment. *Journal of Head Trauma Rehabilitation, 15,* 1000–1021.

Author/Year	Study Objectives	Level/Design/ Participants	Intervention and Outcome Measures	Results	Study Limitations	Implications for Occupational Therapy
Malec (2001)	Determine whether a comprehensive day treatment program would result in positive changes in outcome measures at a level equal to those reported for other postacute rehabilitation programs and with better results than those reported for comparison groups	III—Before and after (pretest–posttest) *N* = 96 (34 in 1st cohort and 62 in 2nd cohort) graduates of the program from 1989–1999 72% with traumatic brain injury; 19% with cerebral vascular accident; 9% had other diagnoses	The Mayo Brain Injury Outpatient program is a comprehensive day treatment, milieu-oriented program that included daily group sessions to build cognitive and behavioral skills through a transdisciplinary approach. The Life Skills group was taught by a recreation therapist and a physical therapist, not an occupational therapist. Individual therapy was provided as needed.	There was significant goal achievement (81% of 552 goals were met at expected or higher level of outcome) and improvement on the MPAI–22 (*t* = 8.35, *p* < .0001). Societal participation at 1-yr. follow-up was increased: 72% living independently, 39% working independently, 10% in transitional placements, and 18% in supported or volunteer work.	No control group; no statistical analysis was reported; patients were in the program at different times during a 10-year span, so that the personnel, design of the program, etc., could have changed. This is a program evaluation study rather than research to investigate the effectiveness of a particular treatment	The roles of the occupational therapist and occupational therapy assistant who participated in this program were not delineated. The Life Skills Group, which one might expect an occupational therapist to run, was run by other professionals. Therefore, this study offers little to practicing occupational therapists. Occupational therapy research needs to demonstrate

	Outcome Measures	Results	Conclusions / Implications
(continued)	*Outcome measures:* ■ Independent Living Scale, which measures independence from 0 to able to live in community without supervision ■ Portland Adaptability Inventory (PAI) or Mayo–Portland Adaptability Inventory (MPAI–22), which measure overall level of disability and impairments ■ Goal Attainment Scaling (GAS), which measures achievement of goals.	On the other hand, 24% of the patients became more depressed and 29% became more irritable as they began to confront and realize their limitations. *Conclusion:* Comprehensive day treatment appears to be effective in improving activity and societal participation, even among persons with a long history of limited participation after brain injury.	the effectiveness of occupational therapy in improving independence in social participation and/or the unique contribution of an occupational therapist within a multidisciplinary team. The likelihood of increased depression and irritability when patients confront their limitations is a good reminder that occupational therapists, who have to engage patients in tasks of everyday life that they were once successfully able to accomplish, should present the tasks with empathy.

Malec, J. F. (2001). Impact of comprehensive day treatment on societal participation for persons with acquired brain injury. *Archives of Physical Medicine and Rehabilitation, 82,* 885–895.

Study	Objective	Design / Participants	Intervention	Results	Limitations	Conclusions
Trombly et al. (2002)	Test the effect of goal-specific outpatient occupational therapy on achievement of self-identified activities of daily living (ADL) and instrumental activities of daily living (IADL) goals, on patients' rating of their performance and satisfaction with their performance of targeted activities, and on their level of participation in non-targeted activities	III—Repeated measures (subjects act as their own controls) *N* = 31 (71% male) persons with mild to moderate traumatic brain injury (TBI), located in 3 different occupational therapy clinics The usual practices of each site concerning patient assignment, treatment, decisions concerning discharge,	All participants received outpatient occupational therapy focused on training in the use of compensatory strategies and environmental adaptation to achieve self-identified ADL and IADL goals. However, each of the sites used its own protocol. Each treatment was approximately 30 minutes. Number of treatments ranged from a mean of 24–63 treatments,	The total number of goals identified by all participants was 149, 81% of which were achieved. 15 participants achieved 100% of their goals, 11 achieved 80%, and 2 achieved 60%. The improvement in GAS scores from admission to discharge was significant ($Z = 7.52$, $p < .001$; combined effect size: $r = .94$). Significant differences were found	Evaluators were not blind to treatment status.	Occupational therapy directed at specific goals valued by the client and using compensatory training and environmental adaptation as intervention to achieve those goals is likely to be successful for persons with mild to moderate TBI. The specific interventions used by the therapists at the three sites were different, but all were compensatory in nature and aimed at

(continued)

EVIDENCE TABLE. FOCUSED QUESTION 2 *(cont.)*

Author/Year	Study Objectives	Level/Design/ Participants	Intervention and Outcome Measures	Results	Study Limitations	Implications for Occupational Therapy
Trombly et al. (2002) *(cont.)*		etc., were used. The data from each site were analyzed separately then combined using meta-analytic procedures.	depending on site. Weeks of no-treatment ranged from 5.8–19.6 weeks. *Outcome measures:* ■ Canadian Occupational Performance Measure (COPM) ■ Community Integration Questionnaire (CIQ) ■ Goal-Attainment Scaling (GAS).	in gain scores for the COPM–Performance ($Z = 4.13$, $p < .001$) and COPM–Satisfaction ($Z = 4.25$, $p < .001$) between the treatment and no-treatment periods, with the greater improvement occurring during the treatment period and no improvement occurring during the no-treatment period. The combined effect sizes were: $r = .71, .76$ respectively. The gain scores of non-targeted skills measured by the CIQ were not significantly different between treatment and no-treatment periods. *Conclusion:* Participants in a goal-specific program of outpatient occupational therapy significantly improved in self-identified ADL and IADL goals. This verified the findings of Phase I of this research.		targeted goals identified by the client in collaboration with the occupational therapist. The effect sizes indicate a strong relationship between occupational therapy and outcome. Non-targeted goals did not improve significantly.

Trombly, C. A., Radomski, M. V., Trexel, C., & Burnett-Smith, S. E. (2002). Occupational therapy and achievement of self-identified goals by adults with acquired brain injury. Phase II. *American Journal of Occupational Therapy, 56,* 489–498.

Author/Year	Study Objectives	Level/Design and Participants	Intervention and Outcome Measures	Results	Study Limitations	Implications for Occupational Therapy
Parish & Oddy (2007)	Determine whether independence can be improved in persons 10 years following acquired brain injury (ABI)	IV—Single subject design $N = 4$ individuals in a continuing rehabilitation center at least 10 years before brain injury (ages 24–46)	*Intervention*: Participants were assessed by an occupational therapist and followed the Giles method (2005) for functional retraining in specific tasks such as meal preparation and showering. Intervention was administered by support staff working under the supervision of the occupational therapist. *Outcome measures*: ▪ Increase in level of independence in the performance of tasks ▪ Wechsler Adult Intelligence Scale III ▪ Supervision Rating Scale ▪ Spot the Word and Speed of Comprehension subtests from the Speed and Capacity of Language Processing Test.	All participants in the program improved in the performance of targeted function activities. Satisfaction with the program was also reported.	Small sample size; lack of baseline measurements; lack of statistical analysis.	Functional improvements can be made over a decade after an individual's initial TBI when provided with task-specific functional training using errorless and procedural learning. Occupational therapists can design and structure such training programs to be carried out by staff and family without professional training. Though generalization of performance is not anticipated, a reduction in caregiver burden may be obtained.

Parish, L., & Oddy, M. (2007). Efficacy of rehabilitation for functional skills more than 10 years after extremely severe brain injury. *Neuropsychological Rehabilitation, 17*, 230–243.

Author/Year	Study Objectives	Level/Design and Participants	Intervention and Outcome Measures	Results	Study Limitations	Implications for Occupational Therapy
Gutman (2000)	Determine whether use of a computer as an environmental facilitator would allow one person with brain injury to resume adult social roles, including developing a greater sense of belonging to his family and resumption of meaningful work	V—Qualitative case study $N = 1$ man with traumatic brain injury (TBI), obsessive-compulsive disorder, and attention-deficit/hyperactivity disorder since childhood; left hemiparesis, left hemianopsia, and	The intervention had three parts: (1) adaptation of computer programs, keyboard, and monitor (see article for specifics); (2) instruction in adapted word processing and e-mailing; and (3) computer-related activities designed to enhance participation	The participant was able to reestablish his roles of brother and adult son; develop and maintain an extended family of others beyond his family of origin; and create a satisfying adult work role that brought greater meaning to his postinjury life. His	There are no controls that allow one to accept with confidence that the treatment caused the outcome. A controlled study would be required to establish that the occupational therapy program (computer adaptation) was the cause of the change	This study of one unique person provides some, but very minimal, evidence of the effectiveness of computer adaptation and instruction aimed at chosen goals. Researchers need to investigate whether the effectiveness of

(continued)

Author/Year	Study Objectives	Level/Design/ Participants	Intervention and Outcome Measures	Results	Study Limitations	Implications for Occupational Therapy
Gutman (2000) *(cont.)*		speech deficits; living in a residential setting	in desired social roles *Outcome measures:* Interview of patient, sister, and mother.	work was creative writing, which he found meaningful whether or not he earned money (previous to treatment, he had been doing piece-work in a shel-tered workshop, which he hated). *Conclusion:* A computer system can be adapted, as implemented in this study, to become an environmental fa-cilitator to reintegrate a person into familial, extended family, and adult worker roles.	in this person and not the attention received from the occupational therapy graduate students who adminis-tered the treatment.	this intervention can be generalized.

Gutman, S. A. (2000). Using a computer as an environmental facilitator to promote post–head injury social role resumption: A case report. *Occupational Therapy in Mental Health, 15,* 71–89.

Author/Year	Study Objectives	Level/Design/ Participants	Intervention and Outcome Measures	Results	Study Limitations	Implications for Occupational Therapy
Kowalske et al. (2000)	Present a treatment program for patients with traumatic brain injury (TBI) that focuses heavily on patient–en-vironment interactions, both during treatment (through environmental simulations in the clinic) and postdis-charge (through build-ing enabling vocational environments)	V—Case studies $N = 3$ (2 male, 1 female) persons with TBI concurrent with ex-tremity bone fractures; with left hemiparesis and left hemianopsia; and/or with seizures	▪ Simulate appropri-ate environment to match each patient's informa-tion processing and executive abilities, starting with low distractibility and progressing to more complex ▪ Guide through tasks by simple commands then gradually withdraw therapist-provided structure ▪ Teach compensa-tory strategies and/ or employ adapted devices	*Case 1:* Research scientist returned to former position; at 6-month follow-up, he reported he was com-pletely reintegrated into the laboratory and had published 2 scien-tific articles. *Case 2:* Student could not pursue a desired health career, but was able to successfully fill a filing position at an insurance company that satisfied her. She remained at the job for 2 years, leaving to be a full-time mother.	There are no controls that allow one to ac-cept with confidence that the treatment caused the outcome. The 3 cases were selected from 57 potential cases on an unknown basis.	All the interventions listed as being used in this treatment program are ones used by oc-cupational therapists. This paper did not provide conclusive evidence of the effec-tiveness of particular interventions or the treatment program as a whole, although it suggests that careful analysis of a patient's problems and careful design of intervention can be successful. There is a need for occupational therapy researchers

to document the effectiveness of similar treatments.

- Use procedural learning (practice to overlearn and chain parts together)
- Develop job facilities appropriate for work environments outside of clinic
- Visit job site to determine environmental obstacles to success
- Modify vocational environment
- Educate family
- Modify behavior to reduce unwanted behaviors

Duration: 7 months

Outcome measures: Description of factors associated with successful return to work.

Case 3: Former mechanical engineer whose family insisted that he return to his job, which he was incapable of doing. Wife arranged with former friend to send him engineering tasks to do at home; she structured his performance using methods she learned in therapy. This satisfied both the family and patient.

Conclusion: "These case studies point out the necessity of specialized treatment that not only focuses on the specific strengths and weaknesses of the individual, but also on extant environmental factors, including the degree of structure or distractions that either reinforce or preclude optimal performance" (p. 989).

Kowalske, K., Plenger, P. M., Lusby, B., & Hayden, M. E. (2000). Vocational reentry following TBI: An enablement model. *Journal of Head Trauma Rehabilitation, 15,* 989–999.

(continued)

EVIDENCE TABLE. FOCUSED QUESTION 2 *(cont.)*

Author/Year	Study Objectives	Level/Design/ Participants	Intervention and Outcome Measures	Results	Study Limitations	Implications for Occupational Therapy
Walker (2002)	Demonstrate the successful incorporation of the strengths of process-specific (remediation) and functional (restorative) treatment approaches within a therapy program for a patient with mild traumatic brain injury (TBI)	V—Case study *N* = 1 male; age 33 years; 1 year post-onset with mild TBI; unable to complete many activities of daily living (ADL) at home due to poor concentration, poor organizational skills, and poor time management skills	• Identify interaction between the patient's cognitive deficits and problematic ADL, using a checklist according to a cognitive framework • Teach the patient compensatory strategies within context of hierarchically arranged ADL • Grade treatment from easiest ADL to most difficult • Develop compensatory strategies for lower level (attention deficits and executive system functioning) and higher level (working memory deficits and reasoning) cognitive deficits • Apply compensatory strategies to tasks within the home, grading from easy to hard tasks • Educate patient and wife concerning the nature of his cognitive deficits Treatment was administered daily for 4 months	The patient consistently used his compensatory strategies to independently complete ADL within the home and community environments that were problematic prior to the receipt of treatment. He was able to adapt his strategies to his work as a bartender 1 year after completing therapy. *Conclusion:* The outcome of this case suggests that a combined approach is beneficial in maximizing the recovery of highly motivated patients with mild traumatic brain injury who have support systems. It is not known whether the therapy program had a direct impact on cognitive abilities because repeat neuropsychological testing was not done.	There are no controls that allow one to accept with confidence that the treatment caused the outcome.	The treatments described in this case study are those that occupational therapists use regularly. As the author said, "developing compensatory strategies for cognitive deficits within the context of real-life tasks that are unique to each patient not only maximizes the number of deficient processes addressed during a specific time frame but also enables the patient to learn his/her new strategies within familiar home and work environments. This increases the number of opportunities a patient has to practice new skills and eliminates the uncertainty of how cognitive processes generalize from abstract to real-life tasks" (p. 624). However, this study does not provide conclusive evidence of the effectiveness of this treatment approach and further, more controlled research is required.

Outcome measures:
Description of ability to
complete activities that
were problematic prior
to treatment because
of cognitive deficits.

Walker, J. P. (2002). Case Study: Functional outcome: A case for mild traumatic brain injury. *Brain Injury, 16,* 611–625.

EVIDENCE TABLE. FOCUSED QUESTION 3.

What is the evidence for the effect of interventions to address psychosocial, behavioral, and social functions on the occupational performance for persons with traumatic brain injury?

Author/Year	Study Objectives	Level/Design/ Participants	Intervention and Outcome Measures	Results	Study Limitations	Implications for Occupational Therapy
Bornhofen & McDonald (2008)	Evaluate whether participation by adults with traumatic brain injury (TBI) can result in the remediation of social perceptional deficits	I—Randomized controlled trial 12 outpatient volunteers with severe, chronic TBI were randomized to treatment (N = 6) and waitlist control (N = 6); ages 20–57, 11 males, 1 female	*Intervention:* Cognitive rehabilitation program to address emotion perception, including recognition of specific patterns of changes in facial features, voice tone, body posture, and movement. Techniques incorporated into the program include errorless learning, self-instruction training, and rehearsal. *Outcome measures:* ■ Facial expression naming task ■ Facial expression matching task ■ Awareness of social inference test ■ Sydney Psychosocial reintegration scale.	Participants in the treatment group had significantly improved accuracy in judging dynamic cues related to basic emotions such as happiness or surprise, as compared to controls. Those in the treatment group also improved in the ability to draw inferences on the basis of emotional cues to determine whether a speaker was being sarcastic, sincere, or deceptive. Participants in the treatment group did not demonstrate improvement in judging static emotional cues in the form of photographed facial expressions. There also was no statistically significant improvement in psychosocial functioning.	Small sample size; treatment and control group compared statistically only at pretest	Impairments in social interactions after a TBI may be in part due to impairments in ability to recognize dynamic emotions in others' faces, voices, or body language and respond appropriately. Intervention focused on monitoring whether physically displayed dynamic emotions and judging the speaker's intent may lead to gains in emotion perception. While the treatment group did not show improvements in psychosocial functioning, the authors do not describe how they directly addressed the application of the emotional perception to social exchanges in role playing or group formats. This area needs additional exploration by occupational therapists.

Bornhofen, C., & McDonald, S. (2008). Treating deficits in emotional perception following traumatic brain injury. *Neuropsychological Rehabilitation, 18,* 22–44.

Boschen et al. (2007)	Evaluate the effectiveness of different family interventions following acquired brain injury (ABI), comparing this with similar literature on other select chronic conditions	I—Systematic review Search conducted in Medline, PsycINFO, CINAHL, Cochrane, and EMBASE. Included articles published since 2000, except for ABI articles, where any qualifying article was included.	Included studies evaluated one or more interventions for family with ABI. Also included were studies of family interventions for persons with dementia, stroke, mental health, and childhood chronic illness. Types of interventions included were education, telerehabilitation, case management, psychotherapeutic intervention or counseling, peer/support group, and multicomponent. *Outcomes measures:* ■ Caregiver strain ■ Burnout ■ Beliefs about caregiving ■ Depression ■ Anxiety ■ Well-being ■ Functional independence.	31 randomized controlled trials (RCTs) were identified. The review included 4 RCTs in ABI, all of which had small sample sizes. At present, there is no strong evidence supporting any specific intervention method for support of family caregivers of individuals with ABI or any other chronic condition.	Small sample sizes, lack of standardized outcome measures, lack of consensus regarding variables to study	While there is no strong evidence to support any particular framework for family intervention, there is evidence that the entire family structure and function is affected by one member's injury. Occupational therapists, as part of the treatment team, should recognize the effect of the brain injury on the entire family and help them access some type of ongoing services. In addition, occupational therapists should collaborate with the team to develop research studies on the long-term outcomes of family intervention after TBI.

Boschen, K., Gargaro, J., Gan, C., Gerber, G., & Brandys, C. (2007). Family interventions after acquired brain injury and other chronic conditions: A critical appraisal of the quality of the evidence. *Neurorehabilitation, 22,* 19–41.

(continued)

EVIDENCE TABLE. FOCUSED QUESTION 3 (cont.)

Author/Year	Study Objectives	Level/Design/ Participants	Intervention and Outcome Measures	Results	Study Limitations	Implications for Occupational Therapy
Dahlberg et. al (2007)	Evaluate the effectiveness of a group intervention program to improve social skills after traumatic brain injury (TBI)	Level I—Randomized clinical trial using a delayed treatment control group Participants were 52 community dwelling clients in the chronic phase of recovery (mean = 9 years postinjury); mean age = 41 years. Over 75% were classified as having a moderate to severe TBI. Participants were randomized equally into the treatment and delayed treatment groups.	Intervention consisted of 12 weekly group sessions of 1.5 hours, each focused on pragmatic language skills, social behaviors, and cognitive abilities needed for successful social interactions. Group sessions involved topics such as starting conversations, problem solving, assertiveness, positive self-talk, social boundaries, conflict resolution, community practice, and videotape feedback. Group size was limited to 8 participants and sessions were held in a living room–type setting. Self-awareness and self-assessment, along with personal goal setting, were used. Homework activities encouraged generalization of group activities to the home and community environments.	Significant improvements were found in social communication skills at follow-up. Participants showed the largest improvements in the scales of the PFIC that measured general participation in conversation and social skills. The treatment group had significantly higher scores on the SCSQ–A, which looked at their level of understanding of social communication and insight regarding communication behaviors. No significant differences were found between the treatment and delayed treatment groups on the secondary outcome measures, except for the Satisfaction With Life Scale, which showed the treatment group had an improved overall life satisfaction sustained during the 9-month-long follow-up.	Clients with past or current psychiatric or substance abuse problems were excluded, strengthening the study but decreasing the study's representation of the TBI population in general. The study population was more educated and less diverse than the TBI population in general, and women represented only 15% of the participants, limiting generalization. Participants were assigned without blinding. There was greater missing data (11 cases) for the PFIC, which was the primary blinded objective measure. The group leaders had extensive experience leading groups and working with the TBI population. The effectiveness of the intervention with less experienced clinicians is not known.	Clients with chronic TBI and social skill impairments may benefit from group intervention focused on pragmatic interaction skills, including cognitive abilities, self-monitoring of social interactions, awareness of social rules and boundaries, and emotional control. Intervention can improve overall social integration in work, school, and leisure environments and improve the client's life satisfaction.

Outcome measures were obtained at 3, 6, and 9 months post-treatment. Primary outcome measures were the Profile of Functional Impairment in Communication (PFIC), and Social Communication Skills Questionnaire–Adapted (SCSQ–A). Secondary outcome measures included Goal Attainment Scales, Craig Handicap Assessment and Reporting Technique–Short Form (social integration and occupation subscales), Community Integration Questionnaire (social integration and productivity subscale), and the Satisfaction With Life Scale.

Secondary measures that assessed community participation did not show significant differences between the groups.

Since the study used a deferred treatment design and did not compare the intervention to an alternative intervention, the outcomes may be due to non-treatment conditions such as socialization.

Dahlberg, C. A., Cusick, C. P., Hawley, L. A., Newman, J. K., Morey, C. E., Harrison-Felix, C. L., et al. (2007). Treatment efficacy of social communication skills training after traumatic brain injury: A randomized treatment and deferred treatment controlled trial. *Archives of Physical Medicine and Rehabilitation, 88,* 1561–1573.

(continued)

Author/Year	Study Objectives	Level/Design/ Participants	Intervention and Outcome Measures	Results	Study Limitations	Implications for Occupational Therapy
Ownsworth et al. (2008)	Compare individual, group, and combined intervention methods for improving psychosocial function and goal attainment	I—Randomized controlled trial with wait-list control group $N = 35$ adults with acquired brain injury (included 21 clients with traumatic brain injury) who were an average of 5 years postinjury, randomized from a convenience sample of 84 participants	Participants divided into 6 groups of the 3 intervention methods (i.e., individual, group, combined) or the wait-list control. Weekly sessions lasted for 3 hours (combined method included 1.5 hours of both individual and group). Outcome measures at pre-, post-, and 3-month follow-up conducted by blinded assessor: ▪ Canadian Occupational Performance Measure (COPM) ▪ Patient Competency Rating Scale ▪ Brain Injury Community Rehabilitation Outcome 39 Scales.	Gains in goal-specific performance were linked to individual intervention; gains in behavioral competency and psychological well-being were associated more frequently with clients who received group and individual intervention; combined intervention supported maintained gains in performance and satisfaction. Pre- and post-assessment changes were completed following the interventions. Due to the small sample size in each group between-group comparison was not completed.	Small sample size for number of conditions; heterogeneity of participants; satisfaction self-ratings on the COPM not stable prior to intervention	Brief intervention formats may be effective in producing psychosocial improvements and goal attainment, but further research is needed to match clients to particular intervention formats.

Ownsworth, T., Fleming, J., Shum, D., Kuipers, P., & Strong, J. (2008). Comparison of individualized, group, and combined intervention formats in a randomized controlled trial for facilitating goal attainment and improving psychosocial function following acquired brain injury. *Journal of Rehabilitation Medicine, 40,* 81–88.

Author/Year	Study Objectives	Level/Design/ Participants	Intervention and Outcome Measures	Results	Study Limitations	Implications for Occupational Therapy
Powell et al. (2002)	Test whether participants randomized to a multidisciplinary community-based outreach program would make significantly greater gains in activities of daily living, social participation, and psychological well-being than those randomized to a control condition of receiving only information about sources of existing help	I—Randomized controlled trial; exploratory $N = 110$, 16 lost to follow-up. 94 followed for 6 months (71 participants male, 23 participants female; mean age = 35 years) Outreach group: $N = 54$ Information-only group: $N = 56$	*Outreach group (E):* Programs were individualized. The treatment was "contracted organised goal setting." Participants worked toward long-term goals that were valued by the clients and their caregivers and considered amenable to intervention by the team via a series of written contracts which specified interim and	Intention to treat analysis. Data gathered at intake and at follow-up 18–40 months postrandomization. *BICRO-39:* 80% of the E group and 70% of the C group improved on the total score. Maximum gain index = 1.5 for E and .5 for C. Mann–Whitney U test on ranked change	Experimental group had more years postinjury than the control group (4.0 years vs. 2.7 years). The control group was significantly less cognitively disabled than the experimental group ($p < 0.02$).	The exact role of occupational therapy and the occupational intervention used in this study were not described. However, we can assume that the occupational therapists used functionally based interventions. "Functionally based rehabilitation shows promise for improving day to day life for people with severe TBI even

Moderate to severe traumatic brain injury (TBI); time since onset ranged from 0.2–20.3 years (mean = 1.3 years)	short-term goals achieved over 6–12 weeks. The methods used to work toward these goals were not reported. Setting was the participant's home or community setting (workplace, college, day center). Treatment was delivered by a team composed of 2 occupational therapists, a physical therapist, a speech–language therapist, a clinical psychologist, and ½-time social worker (2–6 hr/week, twice weekly, for an average of 27 [±19] weeks). *Information-only group (C):* Participants were assessed and given some limited assistance with pursuing referrals to outpatient services. Setting was the participant's home. Treatment was delivered by the team as above. Frequency not reported; treatment given 1 month after discharge from inpatient rehabilitation.	scores = 481, *p* < 0.05. *HADS:* 71% fell within normal range for anxiety and 65% for depression. NS between groups on change from intake to follow-up. *BI:* 60% of participants scored at ceiling at intake, with 14% scoring near ceiling (18 or 19 out of 20). 35% of the E group showed improvement as compared to 20% of the C group. Mann–Whitney U = 831, *p* < 0.05. *FIM+FAM:* 79%, 69%, and 54% of participants scored at ceiling at intake on personal care, mobility, and communication subscales respectively. Modest, similar improvement in both groups. Mann–Whitney U = 1058, *p* = NS. The maximum gain score was significantly greater in the E group than the C group. Mann–Whitney U = 782, *p* < 0.025.	many years after injury" (Dawson, 2002, p. 84). 11% attrition from experimental group, but statistical testing of demographic factors on remaining participants versus control was not significant. 13 experimental and 6 control participants lost to analysis of main outcome measure due to unavailable baseline data. Possible co-intervention bias: Authors report that 6 patients in the E group received less than 6 weeks of treatment while some in the C group "undoubtedly did receive appropriate help from other sources." (p. 201) Floor and ceiling effects for 70%–75% of the participants on some subscales of the outcome measures. Occupational therapist's role not stated.

(continued)

Author/Year	Study Objectives	Level/Design/ Participants	Intervention and Outcome Measures	Results	Study Limitations	Implications for Occupational Therapy
Powell et al. (2002) (cont.)			*Outcome measures:* ■ Brain Injury Community Rehabilitation Outcome (BICRO–39) subscales: Personal care, mobility, self-organization (bill paying, medicine administration, etc.), socializing, productive employment (education, child care, or work), psychological well-being; reliable and valid ■ Hospital Anxiety & Depression Scale (HADS); valid, reliability not reported ■ Barthel Index (BI); reliable and valid ■ Functional Independence/Assessment Measure (FIM+FAM); reliability and validity not reported.	*Conclusion:* "Within this randomised controlled trial, significantly greater gains were made by outreach treated participants [E] than by those given only written information about alternative resources" (p. 199).		

Powell, J., Heslin, J., & Greenwood, R. (2002). Community-based rehabilitation after severe traumatic brain injury: A randomized controlled trial. *Journal of Neurology, Neurosurgery, and Psychiatry, 72,* 193–202.

| McMorrow et al. (1998) | Evaluate the effects of a proactive behavioral-residential treatment program on the functional outcomes of persons with acquired brain injury (ABI) with serious unwanted behaviors that put themselves or others at risk | III—One group, repeated measures design

 N = 71 (90% male, 10% female; age 16–56 years, mean = 30)

 86% had severe brain injury (coma >24 | The program included traditional rehabilitation therapy (occupational therapy, physical therapy, psychological, and speech therapies) plus cognitive, behavioral, and medical approaches. The program consisted of the following: | Measured at referral evaluation, 1 day prior to admission, at discharge, 3 months, 6 months, and 12 months postdischarge. Trained raters were asked to specify one level of functioning in each outcome area during each assessment. Each rater | 23% attrition at 3-month follow-up; 46% attrition at 12-month follow-up.

 Intervention changed partway through the study; the residential continuum was not available for early years. | This study cannot provide occupational therapists with specific guidance for clinical practice because the occupational therapist's role in this program is not identified. However, the practice approach to which all professional staff was said to be committed |

hours or Glasgow Coma Scale rating of 3–8 at time of injury)

Time since onset ranged from 9 days to 20 years (38% were >2 years)

All generally failed to benefit from previous rehabilitation to treat unwanted behaviors

- All staff used the same practice approach that included these commitments: a) use a behavioral approach using positive reinforcement; b) avoid punishment or escape extinction learning operations; c) use minimal effective dosage of medication and avoid as needed usage; d) implement least restriction (residence as well as how treated); e) have no mechanical restraint and no exclusionary or seclusionary procedures; f) keep the person as involved as possible in the life of the community; and g) treat all patients with a high degree of personal dignity and respect
- The interactional style included a) positive interaction; b) early intervention; c) all inclusive (all patients/all the time/all situations); d) reinforce desired behaviors; and e) look for and use teachable moments

presumably reported on his or her area of expertise, but this was not reported, nor was it reported which information was scored from record review, interview, or observation.

From preadmission to discharge evaluations, the percentage of participants scoring at the various levels of achievement showed improvement in all 7 functional outcome areas. All areas except vocational improved to the intermediate level. The group performance attained at discharge was maintained across all 7 functional outcome areas at the 3-month follow-up.

The results for 6- and 12-month follow-up periods are not reported here because of extensive attrition and lack of knowledge concerning what occurred during that time that could have affected the scores (history and maturation threats to validity).

No statistical analyses were done.

The training of the team was not described.

No validity or reliability information for outcome measures reported.

Results not tested statistically.

There was no evidence given about the consistency and commitment of the various staff members to the approach or the delivery of the treatment

The key or required components of the program cannot be identified from this study.

Threats to internal validity (e.g., history, maturation) were not controlled.

Occupational therapy's role was not reported.

is consistent with the philosophy of occupational therapy and provides some weak support for the validity of that philosophy.

(continued)

Author/Year	Study Objectives	Level/Design/Participants	Intervention and Outcome Measures	Results	Study Limitations	Implications for Occupational Therapy
McMorrow et al. (1998) (cont.)			*Residential continuum:* a) reside in place with most to least staff availability; and b) reside in place with greater to lesser emphasis on basic versus complex activities of daily living *Personal intervention planning:* emotional–behavioral self-management through individual and group therapies and ongoing reinforced practice of compensatory strategies to promote successful negotiation of difficult life situations. ■ Personal goal setting (group therapeutic contracting) ■ Functional/integrated cognitive training within context ■ Performance monitoring/weekly feedback ■ Community access review 3 times daily to determine whether the person could be in a less restricted situation	*Conclusion:* "The results of this study suggest that a proactive behavioral-residential treatment program had an important impact on the functional outcomes of a group of persons who had experienced ABI....The post treatment results are strengthened when one considers that they were contrasted to repeated, pretreatment measures that failed to show gains despite the passing of time and inclusion in other forms of treatment during this period" (p. 29).		

Setting: 8-bed community integrated residential setting at first. Later, a continuum of 4 residential options from secure unit to staff-monitored apartment living was added.

Delivered by a rehabilitation/behavioral team, including an occupational therapist.

Frequency: all day, every day; duration: mean length of stay = 7 months.

Outcome measures: 7 functional outcomes were measured:

- Residential status
- Level of independence or freedom from assistance
- Behavioral/emotional status (does the participant intervene on his or her own behalf rather than depend on external help?)
- Level of community participation, with or without assistance
- Level of self-awareness of personal skills and difficulties
- Vocational/higher education/productive activity status

(continued)

EVIDENCE TABLE. FOCUSED QUESTION 3 (cont.)

Author/Year	Study Objectives	Level/Design/ Participants	Intervention and Outcome Measures	Results	Study Limitations	Implications for Occupational Therapy
McMorrow et al. (1998) (cont.)			▪ Level of involvement in productive activity per day and per week. Each of these measures was scored on 5 hierarchical and exclusive levels of performance. No reliability or validity information reported.			

McMorrow, M. J., Braunling-McMorrow, D., & Smith, S. (1998). Evaluation of functional outcomes following proactive behavioral–residential treatment. *Journal of Rehabilitation Outcomes Measurement, 2*, 22–30.

Author/Year	Study Objectives	Level/Design/ Participants	Intervention and Outcome Measures	Results	Study Limitations	Implications for Occupational Therapy
Murrey & Starzinski (2004)	Review the specialized neurorehabilitation program at the Minnesota Neurorehabilitation Hospital (MNH); evaluate the program on persons with traumatic brain injury (TBI) and severe neurobehavioral disorders	III—One group pretest–posttest *N* = 44 (73% male, 27% female; mean age at onset = 23.5 years; mean length of time from onset to MNH admission = 63 months) Rancho Los Amigos cognitive level of 4 or higher *Significant Level I behaviors:* Physical and verbal threatening or aggression, inappropriate sexual behavior, self-injurious behavior, property destruction or other high-risk behaviors post-TBI; multiple failures (>3) in community placements; 89% had a history of	A 4-stage rehabilitation process using an individualized plan and timeline dictated by the patient's abilities and motivation: 1) emotional stabilization (standardized and individualized behavioral programming, environmental management, pharmacological intervention; 2) basic skill acquisition and insight-building (provision of a "tool bag" of various coping strategies and behavioral/emotional regulation techniques and skills while increasing awareness and insight of the maladaptive behaviors and cognitive deficits [see article for specific therapies]);	Evaluated 3 years post-MNH discharge. 30% (13 of 44) had a psychiatric admission; 11% had multiple admissions. LOS ranged from 2 to 1,521 days (mean = 225 days) per admission. 9 participants who had a psychiatric admission returned to initial post-MNH discharge placement site. 18% (6 of 34) were living independently with little or no home support. 59% (20 of 34) were living in specialized TBI foster homes. 50% (17 of 34) were employed (sheltered, supportive, semi-independent, or independent).	The causal relationship between treatment and outcome is shadowed by possible history and maturation effects that could have occurred in the 3 years between treatment and evaluation; designers did not control for these threats to validity. 23% dropout rate (failure to return outcome questionnaires). There was no dropout information on psychiatric or prison admission. Nonstandardized outcome measures; reliability not established. Raters knew the participants were	Because of limitations of measurement and design, and lack of statistical analysis, this study offers little specific guidance to occupational therapy other than the authors' statement that "specialized programmes can produce significant results for persons with TBI who present with very poor prognoses and severe, seemingly ingrained, target behaviors" (p. 529). The sample daily schedule supplied in the appendix includes interventions that occupational therapists are skilled to offer, but what the occupational therapist on the team actually did was not stated.

(continued)

3 or more psychiatric admissions; 86% had mean length of stay (LOS) in psychiatric facility of 263 days; 80% unemployed over a 2-year period prior to MNH admission

3) skills proficiency phase (giving many opportunities to apply various skills and strategies within community settings, including supportive work trials; staff feedback; reality-oriented psychoeducational therapies); 4) community integration or transition phase (moving to a transitional unit or an in-hospital apartment trial program with higher levels of independence).

Delivered by a team (occupational therapist, physical therapist, pastoral counseling, activities director, horticultural therapist, psychologist, art therapist, vocational trainer, nurses), supervised by a behavioral neurologist/medical director. Boundaries between disciplines were transparent.

Frequency: daily from 7 a.m. to 9:30 p.m.; duration not reported.

graduates of the MNH program and why they were being evaluated.

No statistical analyses of data.

Occupational therapist's role not stated.

Conclusion: "Clearly, the combination of the intensive and comprehensive inpatient neurobehavioral program and the specialized/appropriate community support resulted in long-term success on these various measures for the majority of the patients involved" (p. 528).

EVIDENCE TABLE. FOCUSED QUESTION 3 (*cont.*)

Author/Year	Study Objectives	Level/Design/ Participants	Intervention and Outcome Measures	Results	Study Limitations	Implications for Occupational Therapy
Murrey & Starzinski (2004) (*cont.*)			*Outcome measures:* ■ Stability of community placement: current living situation and change of residence since discharge ■ Postdischarge vocational status–employment status ■ Postdischarge psychiatric hospital or correctional facility admissions and LOS Reliability and validity not reported for any measure.			

Murrey, G. J., & Starzinski, D. (2004). An inpatient neurobehavioral rehabilitation programme for persons with traumatic brain injury: Overview of and outcome data for the Minnesota Neurorehabilitation Hospital. *Brain Injury, 18,* 519–531.

Author/Year	Study Objectives	Level/Design/ Participants	Intervention and Outcome Measures	Results	Study Limitations	Implications for Occupational Therapy
Ouellet & Morin (2007)	Evaluate the efficacy of cognitive–behavioral therapy (CBT) on insomnia in persons with traumatic brain injury (TBI)	IV—Single subject design $N = 11$ individuals with mild to severe TBI at an outpatient rehabilitation center who reported insomnia (ages 21–46)	*Intervention:* 8-week CBT program that included stimulus control, sleep restriction, sleep hygiene education, and fatigue management. *Outcome measures:* ■ Total wake time ■ Sleep efficiency ■ Diagnostic criteria for an insomnia syndrome.	Clinically and statistically significant reductions in total wake time and improved sleep efficiency were noted in 8 of 11 participants post treatment. There was an average reduction of 54% in total wake time from pre- to posttest. Progress was maintained at 1- and 3-month follow-up. Improvements in sleep were accompanied by a decrease in general and physical fatigue.	Small sample size While the study sample was similar to age and severity level of those with TBI reported in the literature to have sleep disturbances, the sample was overrepresented by women.	Sleep, a newly identified occupational performance area, can have significant influence on functional performance if its quality is lessened. Clients with TBI are prone to sleep disorders that can impair rehabilitation progress and quality of life. Cognitive–behavioral therapy addressing knowledge, self-awareness and -regulation, environmental assessment, and restructuring performance patterns/habits can improve sleep and reduce daytime fatigue.

Ouellet, M. C., & Morin, C. M. (2007). Efficacy of cognitive–behavioral therapy for insomnia associated with traumatic brain injury: A single-case experimental design. *Archives of Physical Medicine and Rehabilitation, 88,* 1581–1592.

| Schlund & Pace (1999) | Highlight the contribution of focusing on behavior–environment relations (operant conditioning or behavior analysis) for treating and interpreting the effects of feedback on maladaptive behavior exhibited by 3 persons with traumatic brain injury (TBI). | IV—Multiple baseline across subjects

$N = 3$, all male, age 27–48 years (mean = 36)

Diagnosed with TBI and mild depression, 2 with a history of substance abuse

4–9 years (mean = 5.6) posttrauma

All capable of identifying their own primary maladaptive behaviors | Weekly data-based feedback about maladaptive behaviors as part of a behavior analysis or operant psychological approach that used the three-term contingency concept: environmental stimulation, behavior, and consequences. The psychologist reviewed the baseline and weekly frequencies of incidents of the maladaptive behavior with the patient during the treatment period.

Strategies used:
P1: To decrease pseudoseizures, the patient allowed the staff to assist him in expressing himself thoughtfully during group sessions to avoid harassment of others.

P2: To decrease inappropriate sexual behavior, the patient kept his hands down and avoided commenting about others.

P3: To increase compliance of rules of the day program and requests and instructions of the staff, the program rules and procedures were reviewed with him. | P1 reduced target behavior from a mean of twice per week to 0 after one treatment.

P2 reduced target behavior from a mean of 3.6 incidents/week to 1.7/week.

P3 reduced target behavior from a mean of 5.1/week to 0 after 1 treatment. No statistical testing of data between baseline and intervention phases was done.

Conclusion:
"Systematic presentation of data-based feedback decreased maladaptive behaviors exhibited by 3 persons with TBI attending a medical day program" (p. 895). | Social workers and day program staff rated the target behaviors. There is no report of reliability of the raters.

The baselines were unstable for P1 and P2 when treatment was introduced; the baseline for P3 was declining for 5 weeks before treatment began; therefore, no causal relationship between treatment and outcome can be clearly demonstrated. Further, there was no control for concurrent treatment threat to internal validity. | This is a weak study, but, as the authors state, "At the very least, it is plausible to suggest that feedback, as a 'first step' clinical intervention for maladaptive behaviors exhibited by persons with mild psychological and cognitive impairments, may be a worthwhile economical and least restrictive approach in conjunction with other therapeutic techniques" (p. 895). In other words, data-based feedback is unlikely to hurt and more likely to help the patient gain control over his or her social behaviors. |

(continued)

EVIDENCE TABLE. FOCUSED QUESTION 3 *(cont.)*

Author/Year	Study Objectives	Level/Design/ Participants	Intervention and Outcome Measures	Results	Study Limitations	Implications for Occupational Therapy
Schlund & Pace (1999) *(cont.)*			*Setting:* Medical day treatment program. Frequency: Once/week. Duration: 15 weeks (including baseline of 4 weeks for P1, 6 weeks for P2, and 8 weeks for P3). Treatment delivered by a psychologist. *Outcome measures:* Frequency of target behaviors			

Schlund, M. W., & Pace, G. (1999). Relations between traumatic brain injury and the environment: Feedback reduces maladaptive behaviour exhibited by three persons with traumatic brain injury. *Brain Injury, 13,* 889–897.

Author/Year	Study Objectives	Level/Design/ Participants	Intervention and Outcome Measures	Results	Study Limitations	Implications for Occupational Therapy
Zhou et al. (1996)	Test the feasibility of a game format to teach information about acquired brain injury (ABI) to persons experiencing the effects of such injuries; explore whether increased knowledge of residuals influenced participants' behavior outside of the training situation	IV—Multiple baseline experimental design (across residual behavioral categories) *Baseline:* Players could move the game pieces regardless of their answers; no feedback given *Phase I:* Correct answers were required in the behavioral and emotional categories in order to move game pieces. Corrective feedback was given for these categories. Baseline conditions existed for the other categories. *Phase II:* Correct answers were additionally required for cognitive and communication	Training in knowledge about ABI using a game format. The game materials were on the table around which the participants and instructors sat. The primary instructor conducted the sessions while 1 of the 3 auxiliary instructors collected observational data. The game was designed similar to Trivial Pursuit,® with 6 categories of residuals that were targeted: behavior, emotion, cognition, communication, physical, and sensory. Within each category, 18 questions and answers were developed (108 items total). An equal number of questions concerning each category were pre-	All 3 participants increased their percentage of correct responses in the study areas of behavior, emotion, cognition, communication, physical, and sensory residuals. The impact of these improvements on participants' functioning was not consistent. All participants rated themselves lower (less problem) than clinicians. The data were not tested statistically. *Conclusion:* Game format and incentives were effective means in helping the participants to increase their knowledge of	In addition to the game format, the participants received monetary rewards for participating (50 cents), for each correct answer (10 cents), and for winning ($1.00). This contaminated the effect of the intervention, therefore no causal relationship can be assumed between the game format (without monetary rewards) and the outcomes. Participant 1 moved to a new residence and a different clinical staff completed the competency rating scale at follow-up. Occupational therapy was not involved in this therapy, but this study was included because the treatment is similar to	This study is graded at Level IV and involved only 3 persons; therefore, no firm conclusions can be drawn from the study. The results suggest that a game format and game incentives (winning, monetary prizes) can be effective in involving patients in therapy and in helping patients increase their knowledge about their conditions. The results also note that the knowledge did not transfer to real-life situations; therefore, additional therapy would be needed to effect the transition. This study suggests that it would be worthwhile designing a better controlled study involving a greater number

categories. Corrective feedback was directed at the 4 categories. Baseline conditions existed for the physical and sensory categories.

Phase III: Correct answers were required for all 6 categories and feedback was provided. Criterion to change phases was 70% correct for 2 sessions.

N = 3, all male. Age range 30–32. Time since onset ranged from 18 months to 10 years. All were residents of a community-based neurobehavioral program for adults with ABI.

sented at each session. Every participant was asked 3 different questions from each category (18 total per session). Each card also indicated the number of spaces that the player could move on the game board for a correct answer. The objective of the game was to move one's game piece to each of 6 category "headquarters." Answers were scored correct or incorrect according to the predetermined answer or facsimile. There was no time limit for answering. *Setting:* activity room of the residence.

Delivered by a team (graduate students in behavior analysis and therapy), headed by the behavioral analyst (with master's degree). Different members of the team took turns being the lead staff game player. *Frequency:* 1 hour/session, 3 sessions/week. *Duration:* 31 sessions (including 5 sessions for initial baseline).

Outcome measures:
- Knowledge of ABI: percent of correct answers in each residual category; 95% interobserver agreement.

therapies used by occupational therapists.

potential residuals in 6 areas of functioning post-ABI. The game format was an effective means of engaging patients in therapy. The impact of the increased knowledge was not consistently positive in real-life situations.

of participants to test these ideas.

(continued)

Author/Year	Study Objectives	Level/Design/ Participants	Intervention and Outcome Measures	Results	Study Limitations	Implications for Occupational Therapy
Zhou et al. (1996) (cont.)			■ Subjective measure of impairment of daily functioning using a competency rating scale developed for this study: a) participant self-rating and b) staff ratings. The score was the difference between these two ratings. The greater the difference, the less the participant was aware of the effects of the residuals in daily life. Intrarater agreement ranged from 68% to 78% across participants.			

Zhou, J., Chittum, R., Johnston, K., Poppen, R., Guercio, J., & McMorrow, M. J. (1996). The utilization of a game format to increase knowledge of residuals among people with acquired brain injury. *Journal of Head Trauma Rehabilitation, 11,* 51–61.

| Bieman-Copeland & Dywan (2000) | Provide an example of the approach of using implicit memory systems and errorless learning and formation of trusting, nonconfrontational therapeutic relationships | V—Case report

N = 1

Participant: 28-year-old female with severe traumatic brain injury (TBI; coma = 2 weeks); about 22 months postinjury; profound anosognosia (impaired awareness of behavioral limitations); confusion; left-sided weakness; impaired short-term memory; excessive agitation | Nonconfrontational behavioral approach using strategies to make use of implicit memory systems and errorless learning. Targeted behaviors: 1) decrease frequency of phone calling; and 2) decrease frequency of sexually explicit and sexually suggestive behavior.

Strategies: 1) impose time limits (two ½-hour periods)—the participant came to believe that it was more polite to call at certain times; | Phone calls decreased from 175 per week to 25 per week over 3 months. Sexually explicit behaviors decreased from 13 per recording period to 0 after 2 months. Sexually suggestive behaviors decreased from 23 per recording period to <5 per period over 4 months. | No causal relationship was established between treatment and outcome. No controls against threats to validity. No one component of treatment could be identified as the causal factor, even if a causal relationship had been established. | This case report reminds the occupational therapist that the relationship between therapist and patient can be therapeutically effective and its development should be included in the care plan. |

| | | | 2) provide feedback as to how others perceived the sexual behaviors.

Through collaborative negotiation (basis for therapeutic relationship), the participant came to believe that the behaviors were fine in a large city but were not fine in the small town where the rehabilitation facility was located.

Administered by staff; professional discipline that supervised the treatment not reported. | | | |

Bieman-Copland, S., & Dywan, J. (2000). Achieving rehabilitative gains in anosognosia after TBI. *Brain and Cognition, 44*, 1–5.

| DeHope & Finegan (1999) | Report on the use of the self-determination model to address integrated self-awareness in the treatment of individuals with traumatic brain injury (TBI) | V—Case report

N = 3

Case 1: 20-year-old male with severe TBI (coma = 6 days); right hemiplegia; mute; substance abuse; extreme sexual behavior

Case 2: 50-year-old female; acquired brain injury (ABI) secondary to surgical procedure; seizures, occasional incontinence; depression; very limited self-awareness (poor judgment, impulsive in social situations especially with men) as well as other deficits | Self-determination model seeks to increase self-awareness and reentry into the social community. 3 phases: 1) repetitive and consistent education about the brain, brain injury, self-awareness, and self-determination; 2) consistent practice of social skills in therapeutically managed safe situations; and 3) develop opportunities for natural consequences in the community. It is a client-centered and client determined treatment plan. | *Case 1*: Received this therapy for 12 years and continuing. Able to drive, work (plumber), and is married. Still needs to improve self-awareness.

Case 2: Received this therapy for 5 years and is ongoing. Able to manage time 52% of the time; able to work; able to use various strategies (lists of behaviors) for "shower routine," "check your work," etc.

Case 3: Has made some progress; is in process and receives intense assistance from the treatment team. | No causal relationship established between treatment and outcome; no controls against threats to validity; no one component of treatment could be identified as the causal factor, even if a causal relationship had been established | The 3 phases of the treatment are consistent with occupational therapy practice (practice of social skills in occupationally relevant situations). The authors state that the treatment requires 1 year minimum for effectiveness.

Occupational therapists may need to lobby for extended treatment coverage for participants with severe behavioral sequelae post-TBI. |

(continued)

EVIDENCE TABLE. FOCUSED QUESTION 3 (cont.)

Author/Year	Study Objectives	Level/Design/ Participants	Intervention and Outcome Measures	Results	Study Limitations	Implications for Occupational Therapy
DeHope & Finegan (1999) (cont.)		Case 3: 30-year-old male; TBI second-ary to work accident; behavioral dyscontrol, substance abuse, ag-gression, and other negative behaviors	Administered by staff; professional discipline that supervised the treatment not reported.			

DeHope, E., & Finegan, J. (1999). The self-determination model: An approach to develop awareness for survivors of traumatic brain injury. *NeuroRehabilitation, 13*, 3–12.

| Fluharty & Glassman (2001) | Describe behavioral approaches and environmental sup-ports that reduced the agitation of a client with brain injury and facilitated discharge to a group home | V—Case report

N = 1

Participant: 23-year-old male with severe TBI, about 19 months postinjury; increasingly aggressive and un-cooperative behavior; unmanageable; severe cognitive and memory deficits; tactile defen-siveness. The patient had implicit recall of information that was meaningful to him (e.g., location of bathrooms or vending machines). | Decrease sources of agitation through humor, reframing the situation, and diversion of attention antecedent to signs of aggression. Modify environment (cueing for activities of daily living [ADLs], adaptations such as hook-and-fastener closures, use of barber in town to shave and groom, etc.). Reward completed activities with reinforcing ac-tivities (for this patient, walking and snacking). Duration: ~100 days.

Administered by staff; professional discipline that supervised the treatment not reported. | Frequency of ag-gressive behavior diminished markedly. Increased cooperation in carrying out ADLs. Discharged to a group home. | No causal relation-ship was established between treatment and outcome; no controls against threats to validity; no one compo-nent of treatment could be identified as the causal factor, even if a causal relationship had been established. | This case report re-minds occupational therapists that careful, detailed evaluation of the patient's impair-ments and motivations may lead to more ef-fective therapy. In this case, tactile defensive-ness was identified as an underlying cause of problem behavior that could be corrected through adaptations. |

Fluharty, G., & Glassman, N. (2001). Case Study: Use of antecedent control to improve the outcome of rehabilitation for a client with frontal lobe injury and intolerance for auditory and tactile stimuli. *Brain Injury, 15*, 995–1002.

	Objective	Level/Design	Intervention	Results	Comments
Gutman & Leger (1997)	Present clinical guidelines to assist individuals in establishing and maintaining intimate relationships in accordance with community standards for age-appropriate behavior	V—Case report N = 3 Case 1: 26-year-old male, 8 years postinjury Case 2: 22-year-old female, 6 years postinjury Case 3: 36-year-old male, 11 years postinjury	Social training was aimed at enhancing one-to-one interpersonal verbal and nonverbal skills needed to initiate first meetings that may lead to formation of intimate relationships. Treatment also involved strategies to deal with rejection. Treatment included education, observation of others, role playing, graded practice in controlled situations, practice in natural situations, and feedback. The therapy program lasted 6 months. Administered by an occupational therapist.	Case 1: Consistently able to use skills; he formed 2 close relationships through a dating service for people with disabilities Case 2: Able to refrain from greeting other men when with boyfriend; able to handle rejection Case 3: Able to refuse unwanted sexual activity; able to engage in safe sexual activity with those he wanted; respected people's personal space during conversation	Although a causal relationship was not established between treatment and outcome by case reports, such a relationship may be inferred from the close correspondence of the specific treatment and the outcomes reported for these participants. Further study is needed. There were no controls against threats to validity.	"Through role playing, occupational therapists can assist individuals in achievement of their goals to establish friendships with others and to maintain intimate relationships in an appropriate manner" (p. 66).

Gutman, S. A., & Leger, D. L. (1997). Enhancement of one-to-one interpersonal skills necessary to initiate and maintain intimate relationships: A frame of reference for adults having sustained traumatic brain injury. *Occupational Therapy in Mental Health, 13,* 51–67.

	Objective	Level/Design	Intervention	Results	Comments
Rothwell et al. (1999)	Describe an approach based on a comprehensive and individualized behavioral assessment that is used to generate a program focusing on skills training and avoidance of punishment as a treatment principle	V—Case report N = 2 Case 1: 31-year-old male with 2 episodes of brain injury/anoxia; physical aggression Case 2: 40-year-old female with cerebral vascular accident (CVA) with left hemiplegia and left visual neglect, 2 years post-CVA; physical and verbal aggression	Nonaversive behavioral rehabilitation for people with severe behavior problems after acquired brain injury has 5 components: 1) comprehensive behavioral assessment to understand the person and to determine why the person is engaging in the behaviors and how he or she uses these behaviors to solve everyday problems; 2) positive programming—teaching skills necessary to achieve goals without using inappropriate behavior; 3) ecological change—alter social	Case 1: Thorough behavioral assessment indicated aggression was secondary to fear and disorientation. Treatment involved hourly orientation and manipulation of the social environment (female caregivers only). Aggression reduced to 0 immediately and it remained at 0 for 33 months. Case 2: Thorough behavioral assessment indicated aggression was secondary to anxiety that was relieved by social interaction. Anxiety management	No causal relationship established between treatment and outcome; no controls against threats to validity; no one component of treatment could be identified as the causal factor, even if a causal relationship had been established.	This case report reminds occupational therapists that careful, detailed evaluation of the patient's impairments and motivations may lead to more effective therapy. In this case, the psychologist identified the underlying cause of the outward behavior and directed intervention to modify that cause rather than direct therapy to the behavior *per se.*

(continued)

EVIDENCE TABLE. FOCUSED QUESTION 3 (cont.)

Author/Year	Study Objectives	Level/Design/ Participants	Intervention and Outcome Measures	Results	Study Limitations	Implications for Occupational Therapy
Rothwell et al. (1999) (cont.)			environment to accommodate cognitive deficits; 4) focused treatment—use behavioral contingencies to decrease targeted behavior; and 5) reactive strategies—specify actions to be taken to gain short-term control over episodes of bad behavior. Administered by staff; directed by a clinical psychologist.	training as well as other behavioral treatments decreased both physical and verbal aggression over a 22-week period.		

Rothwell, N. A., LaVigna, G. W., & Willis, T. J. (1999). A non-aversive rehabilitation approach for people with severe behavioural problems resulting from brain injury. *Brain Injury, 13,* 521–533.

Author/Year	Study Objectives	Level/Design/ Participants	Intervention and Outcome Measures	Results	Study Limitations	Implications for Occupational Therapy
Sladyk (1992)	Describe the occupational therapy program of a woman with brain injury who exhibited cognitive problems and severe behavioral problems	V—Case report N = 1; 48-year-old female Severe traumatic brain injury (coma = 5 days); 142 days postinjury Unmanageable behavior and attention span of <5 minutes.	Expected behaviors were identified. Positive behaviors were encouraged and praised. Peer feedback was given in twice per day community meetings. Small structured groups met 3 times per week for social skills training and art projects keyed to feelings and behaviors. Computerized cognitive training and cooking and task groups were also used to address cognitive problems. Program lasted 3 weeks; occupational therapy was 1 1/4 to 2 hours per day. Administered by an occupational therapist.	After 58 days of treatment in the neurobehavioral program, the participant showed a great decrease in demanding behavior, no aggressive behavior, controlled behavior without medication, and made her needs known appropriately. Social skills were better than before the accident.	No causal relationship established between treatment and outcome; no controls against threats to validity, especially co-intervention contamination; no one component of treatment could be identified as the causal factor, even if a causal relationship had been established.	The occupational therapy program comprised only 3 out of the 8 weeks of treatment in the program. One cannot say what the exact contribution was that occupational therapy made to this patient's improvement. Further study is needed.

Sladyk, K. (1992). Case Report: Traumatic brain injury, behavioral disorder, and group treatment. *American Journal of Occupational Therapy, 46,* 267–270.

| Yuen (1997) | Illustrate the use of one social skills training technique (positive talk toward others) | V—Case report

N = 1; 43-year-old male, 20 years postinjury with verbally and physically aggressive behaviors | Social interaction skills training to decrease disinhibited interaction behaviors. Positive talk training (verbal statements that contain positive remarks, compliments, and praise directed toward another person) 5 minutes per day within the 1-hour occupational therapy session that focused on cognitive and perceptual training. Conditions of the training were graded in complexity over 4 weeks. Participant also engaged in a 6–8 person group social skills training project run by a behavioral specialist for 1 hr 2–3 times per week.

Administered by an occupational therapist. | Able to make a positive statement when prompted and in new settings. Praise statements included more than tangible characteristics of the other person. Negative statements did not increase. | No causal relationship established between treatment and outcome; no controls against threats to validity, especially co-intervention contamination; no one component of treatment could be identified as the causal factor, even if a causal relationship had been established. | The occupational therapy program comprised <2 hr over the 4 weeks of treatment. On the other hand, behavioral therapy, focusing on similar goals, comprised 2–3 hr per week. One cannot say exactly what contribution occupational therapy made to this patient's improvement. Further study is needed. |

Yuen, H. K. (1997). Positive talk training in an adult with traumatic brain injury. *American Journal of Occupational Therapy, 51*, 780–783.

Reference
Dawson, D. R. (2002). Commentary: A multidisciplinary community-based rehabilitation programme improved social functioning in severe traumatic brain injury. *Evidence-Based Mental Health, 5*, 84.

EVIDENCE TABLE. FOCUSED QUESTION 4.

What is the evidence for the effect of interventions to address cognitive/perceptual functions (attention, memory, executive functions) on the occupational performance for persons with traumatic brain injury?

Author/Year	Study Objectives	Level/Design/ Participants	Intervention and Outcome Measures	Results	Study Limitations	Implications for Occupational Therapy
General						
Cicerone et al. (2000), Cicerone et al. (2005)	Evaluate the effectiveness of cognitive rehabilitation for persons with traumatic brain injury (TBI) or stroke and make recommendations for clinical practice	Level I—Systematic review initially completed in 2000, with an updated review of the literature in 2005 171 studies published between January 1988 and August 1998 were evaluated in the 2000 review, with an additional 87 studies published September 1998–2002 evaluated in the 2005 update. The reviews included experimental (randomized trials, prospective and retrospective controlled trials, single-group interventions) and non-experimental designs (retrospective and case studies).	Interventions were assigned to one of 7 categories: attention, visual perception and constructional abilities, language and memory, communication, problem solving and executive functioning, multi-modal interventions, and comprehensive-holistic cognitive rehabilitation. Recommendations were made for practice standards (at least 1 well-designed Level I study with an adequate sample, with additional Level II or Level III evidence), practice guidelines (supported by 1 or more Level I studies with methodologic limitations, or well-designed Level II studies with adequate samples), and practice options (evidence provided by Level II or III studies).	There is strong evidence supporting two interventions as practice standards: strategy training for attention deficits in postacute clients with TBI and memory strategy training for clients with mild memory impairments. The research suggests such training should include the use of internalized strategies and external memory compensations. Three interventions were classified as practice guidelines: use of external compensations specific to functional activities; training in formal problem-solving strategies during common functional activities; and comprehensive neuropsychological rehabilitation. Several interventions were classified as practice options: self-regulation strategies through self-instruc-	Many of the studies had limited long-term follow-up to determine if gains made with intervention were sustained. Considerable heterogeneity existed with limited details on the components of the intervention, making comparison and classification of interventions difficult.	Occupational therapists should emphasize attentional strategy training during complex functional tasks in the postacute recovery phase rather than the acute rehabilitation period. Memory training for clients with mild traumatic brain injury (MTBI) should incorporate the use of compensatory strategies such as notebooks and external aids. Therapists should incorporate problem-solving and self-regulation training into everyday functional activities used in intervention. Use of repeated exposure and practice on computer-based tasks without therapist involvement is not recommended. The authors state, "Future research should move beyond the simple question of whether cognitive rehabilitation is effective, and examine the therapy factors and patient characteristics that optimize the clinical outcomes

tion and self-monitoring for clients with impairments of emotional self-regulation, or deficits in attention, neglect, and memory; integrated treatment of individualized cognitive; and interpersonal therapies.

of cognitive rehabilitation" (Cicerone et al., 2005, p. 1681).

Outcome measures need to assess clients' recovery at all levels of the World Health Organization's *International Classification of Functioning* (2001; body structure and function, activity, and participation).

Cicerone, K. D., Dahlberg, C., Kalmar, K., Langenbahn, D. M., Malec, J. F., Berquist, T. F., et al. (2000). Evidence-based cognitive rehabilitation: Recommendations for clinical practice. *Archives of Physical Medicine and Rehabilitation, 81*, 1596–1615.

Cicerone, K. D., Dahlberg, C., Malec, J. F., Langenbahn, D. M., Felicetti, T., Kneipp, S., et al. (2005). Evidence-based cognitive rehabilitation: Updated review of the literature from 1998 through 2002. *Archives of Physical Medicine and Rehabilitation, 86*, 1681–1692.

| Rees et al. (2007) | Evaluate the efficacy of cognitive rehabilitation to improve independence following acquired brain injury | I—Systematic review

Searched CINAHL, Medline, EMBASE, PsycINFO from 1980–2006. All published literature related to moderate-to-severe acquired brain injury was included. Bibliographies of selected articles were reviewed as well. Review included experimental (randomized trials, prospective and retrospective controlled trials, single-group interventions) and non-experimental designs (retrospective and case studies). | *Interventions:* Cognitive therapy interventions in the following areas: attention/concentration, learning, and memory.

Outcome measures:
- Tests in the areas listed above
- Functional outcomes
- Psychosocial well-being
- Symptom checklist. | 64 studies were included in the review. There is strong evidence that external aids are effective as compensatory strategies for functional day-to-day memory problems, and strong evidence that the use of internal aids, such as mnemonics, are effective in improving recall for those with mild impairment. The evidence is strong, however, that internal aids are not effective for those with severe impairment. There is moderate evidence for the effect of dual-task training on speed of processing, and goal-management training on improving paper-and-pencil daily activi- | Lack of consensus on the definition of areas of cognition; similar tests used to measure different aspects of cognition; use of outcome measures multiple times may confound practice and treatment effects | Occupational therapists should consider training clients with mild to moderate memory impairments in the use of external aids to improve performance in real-life memory tasks. Training in internal memory strategies should be retained for those clients with mild memory impairments. Cognitive rehabilitation using computerized practice drills to improve attention and memory should be used cautiously as the present evidence does not support their use. Additional research is needed. |

(continued)

Author/Year	Study Objectives	Level/Design/ Participants	Intervention and Outcome Measures	Results	Study Limitations	Implications for Occupational Therapy
Rees et al. (2007) *(cont.)*				ties. There is moderate evidence that drill-and-practice training is not effective for improving attention. There is limited evidence for the effectiveness of general cognitive rehabilitation to improve cognition, exercise to improve visual and verbal learning, and group intervention for executive dysfunction. The evidence is limited that memory training programs and computer-assisted programs are not effective.		

Rees, L., Marshall, S., Hartridge, C., Mackie, D., & Weiser, M. (2007). Cognitive interventions post acquired brain injury. *Brain Injury, 21,* 161–200.

Author/Year	Study Objectives	Level/Design/ Participants	Intervention and Outcome Measures	Results	Study Limitations	Implications for Occupational Therapy
Salazar et al. (2000)	Evaluate the efficacy of inpatient cognitive rehabilitation for patients with moderate to severe traumatic brain injury (TBI), based on the hypothesis that an in-hospital rehabilitation program would yield greater return to work and fitness for duty rates than a limited home program at 1 yr follow-up.	I—Single center, parallel group randomized trial (over 5-year period) N = 107 active duty military personnel with moderate to severe closed head injury, randomly assigned to group	*Group 1:* 8-wk intensive, standardized in-hospital cognitive rehabilitation program. n = 67. Included occupational therapy (work activity), among other professionals. *Group 2:* 8-wk limited, standardized home rehabilitation program with weekly telephone support. n = 53. Whole intervention offered by a psychiatric nurse. *Outcome measures:* Return to gainful employment and fitness for military duty at 1-yr follow-up.	At 1-yr follow-up, there was no significant difference between Groups 1 and 2 in return to employment (90% vs. 94%, respectively) or fitness for duty (73% vs. 66%, respectively). At 1 year, 91% of the hospital group and 93% of the at-home group were working full time. In a post-hoc subset analysis of patients who were unconscious for between 1 and 24 hours (n = 75) follow-ing TBI, the in-hospital group had a significantly greater return-to-duty rate (80% vs. 58%, p = .05, r = .15 [small effect]).	Reliability of outcome measures not reported; pre-study power analysis goals not reached; post-study power analysis indicated N was 1/5 of that required to achieve significance.	The results of this study are not supportive of a major, comprehensive rehabilitation program that includes occupational therapy for restoration of moderate to severe TBI patients to work. Unfortunately, this flawed study may be cited by third-party payers to deny in-hospital intensive therapy. It is imperative that occupational therapists who treat patients with traumatic brain injuries conduct studies of the efficacy and cost-effectiveness of at-home occupational therapy programs to ensure ongoing coverage of

services. Because this study reports such high percentages of return to work that is not common in the brain injury literature, it is imperative that the study be repeated in a non-military, less standardized (more ecological) setting to verify the finding.

Salazar, A. M., Warden, D. L., Schwab, K., Spector, J., Braverman, S., Waler, J., et al. (2000). Cognitive rehabilitation for traumatic brain injury: A randomized trial. *JAMA, 283,* 3075–3081.

| Sohlberg et al. (2007) | Evaluate the effectiveness of different types of prompts delivered via a handheld electronic device for pedestrians with severe cognitive impairments following acquired brain injury (ABI) | II—Nonrandomized controlled design using a within-subjects comparison

N = 20 adults with ABI with the ability to walk or use a mobility device for 1.5 km.; mean age: 47; all participants lived in assisted living facilities and had severe impairments | Participants had four different navigation modes delivered on a wrist-worn navigation device: aerial map images, point-of-view map image, text-based instruction with no image, and audio instructions with no image. Participants walked four equivalent routes. Participants served as their own controls.

Outcome measures:
■ Accuracy
■ Confidence during navigation. | Results indicated that the participants performed significantly better when using the audio-only prompts versus the aerial image or point-of-view prompts. | Small sample size; lack of randomization to prompt mode; study limited to those with severe impairment, making it difficult to generalize to other impairment levels | The need to visually scan and simultaneously move while navigating the environment made speech-based prompts from a handheld electronic device (vs. text or visual displays) more effective in assisting individuals with traumatic brain injury and cognitive impairments travel in their communities. Occupational therapists should explore the use of simple auditory handheld devices (i.e., digital recorders) to assist in community mobility and topographical orientation. |

Sohlberg, M. M., Fickas, S., Hung, P., & Fortier, A. (2007). A comparison of four prompt modes for route finding for community travellers with severe cognitive impairments. *Brain Injury, 21,* 531–538.

(continued)

EVIDENCE TABLE. FOCUSED QUESTION 4 (cont.)

Author/Year	Study Objectives	Level/Design/ Participants	Intervention and Outcome Measures	Results	Study Limitations	Implications for Occupational Therapy
Boman et al. (2007)	Evaluate the effectiveness of the use of electronic aids to daily living (EADL) for persons with memory impairments following acquired brain injury (ABI)	III—Pretest–posttest design *N* = 8 participants with poor to moderate memory impairment and independent or minimal assistance needed for self-care, and no other cognitive impairments such as aphasia. Ages 28–53.	*Intervention:* Participants stayed in two apartments equipped with both basic and advanced EADL for 4–6 months during an intervention time of 2 years. Errorless learning was included in the instruction method. *Outcome measures:* • Canadian Occupational Performance Measure (COPM) • Sickness Impact Profile (SIP) • Structured observations • Self-rating of EADL • Quality of Life Visual Analogue Scale.	There was a significant improvement in the participants' self-perceived abilities to perform the most important activities and self-perceived quality of life between pre- and postintervention. There was also a significant improvement on the body care and psychosocial function subsets of the SIP. Occupational performance was improved as observed by the COPM.	Small sample size; lack of control group; several participants had difficulty completing certain outcome measures.	Occupational therapists should consider using EADLs to facilitate everyday activities and improve satisfaction with occupational performance and quality of life for people with memory impairments. EADLs should be selected and adjusted to meet individual client's needs and residual impairments.

Boman, I-L., Tham, K., Granqvist, A., Bartfai, A., & Hemmingsson, H. (2007). Using electronic aids to daily living after acquired brain injury: A study of the learning process and the usability. *Disability and Rehabilitation: Assistive Technology, 2,* 23–33.

Executive Function

Goverover et al. (2007)	Examine the effects of awareness training on levels of self-awareness and functional performance	I—Randomized controlled trial *N* = 20 persons with moderate to severe traumatic brain injury (TBI) living in the community and attending an outpatient cognitive rehabilitation program, randomized to groups	*Experimental (N* = 10): 6 45-minute sessions over 3 weeks of self-awareness training during the performance of instrumental activities of daily living (IADLs; e.g., birthday gift preparation, pay telephone bill, prepare a birthday cake). Participants predicted performance pre- and posttask and anticipated need for strategies and assistance. Clients wrote journal about performance.	Experimental group significantly improved in IADL performance and self-regulation. No significant difference noted between groups in task-specific self-awareness, general self-awareness, or community integration.	Small sample recruited from only 1 treatment setting, limited number of treatment sessions, limited follow-up	Awareness training may be effective in improving self-awareness during the performance of IADLs. Use of real-world activities provides opportunities to explore current abilities and select compensatory strategies

			Control (N = 10): Conventional therapeutic practice of same IADLs *Outcome measures:* ■ Assessment of Awareness of Disability ■ Self-Regulation Skills Interview ■ Assessment of Motor and Process Skills ■ Awareness Questionnaire ■ Community Integration Questionnaire ■ Satisfaction with quality of care questionnaire.		

Goverover, Y., Johnston, M. V., Toglia, J., & DeLuca, J. (2007). Treatment to improve self-awareness in persons with acquired brain injury. *Brain Injury, 21,* 913–923.

| Levine et al. (2000) | Determine the effectiveness of Goal Management Training (GMT) for persons with traumatic brain injury (TBI) to the frontal lobes | I—Randomized controlled trial

N = 30 persons with moderate TBI, randomized to group | *Experimental:* GMT that includes orienting, selecting goals, partitioning goals into subgoals, encoding and retaining goals and subgoals, monitoring of outcome (match between goal and outcome of action).

Control: Motor skills training (MST) involving reading and tracing mirror-reversed text and designs

Outcome measures: Everyday paper-and-pencil tasks (proofreading, room layout, grouping according to multiple categories). | *Accuracy:* There was a significant difference between groups on proofreading task, but the difference was due to more errors by controls rather than improvement by experimental. The GMT group performed significantly better on the grouping task than did the MST group. Both groups improved on the room layout task; not significant between groups.

Speed: The GMT group slowed significantly on the proofreading task (reflecting increased care and attention) from pretest to posttest as compared to the MST group, which | Task-specific training was shown to cause some improvement in the particular tasks featured in the training in persons who had moderate brain injury of years' standing. However, whether the training can be generalized to non-practiced occupational tasks requires study. Caution must be exercised regarding the authors' conclusion that GMT was effective; the results showed that one difference (proofreading) between groups was because of deterioration of the control group, not improvement of the treatment group. The GMT group outperformed the control

The tasks used to measure were included in the training although the researchers used different versions. The validity and reliability of the outcome measures were not reported. Blinding of evaluator not reported. |

(continued)

EVIDENCE TABLE. FOCUSED QUESTION 4 (cont.)

Author/Year	Study Objectives	Level/Design/ Participants	Intervention and Outcome Measures	Results	Study Limitations	Implications for Occupational Therapy
Levine et al. (2000) (cont.)				did not slow significantly. Both groups reduced time on the room layout and grouping tasks, but not significantly.		group on only one task (grouping) in accuracy and on one task (proofreading) for speed

Levine, B., Robertson, I. H., Clare, L., Carter, G., Hong, J., Wilson, B. A., et al. (2000). Rehabilitation of executive functioning: An experimental–clinical validation of Goal Management Training. *Journal of the International Neuropsychological Society, 6,* 299–312.

Author/Year	Study Objectives	Level/Design/ Participants	Intervention and Outcome Measures	Results	Study Limitations	Implications for Occupational Therapy
Manly et al. (2002)	Examine whether auditory stimuli that interrupt activity would cause patients to pause, evaluate, plan, and change track and thereby improve performance of a complex (multistep) task	I—One group repeated measures crossover design $N = 10$ patients with brain injury (BI; mean age = 32 years; all >1 year posttrauma; mean current IQ = 97) and 24 volunteer controls The controls were used to obtain standard data; the participants with BI were used to test the question.	Subjects were randomly assigned to one of two conditions (alerting to think about present task or control). *Outcome measures:* Six Elements task, Hotel subtest, which was comprised of 6 activities commonly required when running a hotel; this measures the participant's ability to engage and break away from tasks to engage in another task.	There was a significant improvement in the number of tasks started in the alerting condition compared to the control condition. Under the alerted condition, the participants performed time allocation to each task significantly better than under the control condition. There was no significant difference between conditions in time spent in each activity or in time-specific responses or in use of the clock. The alert did not prompt a switch in tasks.	Participants were volunteers, but no information was provided concerning the circumstances of volunteering. Intervention was applied in one 15-min period in a laboratory. Reliability and validity of the outcome measure not reported. Administrator of the outcome measure was not reported.	The use of alerting tones did not interrupt ongoing behavior and focus the patient onto a different task; therefore, this intervention would not be an occupational therapist would choose to use with patients with brain injury. Good information regarding occupational performance can be obtained from simulated "real-life" assessments, which is common to occupational therapy. The improved performance may have occurred due to practice. Although the researchers took care to control for practice effects by changing the versions of the test for the two administrations, they only changed the content, not the processes. Perhaps practice with the process enabled

Manly, T., Hawkins, K., Evans, J., Woldt, K., & Robertson, I. H. (2002). Rehabilitation of executive function: Facilitation of effective goal management on complex tasks using periodic auditory alerts. *Neuropsychologia, 40,* 271–281.

Attention

Novack et al. (1996)	Compare the effects of a focused attention remediation program to an unstructured stimulation program on attentional skills among individuals undergoing acute rehabilitation after traumatic brain injury (TBI) with the expectation that the focused program will promote more extensive recovery; examine functional recovery using the Functional Independence Measure (FIM) with the expectation that improved attentional skills resulting from the focused program will be associated with greater functional independence	I—Matched pairs, randomized controlled trial *N* = 44 persons with acute, severe TBI, matched on age, education, time since injury to when remediation began, and number of remediation sessions; mean age = 27 yrs; mean education = 11.5 yrs; mean onset to intervention ~6 weeks; mean number of sessions prior to selection ~20.5	*Experimental:* Focused stimulation program *Control:* Unstructured stimulation program *Outcome measure:* FIM.	There was no significant difference between groups at admission or at discharge. There was a significant effect for time because the participants performed significantly better at discharge than at admission. This was true for all scores, including the FIM. There was no significant difference between groups on either the motor or cognitive subtests of the FIM at admission or at discharge. Participants made an average improvement of 30 points on the motor portion of the FIM and 10 points on the cognitive portion of the FIM over the treatment period.	Spontaneous recovery is a plausible explanation for the outcome; attrition (FIM used for only 24 subjects) This study offers no guidance for therapy because the effects seen may be accounted for by spontaneous recovery. It indicates that patients with severe TBI can improve in their activities of daily living, although we do not know whether that was due to spontaneous recovery or the assistance of rehabilitation since there was no-treatment group.

Novack, T. A., Caldwell, S. G., Duke, L. W., Bergquist, T. F., & Gage, R. G. (1996). Focused versus unstructured intervention for attention deficits after traumatic brain injury. *Journal of Head Trauma Rehabilitation, 11,* 52–60.

participants to improve regardless of the particular requirements. It is important for occupational therapists to know this because it would support therapeutic use of practice. Occupational therapists need to study the process/content question further under controlled conditions.

(continued)

EVIDENCE TABLE. FOCUSED QUESTION 4 (cont.)

Author/Year	Study Objectives	Level/Design/ Participants	Intervention and Outcome Measures	Results	Study Limitations	Implications for Occupational Therapy
Park & Ingles (2001)	Examine the efficacy of current attention rehabilitation after an acquired brain injury meta-analytically; identify methodological factors that may contribute to the variability reported in the literature; evaluate whether direct-training and specific-skill programs differ in their effectiveness	I—Meta-analysis $N = 30$ studies involving 359 participants and yielded 481 effect size estimates	67% of studies included both auditory and visual exercises; 83% of studies specified that the tasks were graduated in difficulty; 77% of the studies indicated that feedback on training performance was provided. Number of training tasks varied. Mean = 7.7, standard deviation = 8.7, $n = 23$, with 50% of studies providing 5 or more tasks. 89% of programs had a component in which speeded or paced performance was encouraged. In 50% of studies, treatment was via computer. Mean treatment time was 31 hours. *Outcome measure:* Effect size.	All measures of cognitive function (e.g., attention, learning, memory) improved significantly when assessed by pretest–posttest-only type of estimate; however, no measure of cognitive function improved significantly when measured by the pre–post with control estimates. The effect sizes were all <.15 (small effect). The first finding may be attributed to practice effects. The pre–post with control effect size estimates for the different measures of specific skills (e.g., activities of daily living, driving, attention behavior) were all >.49 (moderate effect); driving and attention behavior improved significantly after training. In the 12 studies that investigated the efficacy of direct retraining with control condition, 6 reported no statistically significant improvement set of studies seemed to be more attributable to the acquisition of specific skills rather than to re-training of attention.	None	Training in tasks required in a person's daily life is more likely to result in improved performance than attempts to retrain attentional skills generally. This conclusion supports the advocated practice of occupational therapy, in which emphasis is placed on training of tasks and activities of everyday occupational performance.

Park, N. W., & Ingles, J. L. (2001). Effectiveness of attention rehabilitation after an acquired brain injury: A meta-analysis. *Neuropsychology, 15,* 199–210. Also published in 2000 in *Brain and Cognition, 44,* 1–18.

Source	Purpose	Design/Methodology	Intervention/Outcome measures	Results	Comments
Sohlberg et al. (2000)	Determine whether there are quantitative and/or qualitative differences in the changes reported by participants after Attention Process Therapy (APT) compared to an educational and support method; examine whether responses to APT and the information reveal insights about the effects of practice	I—Two group crossover design with random assignment to group *N* = 14 persons with acquired brain injury, in chronic phase Group 2 (*N* = 7) was 5 yrs older and superior on neuropsychological tests at the start of the study	*Condition A:* Participated in APT, an intervention using hierarchically organized tasks that exercise different components of attention (sustained, selective, alternating, divided) *Condition B:* Received brain injury education, supportive listening, and relaxation training *Outcome measures:* ■ 3 questionnaires assessing perceptions of the impact of attention deficits on daily living, specifically developed to be used with persons who have traumatic brain injury ■ Structured interview.	There was a strong dissociation between cognitive performance (the objective neuropsychological tests) and psychosocial function (the subjective interview). The number of changes in thinking ability reported in interview was significantly greater after APT than education. More memory and attention changes (1.59) were reported than psychosocial functions (.59). The smallest number of changes reported was in everyday functions (.05). More memory and attention changes were reported after APT training than education. More psychosocial changes were reported after education than APT. The results of the study indicate that practice, whether by repeating the assessment tasks or from participating in the training of general processes using APT, improves performance	Unequal group characteristics at start of study, despite random assignment to group. Experimental treatment administered at 2½ times intensity of control treatment. Occupational therapists use structured interview as an assessment measure. In this study, the structured interview was found to be a valuable evaluation procedure to ascertain how attention was employed in day-to-day life and the nature of the impact of attentional deficits in daily life. Practice was important to improve performance within the cognitive realm, but the changes did not transfer to daily life.

Sohlberg, M. M., McLaughlin, K. A., Pavese, A., Heidrich, A., & Posner, M. I. (2000). Evaluation of attention process training and brain injury education in persons with acquired brain injury. *Journal of Clinical and Experimental Neuropsychology, 22,* 656–676.

(continued)

EVIDENCE TABLE. FOCUSED QUESTION 4 (cont.)

Author/Year	Study Objectives	Level/Design/ Participants	Intervention and Outcome Measures	Results	Study Limitations	Implications for Occupational Therapy
Memory						
Hart et al. (2002)	Determine whether use of an electronic device (a voice organizer) could help clients with traumatic brain injury (TBI) remember and articulate therapy goals	I—One group, repeated measures design with conditions randomized $N = 10$ persons with moderate to severe TBI; mean age = 31.5 (range = 19–45); 9 > 1-year postinjury, 1 at 3-mos postinjury; all engaged in postacute therapies for 1 to 43 months (mean = 11.8)	*Experimental:* Use of a personal digital assistant (PDA) to remind the participant about therapy goals. The PDA (Parrot Voice Mate III) reminded the client several times a day about 3 of the 6 goals, randomly chosen. *Control:* Remember 3 randomly chosen goals without aid of PDA or other orthosis. *Outcome measures:* Recall of 6 goals under 2 conditions: free recall and cued recall.	There was no resistance to use of the device. No participant missed a full day's worth of listening episodes. The results showed that using a voice organizer to listen to recorded goals at multiple, consistent times each day was effective in enhancing recall of goals at the verbal level, with and without the addition of brief reminder cues. All 10 participants liked using the device.	None	Occupational therapists can join in the continued research of this promising intervention to evaluate what effect, if any, recall of goals supported by a PDA has on behavior of persons with moderate to severe TBI and whether a device like a PDA can be used to influence important behaviors more directly through reminders throughout the day. The design of the research reported in this study offers occupational therapists a good model to use in clinical research, where participants are few and heterogeneous.

Hart, T., Hawkey, K.., & Whyte, J. (2002). Use of a portable voice organizer to remember therapy goals in traumatic brain injury rehabilitation: A within-subjects trial. *Journal of Head Trauma Rehabilitation, 17,* 556–570.

Kessels & de Haan (2003)	Quantitatively investigate the effects of vanishing cues and errorless learning in persons with memory impairments and amnesia and discuss the outcome and applicability to memory rehabilitation	I—Meta-analysis $N =$ Literature search in Medline (1996–2002), PsychINFO (1887–2002), and reference lists of identified studies; 27 studies were identified, 11 met criteria	Vanishing cues method of teaching persons with memory disorders and errorless learning method of teaching patients versus control conditions, usually trial-and-error learning *Outcome measures:* Weighted (by sample size) effect size (e.g., the difference between intervention and control performance divided by the pooled standard deviation).	Overall effect sizes for errorless learning or vanishing cues compared to errorful learning or standard anticipation (control conditions) was 0.59 (a moderate effect). Effect size for errorless learning compared to trial and error learning was 0.87 (large effect). Effect size for vanishing cues compared to trial and error learning was 0.27 (small effect).	None	This meta-analysis suggests that the use of the principle of errorless learning in relearning habitual occupational performance tasks would be an effective method of teaching patients with severe memory impairments. Because the material to be learned in the studies of this meta-analysis was lists of names and other laboratory tasks,

further research by occupational therapists is needed using habitual occupational tasks as the material to be learned.

Kessels, R. P. C., & de Haan, E. H. F. (2003). Implicit learning in memory rehabilitation: A meta-analysis on errorless learning and vanishing cue methods. *Journal of Clinical and Experimental Neuropsychology, 25,* 805–814.

| Loya (1999) | Quantitatively determine the magnitude and efficacy of memory rehabilitation in moderate to severe traumatic brain injury (TBI); identify the most efficacious treatment strategies for improving postinjury memory functioning; identify moderating variables that facilitate the rehabilitation process | I—Meta-analysis

N = Electronic databases and 54 journals from 1970 through 1999 pertinent to memory rehabilitation were searched; 117 articles retrieved, 14 met inclusion criteria | Emphases of cognitive rehabilitation: restorative (visualization, mnemonics); compensatory (internal mnemonics and external memory aids); and external change/adapt environment

Outcome measures:
■ Weighted effect size *d*
■ Test of homogeneity
■ File drawer calculation. | 9/14 studies used various forms of visual and/or verbal imagery, with a grand mean weighted effect size for between-group studies of .47. There was a significant, positive outcome resulting from memory rehabilitation among TBI survivors. Homogeneity of effect size estimates obviated further analyses to rank order treatments by their effectiveness or to identify moderator variables. The attribution of superiority of one intervention over another cannot be justified on the basis of available research. | None | Restorative and compensatory treatment that involves verbal and visual imagery, as well as other treatments to remind the person about upcoming events, and treatments that focus on altering the environment to prompt remembering by the patient have been found to be efficacious for adolescents and adults with moderate to severe traumatic brain injury and can be validly included into practice. This meta-analysis provides support for the coverage of payment for occupational therapy services that include these treatments. The meta-analysis further provides support for inclusion of planning for, carrying out, and evaluating these treatments in the education and training of occupational therapy students. |

Loya, G. J. (1999). *Efficacy of memory rehabilitation among adolescent and adult TBI survivors: A meta-analysis.* Unpublished doctoral dissertation, University of Nebraska, Lincoln.

(continued)

EVIDENCE TABLE. FOCUSED QUESTION 4 *(cont.)*

Author/Year	Study Objectives	Level/Design/ Participants	Intervention and Outcome Measures	Results	Study Limitations	Implications for Occupational Therapy
Paniak et al. (1998)	Determine whether extensive treatment (treatment-as-needed; TAN) was significantly more effective than a single session (SS) of educational and emotionally reassuring intervention	I—Randomized controlled trial *N* = 119 persons with mild traumatic brain injury (MTBI) enrolled. 111 participants completed the study (52 men, 59 women); mean age = 32.7 for SS and 33.6 for TAN; education = 13.7 yrs for SS and 14.1 yrs for TAN	*SS:* Met with the primary investigator and discussed any concerns about head injury; read *The Unseen Injury—Minor Head Trauma* (Kay, 1986) and discussed any comments or questions *TAN:* The same treatment as SS, but also had a 3–4 hr neuropsychological and personality assessment and feedback, a consultation with a physical therapist, and further treatment-as-needed for MTBI complaints *Outcome measures:* ■ Community Reintegration Questionnaire (CIQ) ■ Problem Checklist (PCL) ■ SF–36 (Short Form).	*CIQ:* No statistically significant effect for time, group, or group by time interaction. *Occupational status:* Statistically significant effect for time but not for treatment group or treatment by time interaction. Mean number of days before return to full-time pre-injury vocational activity averaged 28.7 days and did not differ between groups. *SF–36:* Statistically significant effect for time, but not group or time by group interaction. *PCL:* Statistically significant effect for time, but not group or time by group interaction. No significant difference between groups in satisfaction with treatment scores.	The independent variable (amount of therapy) may have been compromised (equalized between groups) because the TAN group reported a median of only 1 further treatment after the initial educational treatment. No reliability or validity information given for 3 outcome measures. No information was given concerning ceiling effects on the CIQ, which are likely in this population.	Neither group improved in community integration (occupational performance) as a result of either of these treatments. In light of this, occupational therapists should investigate what the minimal effective therapy is for patients they see with MTBI; document the improvements in occupational performance as a result of this therapy; and ascertain the profile of patients who are satisfactorily helped to recover in all areas of their occupational performance by a brief engagement in occupational therapy and those who require more therapy aimed at organizational and other executive skills that may be deficient secondary to MTBI.

Paniak, C., Toller-Lobe, G., Durand, A., & Nagy, J. (1998). A randomized trial of two treatments for mild traumatic brain injury. *Brain Injury, 12,* 1011–1023.

| Paniak et al. (2000) | Test the hypothesis that differences between treatment groups on the outcome measures would continue to be negligible in size at the 12-month follow-up and that gains shown at 3 months postinjury would be maintained at 12 months | I—Randomized trial

$N = 105$ persons with mild traumatic brain injury (MTBI), 12 months postinjury, randomized to group

Single session (SS) group = 53

Treat-as-needed (TAN) group = 52 | SS: Aims of the one-time-only intervention were to legitimize the participants' experience as being "real" and educate them regarding common complaints following MTBI.

TAN: The same treatment as SS, but also had a neuropsychological and personality assessment and feedback, a consultation with a physical therapist, and further treatment-as-needed for MTBI complaints.

Outcome measures:
■ Problem checklist (PCL)
■ Community Integration Questionnaire (CIQ); 13 items regarding home, social role, and productive activity
■ SF–36: Self-rating scale to determine perceptions of one's mental health and physical health. | There were no significant changes in the PCL, CIQ, or SF–36 between 3 and 12 months postinjury and there were no significant differences between groups. | Information that would allow determination of threats to internal validity was not included in this report. Validity and reliability of the outcome measures were not reported. Outcomes were obtained via telephone at 3 months and 12 months postinjury. | This study indicates that persons with mild traumatic brain injury can benefit from a well-designed intervention offered early in recovery that educates the patient concerning what he or she can expect in terms of functioning, reassures him or her about recovery, and, although not mentioned in this article, offers suggestions of strategies to circumvent anticipated problems as recovery occurs. Occupational therapists can provide this service economically because they address daily functioning, should be included when this intervention is offered to patients. |

Paniak, C., Toller-Lobe, G., Reynolds, S., Melnyk, A., & Nagy, J. (2000). A randomized trial of two treatments for mild traumatic brain injury: 1 year follow-up. *Brain Injury, 14,* 219–226.

(continued)

EVIDENCE TABLE. FOCUSED QUESTION 4 (cont.)

Author/Year	Study Objectives	Level/Design/ Participants	Intervention and Outcome Measures	Results	Study Limitations	Implications for Occupational Therapy
Thickpenny-Davis & Barker-Collo (2007)	Evaluate the effectiveness of a memory rehabilitation program on impaired memory functioning	I—Randomized controlled trial *N* = 12 adults (10 with traumatic brain injury [TBI], 2 with cerebral vascular accidents) randomized to treatment (*n* = 6) or waitlist control (*n* = 6)	Eight learning modules, 1 hour, twice per week for 4 weeks, including didactic information about memory and memory strategies, small group activities, discussion, and inclusion of errorless learning techniques. *Outcome measures:* ■ California Verbal Learning Test ■ Wechsler Memory Scale–Revised, Logical Memory Subtest ■ Visual Paired Associates ■ Memory in everyday life and aids and strategies questionnaire ■ Behavioral indices of memory impairment checklist.	Participants in the memory intervention group had significant improvement at 1-month follow-up than wait-list controls on knowledge of memory and memory strategies, use of memory aids and strategies, decreased behaviors indicative of memory impairment, and a positive effect on neuropsychological assessments of memory.	Small sample size. As the sample had mostly severe TBI, it is difficult to generalize to mild or moderate TBI. Limited length of follow-up	While the role of occupational therapy is not detailed in this study, the intervention described falls within the scope of occupational therapy practice. Occupational therapists should consider engaging clients with memory impairments in group-based intervention focused on learning strategies, memory aids, and errorless learning techniques.

Thickpenny-Davis, K. L., & Barker-Collo, S. L. (2007). Evaluation of a structured group format memory rehabilitation program for adults following brain injury. *Journal of Head Trauma Rehabilitation, 22,* 303–313.

| Watanabe et al. (1998) | Examine the relationship among age, injury severity, and use of calendar on emergence from posttraumatic amnesia (PTA) | I—Randomized trial. $N = 32$ persons with PTA secondary to traumatic brain injury (TBI; 50%) or other brain disorders. There were equal numbers of TBI patients in each group. Randomized to condition by room assignment. | *Experimental:* Presence of an 8½-x-11 inch, boldly printed calendar in the patient's room, easily visible to the patient. *Control:* No calendar. *Outcome measure:* Temporal Orientation Test (TOT) administered daily while the patient had access to calendar if in experimental group; which measures orientation to time. Scoring not reported. Discontinued when patient accurate 2 consecutive days or discharged. | Presence of a calendar was not significantly associated with emergence from PTA (answers a different question than that proposed as research objective). | Possible contamination of the control group, who probably received orientation information from other staff or visitors. Details of intervention not included. Validity and reliability of the TOT not reported. Not adequately powered. Statistical analysis changed from planned test of differences between groups to regression analysis because too few participants emerged from PTA. Report of statistical outcomes was incomplete. | This study lacked rigor to establish a causal relationship between use of a calendar and recovery of temporal reorientation. Therapists cannot conclude that calendars are useful or not useful from this study. |

Watanabe, T. K., Black, K. L., Zafonte, R. D., Millis, S. R., & Mann, N. R. (1998). Do calendars enhance posttraumatic temporal orientation? A pilot study. *Brain Injury, 12,* 81–85.

| Wilson, Emslie, et al. (2001) | Determine whether a paging system enabled people with memory and planning problems after brain injury to carry out everyday tasks; answer whether the kind of impairment (e.g., memory or executive functions), the degree of impairment (e.g., mild, moderate, or severe), or both influence the effectiveness of the paging system | I—Randomized control trial, crossover. $N = 143$ persons with brain injury of various types; 44% traumatic brain injury (TBI), 25% stroke. Mean age = 38 yrs, 72% living at home, 73% male. Randomized to group. | *Pager condition:* Carried out in the home and community for 7 weeks. Participants were involved in establishing target behaviors to be monitored throughout the trial. *Wait-list condition:* No therapy for 7 weeks. *Group A:* Pager first, nothing second. *Group B:* Wait list (no treatment) first, pager second. | The results indicate that this particular paging system significantly reduces everyday failures of memory and planning and enables people with brain injury to carry out more everyday tasks at relatively low cost. Less than 50% of the target behaviors were achieved without the pager; 76% were achieved with the pager. 7 weeks after the pager was removed, ~62% | The outcome measure was self-report and left to the patient to fill out daily. No reliability information or compliance information given. | Because of this relatively well-controlled study, occupational therapists can feel relatively confident in recommending the use of a pager system to patients with brain injury who have some insight into their memory and planning problems, can read the pager, and can respond by pushing the correct button on the pager. |

(continued)

Author/Year	Study Objectives	Level/Design/Participants	Intervention and Outcome Measures	Results	Study Limitations	Implications for Occupational Therapy
Wilson, Emslie, et al. (2001) (cont.)			*Outcome measures:* 4–7 item questionnaire devised for each participant to fill out daily to determine whether the person had remembered to do targeted tasks without being reminded.	of the behaviors were achieved, still significantly more than at baseline. Minimal training was needed.		

Wilson, B. A., Emslie, H. C., Quirk, K., & Evans, J. J. (2001). Reducing everyday memory and planning problems by means of a paging system: A randomized control crossover design. *Journal of Neurology, Neurosurgery, and Psychiatry, 70,* 477–482.

Burke et al. (2001)	Test a tracking system for patients with traumatic brain injury (TBI) that couples the indoor fluorescent light fixture-based location system ("Talking Lights") with handheld computer technology to provide greater independence in patients' adherence to therapy schedules without staff prompting; compare a manual staffing intervention strategy using a reminder notebook and verbal prompts from the staff with the automated strategy	II—Two condition, non-randomized, repeated measures design N = 5 persons with brain damage; 3 acquired brain injury, 2 subarachnoid hemorrhage secondary to clipped intracerebral aneurysms; mean age: 50 yrs (range: 20–72)	*Experimental condition:* The patient locator and minder (PLAM) is a system that includes a handheld computer and indoor fluorescent light fixture-based location system ("Talking Lights"). It provides verbal cues that seize the patients' attention and trigger their memory to begin traveling to a destination. The PLAM also provides feedback regarding how well the patient is doing in traveling toward the destination and redirects him or her if necessary. *Control condition:* Manual staffing intervention—Use of a reminder notebook and verbal prompts from staff. Notebook had schedule of the day, including therapies, meals, and medications.	With the PLAM system, the average number of human prompts dropped more than 50%. The number of sessions requiring no prompting increased from 7% to 44%, a significant increase. During the baseline condition, the patients arrived at their activities on average 4.8 min late (range 2–7 min) while they arrived an average of 1.3 min *early* (range 4.6 min early to 2.9 min late) during the experimental condition, an improvement of 6.1 min over the human prompt system.	Only 3 of the 5 participants had traumatic brain injury. Sampling process not described. The two conditions were of different durations: 3 days (experimental) versus 1 week (control). The reliability of the outcome measure was not reported, nor was the training given to the staff who recorded the data. Statistical analytical methods are questionable. Statistic not reported. Their conclusion regarding the PLAM prompting facilitated learning exceeded their data—they did not measure learning.	This exploratory study indicates that computerized cognitive orthoses can be more effective than the common occupational therapy intervention of a notebook memory aid.

Outcome measures: Number of human prompts necessary to direct a patient to, and ensure arrival at, a scheduled therapy destination. Proportion of therapy sessions requiring no prompting.

Burke, D. T., Leeb, S. B., Hinman, R. T., Lupton, E. C., Burke, J., Schneider, J. C., et al. (2001). Using Talking Lights to assist brain-injured patients with daily inpatient therapeutic schedule. *Journal of Head Trauma Rehabilitation, 16,* 284–291.

Cicerone et al. (2004)	Compare the effectiveness relative to community integration of a program of holistic, intensive, cognitive rehabilitation with conventional rehabilitation for persons with traumatic brain injury (TBI); assess participants' satisfaction with their functioning after treatment	II—Two-group, pretest–posttest nonrandomized design *N* = 56—40 men, 16 women; admitted between January 1997 and December 1998; mean age: 37; mean yrs of education: 13; 89% competitively employed before injury; 89% with moderate to severe TBI, 11% mild	*Experimental:* Intensive Cognitive Rehabilitation Program (ICRP); *n* = 27. Administered by neuropsychologists. *Control:* Standard Rehabilitation Program (SRP); *n* = 29. Administered by a physical therapist, occupational therapist, speech therapist, and neuropsychologist *Outcome measures:* ■ Community Integration Questionnaire (CIQ) ■ Quality of Community Integration Questionnaire (QCIQ). ■ Subscale of QCIQ addressing participants' satisfaction with cognitive functioning (QCOG)	Both groups showed significant improvement on the CIQ, with the ICRP group exhibiting a significant treatment effect compared to the SRP group. Among the participants receiving ICRP, 52% showed clinically significant improvement on the CIQ compared with 31% of those receiving SRP. Among SRP participants, 7% showed clinically significant decline on the CIQ, whereas none of the ICRP participants showed decline. SRP participants expressed significantly greater satisfaction with their community functioning than did the ICRP group. The SRP group also	Members of the SRP group were significantly more acutely injured than the ICRP group, providing an alternate explanation for outcome (spontaneous recovery). Intervention contamination may have occurred; no information was supplied regarding control for this. Because the sampling bias provides an alternate explanation for the outcome, this study does not offer clear direction for therapy for patients post-TBI. Neither program presented in this study was ineffective; each had a different goal (one community reintegration and the other neurorehabilitation). Patients in both groups improved significantly on the CIQ, whereas only those in the ICRP program were reported to have received actual training in applying their therapeutic gains to everyday community living. Other outcomes expected from the neurorehabilitation program were not measured.

(continued)

Author/Year	Study Objectives	Level/Design/ Participants	Intervention and Outcome Measures	Results	Study Limitations	Implications for Occupational Therapy
Cicerone et al. (2004) *(cont.)*				reported greater satisfaction with their cognitive functioning, but the overall difference between groups on the QCIQ was not significant.		Although the participants in the SRP group were significantly more satisfied with their community integration and cognitive skills applied to daily life, this probably reflects that their injuries were recent and a lack of time living with the disability. A randomized controlled study of two different rehabilitation programs with the same outcome goal is needed to measure the relative effectiveness of the intensive cognitive rehabilitation program.

Cicerone, K. D., Mott, T., Azulay, J., & Friel, J. C. (2004). Community integration and satisfaction with functioning after intensive cognitive rehabilitation for traumatic brain injury. *Archives of Physical Medicine and Rehabilitation, 85,* 943–950.

| Freeman et al. (1992) | Investigate the efficacy of memory retraining in patients with traumatic brain injury (TBI) using executive and compensatory memory retraining strategies | II—Two group pretest-posttest

N = 12 persons with acquired head injury with cognitive deficit

Treatment group = 6 persons referred for cognitive treatment

Control = 6 persons referred for neuropsychological evaluation | Memory retraining consisting of read aloud paragraph retention. Techniques to enhance retention included note taking in a memory notebook; self-monitoring skills; prompting from staff; restating presented material in own words; using imagery; and providing specific feedback concerning success.
Control: No treatment.

Outcome measure:
Paragraph Memory Task—Score of ideas and details identified for a total of 100 points per paragraph. | The treatment group performed significantly better than the control at posttest and the effect was strong ($t_{(10)}$ = 2.32, p = 0.02, r = .59).

The authors concluded that the inclusion of memory retraining in cognitive remediation programs can improve memory function in patients with TBI. Because members of the treatment group were in the chronic stage of recovery, the significant recovery can be attributed to the treatment rather than spontaneous recovery. | The groups were referred for different reasons and could therefore have differed in some way, although they were not significantly different in IQ or memory deficit. The treatment group was significantly more chronic than the control group (33 months post vs. 12 months post). Reliability and validity of outcome measure not reported. Binding of evaluator was not reported. | Task-specific training was shown to cause improvement in the particular tasks that were practiced in persons with longstanding TBI. However, whether the improvement generalizes to everyday tasks cannot be determined from this study. |

Freeman, M. R., Mittenberg, W., Dicowden, M., & Bat-ami, M. (1992). Executive and compensatory memory retraining in traumatic brain injury. *Brain Injury, 6,* 65–70.

| Tam & Man (2004) | Compare the effectiveness of four different computer-assisted memory training strategies based on the behavioral approach | II—Five group, pretest–posttest design

Subjects randomly assigned to 1 of 4 experimental groups, but control subjects "chosen." Analysis was on pretest to posttest, not across groups.

$N = 32$; 24 experimental and 8 control; Hong Kong Chinese; 18 male, 14 female; memory deficits secondary to closed head injury

Experimental mean age: 36.5 yrs; control mean age: 45 yrs. | Each program included 4 modules that were similar across programs and related to important daily functions: remembering names and faces, remembering to do something, remembering what people say, and remembering where something was put.

Group 1: Self-paced practice; $n = 6$ or 7

Group 2: Visual presentation; $n = 6$

Group 3: Multisensory feedback; $n = 6$ or 7

Group 4: Personalized training content; $n = 6$

Group 5: No treatment control; $n = 8$

Outcome measures:
■ Self-efficacy rating scale
■ Rivermead Behavioural Memory Test (RBMT). | No significant improvement on the RBMT by any of the groups. The feedback group showed a significant ($p < 0.05$) gain in self-efficacy score; no other group improved significantly.

All 4 computer groups improved significantly ($p < 0.05$) on the computer quiz scores using their own module as compared to before treatment.

Authors' conclusion: The results of the present study evidenced the effectiveness of using computers in patients' cognitive rehabilitation. The feedback group showed the greatest percentage of improvement of self-efficacy; this implies that feedback is a crucial factor to improve self-efficacy. | Did not compare across groups to determine whether any one of the treatments is significantly better than another. Repeated t tests without correction were used to test pre–posttest effects. No information to allow judgment of threats to validity of independent variable.

The first conclusion is inaccurate; there was no significant improvement on a standardized test of memory. | The outcome of this study verifies to therapists that clear, consistent, nonjudgmental feedback is likely to increase a person's self-efficacy if the tasks being learned are within the person's capabilities, even if challenging. It does not support the effectiveness of computer-assisted programs to improve memory. |

Tam, S-F., & Man, W-K. (2004). Evaluating computer-assisted memory retraining programmes for people with post-head injury amnesia. *Brain Injury, 18,* 461–470.

(continued)

EVIDENCE TABLE. FOCUSED QUESTION 4 *(cont.)*

Author/Year	Study Objectives	Level/Design/ Participants	Intervention and Outcome Measures	Results	Study Limitations	Implications for Occupational Therapy
Wright, Rogers, Hall, Wilson, Evans, & Emslie (2001)	Replicate previous work; examine the hypothesis that encouraging people to use a pocket computer more often for other activities, such as games, will increase the use of the memory aids	II—One group, repeated measures, counter-balanced design $N = 12$; 10 male, 2 female; 9 with traumatic brain injury (TBI), 2 with subarachnoid hemorrhage; 1 not classified; mean age: 39 yrs (range 19–57); mean duration since injury: 3 yrs (range 1–10 yrs). Two had previously used NeuroPage.	Both computers (Hewlett Packard [HP] 360LX and Casio E10) had an appointment diary and notebook. These were linked so that from a diary entry, participants could link to a notebook page containing details about the situation of the diary entry. A memory aid to-do list was added and three games chosen to encourage planning and remembering were included in each computer. Pairs, Hangman, and Mosaic were added to one computer. Chess, Crosswords, and Solitaire were added to the second. *Outcome measures:* Attitude toward ease of use of computers on a 1–10 point scale; usage by time-stamped computer log file of entries made.	All participants could use the computers and 83% (10/12) found them useful. Mean attitude ratings (maximum = 10) for appointment diary = 7.3; notebook = 5–6.7; to-do list = 5.8. Frequency games played = 5.4. The mean number of new entries made to each computer was Casio = 37 ($\pm$33) and HP = 47 ($\pm$43). The diary features used most often were auditory alarms (54% total entries) and repeated entries (46% total entries). People categorized as high users made significantly more new diary entries than people who were not. The use of games did not correlate with computer usage as memory aid.	Sample and sampling procedures not fully explained. No standardized outcome measures with established reliability. Little detail concerning possible threats to internal validity (e.g., blinded evaluation, contamination or co-intervention).	This study confirms the previous study. Although all participants were able to use the computers after training, only 83% (10/12) found them useful, indicating personal preferences affect choice of memory prosthetic appropriate for particular patients. There was no measure of effectiveness of the memory aids on occupational performance (e.g., medications, keeping appointments), which should be studied.

Wright, P., Rogers, N., Hall, C., Wilson, B., Evans, J., & Emslie, H. (2001). Enhancing an appointment diary on a pocket computer for use by people after brain injury. *International Journal of Rehabilitation Research, 24*, 299–308.

| Wright, Rogers, Hall, Wilson, Evans, Emslie, et al. (2001) | Test whether an interface could be designed for memory aids on pocket computers, including an appointment diary and notebook that could be easily mastered by people with memory problems; compare people's attitudes to and use of pocket computer memory aids when essentially the same interface is made available on a handheld computer with a keyboard (HP) and on a palm-size computer (Casio) having a touch-screen keyboard | II—One group, repeated measures, counterbalanced design

$N = 12$ original + 12 (data-producing group further recruited after large drop out [51%] of first 12 participants); 6 male, 6 female; non-progressive closed head brain injury—most traumatic brain injury (TBI); mean age: 34 yrs (range: 22–54 yrs). Mean duration since injury: 6 yrs (range: 2–12 yrs). 4 had previously used NeuroPage. | Same as above with the exception of the memory aid to-do list and three games.

Outcome measures: Same as above | All participants could use the computers and 83% found them helpful. Amount of use varied widely. The diary was considered more useful than the notebook by 10 out of 12 people (mean scores of 7.6 [out of possible 10] versus 4.8). 9 versus 2 people rated the Casio higher than the HP.

Performance Data (computer logs of actual use): 3 total entries/day, with 1 new entry/day. On average, more diary and notebook entries were made with the Casio than the HP, with wide variation. High use subgroup used HP more to make entries than Casio ($t_{(4} = 2.48$, $p < 0.07$, $r = .77$). Low users made twice as many entries with the Casio than the HP ($t_{(6)} = 4.97$, $p < 0.01$, $r = .89$).

The only statistically reliable difference between the pocket computers was the greater use of alarms for diary entries when using the HP ($t_{(11)} = 2.38$, $p < 0.04$, $r = .58$). | Same as above | This study provides evidence that memory aids (diary, notebook, and links between) on a handheld computer that has a custom-designed interface to allow patients with brain injury to use the system by ticking off choices (problem-solving skills) rather than memory can be useful for some persons with brain injury. Although all participants were able to use the computers after training, only 83% (10/12) found them useful, indicating personal preferences affect choice of memory prosthetic appropriate for particular patients. There was no measure of effectiveness of the memory aids on occupational performance (e.g., medications, keeping appointments), which should be studied. |

Wright, P., Rogers, N., Hall, C., Wilson, B., Evans, J., Emslie, H., et al. (2001). Comparison of pocket-computer memory aids for people with brain injury. *Brain Injury, 15,* 787–800.

(continued)

Author/Year	Study Objectives	Level/Design/ Participants	Intervention and Outcome Measures	Results	Study Limitations	Implications for Occupational Therapy
Braverman et al. (1999)	Describe a multidisciplinary rehabilitation program for active duty military service members with moderate head injuries	III—Treatment arm of a randomized control trial; this arm used a one-group pretest–posttest design $N = 67$ persons with moderate traumatic brain injury (TBI); mean age: 24.7 yrs; 32% married; 61% high school graduates; 72% junior enlisted rank in military	Multidisciplinary program. Role of occupational therapy (some group therapies were co-led with other professionals): Cognitive skills group, planning and organization group, individual therapy, work therapy, work skills group, community reentry outings several hours per week. *Outcome measure:* Return to work	At 1-year follow-up, 64 (95.5%) were able to work or were enrolled in college. 44 (66%) remained on active duty or remained fit for duty, but were discharged from military for nonmedical reasons.	No control group; one-group observational study only; outcome may have occurred for a reason other than the intervention; no description of sampling procedure; no description of how return to work was measured or its reliability; no statistical testing.	This study describes a program in which occupational therapy played a major role. In terms of return to work for these patients with moderate brain injuries, it was successful. The amount of occupational therapy given was extensive (~10–12 hrs/week). Although the study is weak, it does describe a viable program that occupational therapists could use as a guideline.

Braverman, S. E., Spector, J., Warden, D. L., Wilson, B. C., Ellis, T. E., Bamdad, M. J., et al. (1999). A multidisciplinary TBI inpatient rehabilitation programme for active duty service members as part of a randomized clinical trial. *Brain Injury, 13*, 405–415.

Author/Year	Study Objectives	Level/Design/ Participants	Intervention and Outcome Measures	Results	Study Limitations	Implications for Occupational Therapy
Egan et al. (2005)	Determine whether people with acquired cognitive–linguistic impairments following traumatic brain injury (TBI) could learn to use the Internet using specialized training materials, which had been successfully trialed with people with aphasia; evaluate whether these "aphasia-friendly" materials would need to be modified to suit the training needs of people with a TBI.	III—One group, pretest–posttest design $N = 7$ persons with cognitive–linguistic deficits secondary to TBI; mean age: 46 (range 20–81); mean duration of injury: 8 yrs (range 1–35 yrs); all were unemployed; 6/7 lived with family members	Internet training materials used in conjunction with a volunteer, nonprofessional, tutor. 4 modules were taught over 6 lessons, with the option of additional lessons. The 4 modules incorporated 12 Internet tasks. *Outcome measure:* The Internet skills assessment measured.	The majority (6/7) had rarely or never used the Internet and another used it once or twice a week. 6 had Internet access at home and 1 had access at the library. Internet skills assessment: Group means show a posttest rating of moderate-to-total independence on all tasks. Six participants demonstrated significant gains in independence ($Z =$	No information was given regarding whether the independent variable was contaminated (by participant or tutor) with activity outside of the research. The treatment was administered by tutors with a range of computer and teaching skills. The evaluators were not blind to participation or content of the teaching modules.	This study supports the idea that with structured, intensive training, patients with cognitive problems secondary to TBI can learn to engage in occupational performance tasks of some complexity. The study serves as a model for occupational therapists to modify their training materials if necessary, and to test the effectiveness of the training provided in occupational therapy. The

			the participant's ability to do the 12 Internet tasks. Scored on a 5-point scale of independence from totally independent (1) to not at all independent (5).	2.20, $p = 0.028$, $r = .78$). Participants achieved higher levels of independence in more concrete tasks that had fewer steps and required less abstract reasoning.	authors of the study made their training materials available free of charge online at http://www.shrs.uq.edu.au/cdaru/aphasiagroups/.

Egan, J., Worrall, L., & Oxenham, D. (2005). An internet training intervention for people with traumatic brain injury: Barriers and outcomes. *Brain Injury, 19,* 555–568.

Gentry et al. (2008)	Examine the efficacy of personal digital assistants (PDAs) as cognitive aids	III—One-group pretest–posttest design $N = 23$ individuals living in the community who were a minimum of 1 year after a severe traumatic brain injury (TBI)	Intervention consisted of one-to-one training in the use of the PDA during 3–6 90-minute home visits over a 30-day period. Participants asked to use the PDA for 8-week period with investigator available by e-mail or phone contact only if initiated by the participant. ■ *Outcome measures:* Canadian Occupational Performance Measure (COPM) and Craig Handicap Assessment and Rating Technique–Revised (CHART) Used before and 8 weeks after training.	Significant improvement in satisfaction and self-estimation of occupational performance (COPM) and self-ratings of participation (CHART).	Small sample size not representative of severe TBI population as a whole. No separate statistical analysis of the 7 participants who had additional phone or e-mail contact to determine if they performed any differently. Short follow-up period. Brief training intervention in the use of PDAs as cognitive aids can improve self-ratings in everyday tasks.

Gentry, T., Wallace, J., Kvarfordt, C., & Lynch, K. B. (2008). Personal digital assistants as cognitive aids for individuals with severe traumatic brain injury: A community-based trial. *Brain Injury, 22,* 19–24.

(continued)

EVIDENCE TABLE. FOCUSED QUESTION 4 (cont.)

Author/Year	Study Objectives	Level/Design/ Participants	Intervention and Outcome Measures	Results	Study Limitations	Implications for Occupational Therapy
Ho & Bennett (1997)	Test the efficacy of a cognitive rehabilitation program using strict inclusion criteria; demonstrate that cognitive functioning, as measured by neuropsychological test scores, would improve following a specific program of remediational and compensatory therapies; demonstrate that these improvements in neuropsychological scores would reflect improvements in ratings of functioning in activities of daily living	III—One group, pretest–posttest design *N* = 36 persons with mild to moderate traumatic brain injury (TBI) secondary to motor vehicle accident; 3–38 months postinjury (median = 7 months)	Each person's intervention was individually developed but contained the following 2 aspects. Frequency and duration varied according to individual needs. Formal cognitive remediation to redevelop previous skills; deficits identified by neuropsychological testing. Compensatory training to develop skills to compensate for cognitive deficits within everyday life settings by direct utilization of the skills in the patient's normal environment and activities (occupational performance). *Outcome measures:* ■ Halstead Reitan Neuropsychological Battery (selected subtests): attention, speed of processing, learning and memory, executive functions/conceptual skills/flexibility of thinking, and general intellectual functioning ■ Activities of Daily Living Scales modified from Acimovic & Keatley (1991)[1] using a 4-point Likert scale	There was a significant improvement in the pre- and postrehabilitation scores for almost all neuropsychological test scores. There was significant improvement in functional performance as measured by the modified Acimovic–Keatley subtests, as well as the total scores.	Pretest data were obtained from records; although not stated, this appears to be a retrospective, not prospective, study. No information is provided to judge whether there was contamination of the independent variable or whether co-intervention took place. Timing bias may have existed because some participants were in treatment for 1½ yr, during which procedures and therapists could have changed or spontaneous recovery could have occurred. The validity and reliability of the outcome measures were not reported. The person who accessed the records probably was not blind to outcome; this is not reported. There was no measure included of actual occupational performance.	We can assume that occupational therapists were the professionals responsible for the application of compensatory strategies to everyday life in this study. The actual improvements in occupational functioning were not measured or reported, although improvements in the so-called functional subtests were significant. Although it provides vague support for efficacy of occupational therapy in restoring occupational functioning after TBI, this study does suggest that occupational therapy may be effective and is not detrimental. This study points out the need for occupational therapists to research the efficacy of their own interventions. A comment made by the authors is important: According to the authors, because there was no significant correlation between the neuropsychological test scores and the modified activities of daily living scales, the latter may be measuring aspects of cognitive

functioning that are not the same as aspects of cognitive functioning that are reflected in neuropsychological test scores. This indicates the importance of occupational therapy assessment of effectiveness of interventions for patients with TBI. Occupational therapists should emphasize their contributions to TBI and cognitive rehabilitation through research-based publications in journals that currently contain numerous contributions from psychologists measuring the effect of occupational therapy and calling it "cognitive rehabilitation" (the domain of neuropsychologists)

Ho, M. R., & Bennett, T. L. (1997). Efficacy of neuropsychological rehabilitation for mild–moderate traumatic brain injury. *Archives of Clinical Neuropsychology, 12,* 1–11.

| Mills et al. (1992) | Report functional outcomes of patients with traumatic brain injury (TBI) in an outpatient community, postacute program that used a functional retraining approach | III—One group, pretest–posttest

$N = 42$

Prior to injury, all patients were involved in productive activities—30 employed, 12 in school. At time of enrollment, none were successfully | Structured community-based rehabilitation program that emphasized improvement of the patient's real-life functional abilities (occupational performance) and psychological support. A functional rather than cognitive remediational approach was used. | There was a significant improvement in functional evaluation pre- and posttreatment. The average overall percentage of treatment goals achieved was 67.5% ($n = 41$); range: 25%–93.7%. The majority of patients ($n = 32$) maintained or improved their | It is unknown who provided the therapy. The reliability of the percentage of goals outcome measure was not reported. Evaluators probably were not blinded, but this was not reported. There may have been a memory bias regarding | As the authors stated, late programs of rehabilitation should provide structured and paced learning opportunities, emphasize individual needs, and focus on expected real-world function to maximize successful outcomes. Client-centered occupational |

(continued)

Author/Year	Study Objectives	Level/Design/ Participants	Intervention and Outcome Measures	Results	Study Limitations	Implications for Occupational Therapy
Mills et al. (1992) (cont.)		employed or engaged in any productive school, recreational, or volunteer activities.	Eight treatment goals were individually established by the treatment team, which included the patient and appropriate family member or friend. The goals were variously in-home, community, leisure, or vocational domains. Treatment discontinued when functional goals were achieved, when progress toward goals did not show progress in a reasonable amount of time (6–8 wk), or when patient decided goal was achieved and self-discharged. *Outcome measures:* Functional assessment of performance in the clinic, at home, and in the community. Percentage of achievement of identified goals, individually determined.	overall status in the home (87.5%), community (87.5%), leisure (90%), and vocational function (90%) 6 months postdischarge. These gains continued to be maintained or improved at 12 months (*n* = 13): home, 84.6%; community, 92.3%; leisure, 92.3%; vocational, 61.5%; and 18 months (*n* = 18): home, 88.8%; community, 88.8%; leisure, 72.2%; and vocational, 77.7%. There was no significant improvement in cognitive abilities after treatment.	maintenance of goal performance because it was evaluated by interviewing patient and family members who had to remember immediate past performance. It would have been better to use goal attainment scaling (observational) for an outcome measure rather than interview of patient and family (subjective, remembered estimate of performance). The statistical analysis regarding the correlations of outcome with demographic factors mentioned in results were not reported.	therapy, which aims to increase the participation of patients in their desired life roles, offers all these components of therapy. Whether occupational therapy was part of this particular program was not reported. It is imperative for occupational therapists to document the outcomes of occupational therapy intervention in order to inform the medical community, insurers, and the public that occupational therapy is an essential service for patients with TBI. Other disciplines report programs, such as the one reported here, that are in fact occupational therapy without identifying the program as occupational therapy or without involving an occupational therapist.

Mills, V. M., Nesbeda, T., Katz, D. I., & Alexander, M. P. (1992). Outcomes for traumatically brain-injured patients following post-acute rehabilitation programmes. *Brain Injury, 6,* 219–228.

Author (Year)	Purpose	Design & Level of Evidence	Intervention/Outcome Measures	Results	Comments
Parente & Stapleton (1999)	Evaluate the effectiveness of group thinking skills training as a precursor to vocational placement and reentry into the work world, measured by client's success in training, return to work, and job longevity	III—Two-group observational study; data for control group from retrospective records. $N = 33$ patients diagnosed with brain injury in the Cognitive Skills Group (CSG; experimental) with attrition to 13. Baseline (control) group: 568 records reviewed, 64 chosen as comparable to CSG group. Mean age both groups: 32 yrs; mean education both groups: 12 yrs	CSG (Cognitive Skills Training Model): Once per week for 2 months to 1 year (mean: 4 months). Control: Baseline group. Outcome measures: Employment rate, job longevity, job reentry, performance in training	10/13 clients of CSG group currently working full time (rehabilitation rate of 76%). The rehabilitation rate for the baseline group was 58%. All employed CSG group clients were employed >60 days; no data for baseline group. Grade point averages for CSG group ranged from 2.5–3.5.	The authors' conclusion that the CSG is a cost-effective method cannot be made because the cost effectiveness of the program was not studied. Little information is given concerning sampling procedure. No information concerning severity or chronicity of brain injury. The two groups received therapy from different types of therapists/educators at different places. Reliability of outcome measures not reported.	This is a very weak study that indicates training in a variety of thinking skills is useful to "brain injured" patients. The authors do not include the severity of the brain injury, the time postinjury, or the thinking deficits the patients had going into the experimental training. The program is best applied to certain patients, but we do not know enough about the participants to know who those people are or what the discharge criteria were. This report does not give enough information concerning efficacy or cost effectiveness to be useful as a guide for cognitive rehabilitation therapy.

Parente, R., & Stapleton, M. (1999). Development of a cognitive strategies group for vocational training after traumatic brain injury. *NeuroRehabilitation, 13,* 13–20.

Author (Year)	Purpose	Design & Level of Evidence	Intervention/Outcome Measures	Results	Comments
Quemada et al. (2003)	Assess the effectiveness of a memory rehabilitation program on patients with traumatic brain injury (TBI) and compare different instruments, such as neuropsychological tests and memory failure questionnaires, as outcome measures	III—One group, pretest–posttest design. $N = 12$ persons with TBI; mean age: 33 (range: 15–65); 8 were ≤6 months posttrauma, 4 ≥24 months; initial mean Glasgow Coma Scale score: 5.7 (range: 3–9); posttraumatic amnesia was >28 days in all patients	Memory rehabilitation using Wilson's structured behavioral memory program (1996), which includes behavioral compensation techniques and mnemonic strategies. Included environmental adaptations to reduce environmental demands (e.g., lines on floor, labels, painting doors different colors); external aids to help	No significant changes between baseline and posttreatment scores for any of the tests, including the RBMT and the Memory Failures in Everyday Memory. After treatment, 9 patients were able to travel around their town without supervision. 6 relearned how to use public transportation indepen-	The treatments described in this study are ones that occupational therapists use in the treatment of persons with cognitive disorders. Spontaneous recovery, which could explain the improvement reported, was not controlled for in this study. However, because there was no significant improvement in memory

(continued)

Author/Year	Study Objectives	Level/Design/ Participants	Intervention and Outcome Measures	Results	Study Limitations	Implications for Occupational Therapy
Quemada et al. (2003) (cont.)			coding, storing, and retrieving information (e.g., tape recorders, notebooks, diary schedules, maps); and reality orientation. Reorganization and restoration techniques were also used for 11 persons. Internal aids, such as mnemonic strategies, and nonverbal strategies, such as visualization and association, were included. Additional therapies were offered as needed (10 persons), including social skills training and problem solving training. Treatment was individualized. Daily 50-min sessions for 6 mos, reduced to 3 times/wk in the last month. *Outcome measures:* Several neuropsychological tests. Of interest to this review: ■ Rivermead Behavioural Memory Test (RBMT), which measures impairments of everyday memory in ADL ■ Memory Failures in Everyday Memory Questionnaire (patient version and caregiver version), which is a self-	dently and regularly used it. 4 redeveloped basic shopping and cooking skills. In the 3 most severely affected patients, functional gain was limited to improvements in dressing, personal hygiene, and organizing their daily routines to require less supervision. These functional gains were not detected by the RBMT, probably because therapy was aimed at behavioral adaptation, situation-specific procedural training, or family intervention, which did not affect performance for remembering names, faces, or appointments, and did not transfer to these skills measured by the RBMT. In this study, neither patients nor families felt that memory had improved after treatment (did not meet expectations of effect of therapy).	in a head trauma unit for 6 mos and this program only required 1 hr per day; it is likely that the co-intervention produced the improvement in occupational performance reported. No functional assessment was included.	processes during the treatment period, we can assume that the intervention resulted in the outcomes reported. This study indicates that occupational therapy practitioners can emphasize to the patient, the family, colleagues, and the medical community that recovery of occupational performance occurs as a result of behavioral and environmental compensation therapy, which can be demonstrated by activities of daily living (ADL) and instrumental activities of daily living (IADL) evaluations, but not by evaluations of memory processes. Changes or lack of changes in memory processes do not explain changes in occupational performance. The development of a sensitive ADL/IADL scale for use with patients with cognitive impairments would be a benefit to occupational therapy practice and research.

appraisal of memory performance on a 3-point Likert scale.

Quemada, J. I., Cespedes, J. M. M., Ezkerra, J., Ballesteros, J., Ibarra, N., & Urruticoechea, I. (2003). Outcome of memory rehabilitation in traumatic brain injury assessed by neuropsychological tests and questionnaires. *Journal of Head Trauma Rehabilitation, 18,* 532–540.

Bergman (2000)	Describe a cognitive orthotic (CO) and the ease with which a heterogeneous group of individuals with traumatic brain injury demonstrated mastery when given the opportunity to try the CO	Uncategorized—Observational posttest only *N* = 41; mean age: 33.5 years (range 12–72 years); 44.7% with moderate-to-severe memory impairment. All participants had tried, without success, conventional strategies and materials, such as notebooks, sticky note reminders, wall calendars, or mnemonic devices.	Cognitive orthotic, the design objectives of which were error-free learning, rapid system learning, and skill acquisition, and facilitated generalization. The CO is highly simplified and provides on-screen structure, sequencing, and cueing that people with significant memory deficits need. The display of only relevant cues and functions promotes error-free learning. Organization of display is consistent across the various activities to promote transfer of training. *Outcome measures:* Success defined as mastery (unassisted reliable completion of a targeted task) of 4 or more modules as determined by 1 independent evaluator and the author from a videotape.	Of the 41 participants provided with a CO, 36 (88%) achieved mastery of 4 or more activity modules, and therefore were considered successful users. 39 (95%) mastered the first module (the Journal) within minutes; 91% (31 of 34) achieved mastery of the Telephone Log within minutes; 100% (10 of 10) participants mastered Directory; 97% (33 of 34) mastered Savings Deposit/Withdrawal; 87% (27 of 31) mastered Check Writing; and 91% (32 of 35) mastered Appointment Scheduling. 5 participants were unsuccessful, suggesting that some minimal level of intellectual functioning, orientation, initiation, perception, and	No control group or condition; no pretest or pretreatment baseline; inclusion and exclusion criteria were not reported; none of the particulars about setting, administrator, frequency, or duration of intervention were reported; the role of multiple "examiners," depending on site, was not delineated; no reliability or validity of outcome measure reported; process of measuring outcome was not fully explained; no statistical analysis.	Although this study is not definitive evidence for the effectiveness of cognitive orthoses, it suggests three ideas for occupational therapy practitioners to consider: ■ Patients with a constellation of poor cognitive functions are not likely to benefit from direct therapy to compensate for deficient memory function (all the participants in this study had failed to benefit from conventional memory orthoses before using the computerized CO; those with poor cognitive functioning failed to benefit from the computerized CO). Therapy for those patients is better directed toward the caregiver and environmental modification to promote

(continued)

EVIDENCE TABLE. FOCUSED QUESTION 4. *(cont.)*

Author/Year	Study Objectives	Level/Design/ Participants	Intervention and Outcome Measures	Results	Study Limitations	Implications for Occupational Therapy
Bergman (2000) *(cont.)*				reasoning are required for success with this CO.		some occupational participation. ■ Patients with adequate cognitive functioning can benefit from structured, consistent, low memory–demand cognitive orthoses and can regain performance of some occupational tasks that increase their independent participation. Therapists can be advocates for their patients to obtain such orthoses. ■ Structured, consistent, low memory–demand therapy situations in which the patient is guided to discover the correct response and receives consistent feedback promote learning and performance in patients with memory impairment after traumatic brain injury.

Bergman, M. M. (2000). Successful mastery with a cognitive orthotic in people with traumatic brain injury. *Applied Neuropsychology, 7,* 76–82.

[1]Acimovic, M. L., & Keatley, M. A. (1991, October). *Cognitive brain injury descriptor scale. Automated program evaluation.* Presented at the meeting of the Colorado Head Injury Foundation, Boulder.

Reference

Kay, T. (1986). *The unseen injury—Minor head trauma.* Framingham, MA: National Head Injury Foundation.

EVIDENCE TABLE. LEVEL IV (EXPERIMENTAL SINGLE-CASE STUDY[1]) FOR FOCUSED QUESTION 4.

What is the evidence for the effect of interventions to address cognitive/perceptual functions (a) attention, (b) memory, (c) executive functions on the occupational performance for persons with traumatic brain injury?

Author/Year	Study Objectives	Level/Design/ Participants	Intervention and Outcome Measures	Results	Study Limitations	Implications for Occupational Therapy
General						
Kirsch, Shenton, Spirl, et al. (2004)	Present case studies as examples of assistive technology for cognition (ATC) interventions that use some Web-based features as the basis for interventions that address moderately complex sequential functional tasks	IV—ABA[1] design (baseline, intervention, withdrawal) for TD and extended ABAB design for CO in which the intervention (A) and nonintervention (B) phases were alternated for a total of 11 trials. $N = 2$; 19-year-old man (TD) with traumatic brain injury (TBI) with severe impairments of all memory components, executive reasoning skills, and topographic gnosis. 71-year-old woman (CO) 1 year post-TBI with a sleep disorder and severe memory and reasoning impairments	ATC, which is any technologically oriented intervention designed to facilitate performance of functional activities that would otherwise require human intervention. The ATC tested here consisted of a series of Web pages created to provide interactive assistance to each participant regarding performance of a targeted functional activity. *Baseline:* A speech–language pathologist (SLP) or occupational therapist (OT) informed the patient that an error had occurred in his or her attempts to do the targeted activity and should be corrected. 5 min time limit. *Treatment phase:* 5 min. duration of each trial. During treatment phases, the therapists would tell the patient when an error was made and advise use of the computer to correct it.	*TD:* During baseline, mean errors across trial days were 3.72; he was unable to achieve any navigational goal successfully. During B phase, the mean errors dropped to 0.93. During the A phase, mean errors rose to 1.14, lower than baseline, indicating that some learning had occurred. *CO:* Mean errors were 0.33 for treatment trials and 2.23 for nonintervention trials. During each treatment trial, CO was able to complete all 6 steps of the alarm clock task within the allotted time, which she could not do during non-cued trials. After intervention withdrawal, there was evidence of modest improvement in both subjects for independent performance of the targeted task, but this learning appeared to be fragile.	No explanation for sampling given (how the subjects were chosen, whether they were the only ones chosen, etc.). The SLP and OT rated performance, but no reliability was reported and these evaluators were not blind to condition. No statistical analysis of outcome data, and no control for intervening variables.	This intervention uses Web-based programming within a wireless Internet infrastructure. The education of occupational therapists needs to include basic computer and Internet programming and usage skills if this study signals a viable future trend. As ATC interventions become more specialized, greater technical expertise will be needed for both development and maintenance, which will involve rehabilitation engineers. It will be important for occupational therapists to learn to collaborate with these professionals.

(continued)

EVIDENCE TABLE. LEVEL IV (EXPERIMENTAL SINGLE-CASE STUDY[1]) FOR FOCUSED QUESTION 4 (*cont.*)

Author/Year	Study Objectives	Level/Design/ Participants	Intervention and Outcome Measures	Results	Study Limitations	Implications for Occupational Therapy
Kirsch, Shenton, Spirl, et al. (2004) (*cont.*)			*Outcome measures:* All ratings by the SLP or OT. TD was measured on average number of errors per route per day. CO was measured on the average number of errors per task substep attempted. Error was defined as any deviation from correct task performance.			

Kirsch, N. L., Shenton, M., Spirl, E., Rowan, J., Simpson, R., Schreckengost, D., et al. (2004). Web-based assistive technology interventions for cognitive impairments after traumatic brain injury: A selective review and two case studies. *Rehabilitation Psychology, 49,* 200–212.

Author/Year	Study Objectives	Level/Design/ Participants	Intervention and Outcome Measures	Results	Study Limitations	Implications for Occupational Therapy
Tam et al. (2003)	Evaluate the effectiveness and perceived efficacy of a customized tele-cognitive rehabilitation program. [Online rehabilitation offering the same experiences as receiving computer-assisted training in front of a clinic-based computer.]	IV—ABA single case experimental design (no intervention [A], intervention [B], and no intervention withdrawal phase [A]) *Participants:* 2 persons with traumatic brain injury (TBI) and 1 postsurgical repair of arteriovenous malformation (AVM). 37-year-old male (TM) with language deficits and 20-year-old male (KW) with impaired memory of routine daily tasks (prospective memory). 20-year-old woman with AVM—not reported here.	Online presentation of remedial computer programs. The therapist shared the control of the patient's computer screen and provided demonstrations or cues or opened additional programs to assist the patient. TM's goal was to recognize and pronounce 60 Chinese characters; KW's goal was to improve memorization of daily tasks *Outcome measures:* 5-point Likert scale to rate efficacy of tele-cognitive training program and confidence at solving daily living problems. TM was measured	The relationships among the three phases were analyzed visually and by trend line analysis using the split-middle method. Both subjects showed improvement during the treatment phase (TM: gradient changed from +0.3 to +0.42; KW: gradient changed from −0.14 to +0.14). In both A phases, there were decreasing trends; in the 2nd A phase, gradients changed as follows: TM = +0.42 to −0.3; KW = +0.14 to −0.43. Self-confidence improved ~10% (TM) or ~40% (KW). All users gave positive feedback on tele-cognitive rehabilitation.	The results do not generalize to other behaviors or to other persons; the evaluators were not blind to participation; no intervening variables were controlled; no information was given concerning how computer-savvy the participants or the therapists were, or had to be.	This is one of the few occupational therapy research studies reported. The basic assumption of the program was that remedial therapy would be effective in changing occupational performance. Other studies have shown this not to be true. However, this study measured outcome on the same tasks as being trained and did show an improvement. It would be interesting to adapt this method of delivering service to compensatory therapy found in other studies to be more effective than remedial therapy. Tele-rehabilitation requires therapists to be very skilled in computer hardware

and software usage and adaptation; this suggests that educational programs need to include criterion for this skill in their curricula.

on number of words recognized; KW was measured on number of 5 different timed tasks memorized and carried out during each phase.

Tam, S.-F., Man, W. K., Hui-Chan, C. W. Y., Lau, A., Yip, B., & Cheung, W. (2003). Evaluating the efficacy of tele-cognitive rehabilitation for functional performance in three case studies. *Occupational Therapy International, 10*(1), 20–38.

Executive Function

Ownsworth et al. (2006)	Investigate neurocognitive, psychological, and socioenvironmental factors underlying unawareness for an individual with severe awareness deficits and develop an associated treatment rationale; evaluate a theory-driven intervention to promote functional gains	IV—Single-case experimental study with multiple baselines across settings *Participant:* 46-year-old man with very severe traumatic brain injury (TBI) who demonstrated long-term awareness deficits. 4 years postinjury. Posttraumatic amnesia >6 months. Left-sided neglect and left upper extremity hemiparesis. Had 18 months of occupational and physical therapy. 2 years postinjury, vocational assessment concluded that he was unemployable.	Metacognitive contextual intervention based on guidelines for neurocognitive and socioenvironmental interventions. Systematic feedback approach was used to target error behavior (i.e., self-monitoring and correction) on functional tasks to achieve his goals of cooking and paid employment. The intervention included education for the participant's social supports and demonstrated the use of effective feedback and prompting during his performance on cooking and work tasks. Targeted error awareness and self-correction in two real life settings: 1) cooking at home; 2) volunteer work. 1st treatment: Role reversal technique	During the 4-week baseline period in cooking setting, average of 21 errors, with a decline in errors over the baseline period. During the 8-week treatment period in the cooking setting, a 44% reduction in error frequency (11.8) was recorded. The average error frequency (11.0) in the maintenance period indicated that the treatment effect was maintained. No spontaneous generalization to volunteer work. With specific training, error frequency in work setting: 12-week baseline = mean of 12.3, with no trend; treatment = mean of 7.5 (39% reduction). No appreciable improvement was observed in general awareness of deficits. 3 weeks after the intervention, he gained	Baseline of cooking setting was descending without treatment; self-correction may have occurred as a result of practice, rather than the feedback intervention; there were no controls for intervening variables; sample of 1 does not allow generalizing to other persons; no statistical analysis of data; evaluators were involved in the intervention.	This study is authored by occupational therapists and tests an occupational therapy–psychological intervention. The outcome for 1 patient in 2 settings was positive. Although this study only provides weak evidence of efficacy, the intervention may be useful for others. Enough detail is provided in the report for other occupational therapy practitioners to try this intervention in their practices.

(continued)

EVIDENCE TABLE. LEVEL IV (EXPERIMENTAL SINGLE-CASE STUDY[1]) FOR FOCUSED QUESTION 4 (*cont.*)

Author/Year	Study Objectives	Level/Design/ Participants	Intervention and Outcome Measures	Results	Study Limitations	Implications for Occupational Therapy
Ownsworth et al. (2006) *(cont.)*			used for the participant, with therapists' prompting, to correct his mother's cooking procedure, deliberately in error. 2nd treatment: Observation of video of own cooking with identification of errors. Next treatments: Use of timer (to prompt looking at recipe), precooking discussion with feedback, and a post-cooking feedback discussion. During the 4-week maintenance period, the timer and therapist feedback were withdrawn. Mother still offered feedback. *Outcome measures:* 1) Error frequency (interrater agreement = 83% cooking, 91% work). Scored by therapist and mother or supervisor. 2) Error behavior using the "Pause, Prompt (general and specific), Praise" technique (interrater agreement = 88% for cooking and 94% for work).	paid employment with the use of a job coach (trained by the therapists) for 1 month.		

Ownsworth, T., Fleming, J., Desbois, J., Strong, J., & Kuipers, P. (2006). A metacognitive contextual intervention to enhance error awareness and functional outcome following traumatic brain injury: A single-case experimental design. *Journal of the International Neuropsychological Society, 12,* 54–63.

| Turkstra & Flora (2002) | Demonstrate the effectiveness of compensatory strategies for ameliorating impairments of executive function; the strategies were designed to enable 1 client with traumatic brain injury (TBI) to obtain professional employment | IV—Single case, pre–post experimental design (ABA) *Participant:* 1 49-year-old male with history of multiple prior head injuries and substance abuse. Severe brain injury at age 26. Abstinent since age 38. Disabling level of anxiety when faced with professional documentation tasks. | *Treatment condition:* Facilitation of organization using supports to reduce memory demands: structured format (carrier phrases and SOAP note format), computer-based intake assessment program readily available in employment situations. *Control condition:* No treatment. *Outcome measures:*
■ Report accuracy—accuracy of reports compared to actual situation under controlled conditions
■ Spelling accuracy—number of spelling errors
■ Discourse cohesion—number of complete, incomplete, and erroneous/ambiguous cohesive ties (obvious referent for pronouns) | Significant improvement in report accuracy. Modest increases in number of facts reported, but greater improvement in eliminating extraneous and erroneous information. No significant changes from pretest to posttest in Spelling or Cohesion tests. Patient reported that the stress of report writing was virtually eliminated. After much job searching and failed application, he obtained a full-time position (with a job coach accommodation) as a chemical dependency counselor in an outpatient clinic. | Single-subject design does not allow generalization, but suggests an intervention to try. How or why this particular participant was chosen was not reported. Both authors acted as assessors and treaters, therefore were not blind to assignment. | The guidelines these authors used in designing this successful intervention are the same as used by occupational therapists: 1) personally relevant occupation as therapy; 2) structuring the environment or circumstances to enable performance when an impairment cannot be remediated; 3) client-centered therapy—goals set by client; 4) providing opportunity for success (mentoring, scaffolding); 5) prioritizing goals and work on a key, one which may result in improvement in other goals without direct intervention. |

Turkstra, L. S., & Flora, T. L. (2002). Compensating for executive function impairments after TBI: A single case study of functional intervention. *Journal of Communication Disorders, 35,* 467–482.

(continued)

EVIDENCE TABLE. LEVEL IV (EXPERIMENTAL SINGLE-CASE STUDY¹) FOR FOCUSED QUESTION 4 (cont.)

Author/Year	Study Objectives	Level/Design/ Participants	Intervention and Outcome Measures	Results	Study Limitations	Implications for Occupational Therapy
Attention						
Shimelman & Hinojosa (1995)	Examine the result of gross motor activities on the attention behavior of 3 adults with brain injury as measured by their performance on letter cancellation tasks	IV—Single-subject, ABA reversal design *Participants:* 3 persons, 1 with stroke and 2 with traumatic brain injury	*Treatment (B):* 7 sessions of 15 min of gross motor activity consisting of 5 min each of throwing and catching a ball, tossing a balloon, and throwing bean bags into a container. *Control (A):* Individualized occupational therapy that included activities of daily living and tabletop activities. 4–7 sessions first baseline, 4-session second baseline. *Outcome measure:* 6-letter cancellation task devised for the study.	Visual inspection of graphs indicate no clear changes in trend or level of performance in the 3 phases of the study, nor in the 6 test tasks. Observation notes indicate changes in scanning style of all 3 subjects starting 2 to 3 weeks after treatment was started. *Conclusion:* Gross motor activity did not influence the performance of 3 adults with brain injury in 6 tasks involving attention.	Therapy not theory-based; no information concerning participants, other than age, provided; exact amount of therapy not reported; validity of outcome measure not reported; possible practice effects on retesting; no statistical analysis of data.	This atheoretical occupational therapy treatment based on previous observations by one of the authors—15 min of gross motor upper extremity activity twice a week for 3 weeks—did not improve performance on a 6-letter cancellation task, presumed to measure various aspects of attention.

Shimelman, A., & Hinojosa, J. (1995). Gross motor activity and attention in three adults with brain injury. *American Journal of Occupational Therapy, 49*, 973–979.

Author/Year	Study Objectives	Level/Design/ Participants	Intervention and Outcome Measures	Results	Study Limitations	Implications for Occupational Therapy
Wilson & Manly (2003)	Determine the effect of sustained attention training (SAT) in conjunction with errorless learning on self-care performance and deficits in spatial awareness in a densely amnesic patient with unusual enduring ipsilesional personal and extrapersonal neglect	IV—Single-case, time series design (ABA) *Participant:* 40-year-old woman, 2 yr postonset; dependent in all activities of daily living (ADL); left hemi-inattention secondary to middle cerebral artery occlusion and subdural hematoma following a severe head injury obtained in a fall	*Intervention: Treatment (B):* SAT + fixed order ADL training. 2 min per day just prior to ADL training for 10 days. *Control (A):* Fixed order ADL training for 10 days prior to experimental treatment and 10 days after. *Outcome measure:* Self-care performance (number of prompts required to complete ADL without errors).	Serial dependency was statistically removed. The number of prompts required to finish the ADL program was significantly lower during the SAT phase relative to baseline (mean total prompts = 14 for SAT and 39.6 for preintervention baseline). No statistical effect between SAT and postintervention phase. The number of prompts required continued to improve (total prompts	Statistics not reported, only *p* level. Although prompts required decreased, the actual level of impendence was not measured after treatment. The explanation of the Baking Tray Task as part of treatment and/or outcome was inadequate. No score or statistic given for one outcome measure: Comb and Razor/Compact Test. Frequency of mea-	This study provides weak evidence that a sustained attention training procedure may improve performance of persons with hemiattention disorder. Further controlled study is required before adopting this as a recommendation.

Study	Purpose	Level/Design	Method/Outcome measures	Results	Conclusions
			Comb and Razor/Compact Test, a measure of neglect of personal space.	during SAT = 14 and during postintervention phase = 10.9).	surement of outcome not clear. Validity and reliability of outcome measures not reported.

Wilson, F. C., & Manly, T. (2003). Sustained attention training and errorless learning facilitates self-care functioning in chronic ipsilesional neglect following severe traumatic brain injury. *Neuropsychological Rehabilitation, 13*, 537–548.

Memory

Study	Purpose	Level/Design	Method/Outcome measures	Results	Conclusions
Campbell et al. (2007)	Examine the effectiveness of errorless learning in reducing frequency of everyday memory problems	IV—Multiple baseline (8 datapoints per day for a 10 day baseline period), single-case experimental design study of errorless learning in a patient with severe memory impairment following traumatic brain injury, 6 years postinjury	Client's caregiver (i.e., mother) was trained to facilitate errorless learning in the home environment with client-generated cues. Intervention focused on recording entries in his memory notebook and walking his dog. *Outcome measures:* ■ Daily frequency counts of everyday memory problems as an index of change ■ Caregiver Strain Index ■ Rivermead Behavioural Memory Test ■ Dysexecutive Questionnaire from the Behavioural Assessment of Dysexecutive Syndrome.	Statistically significant change (*p* < 0.001) in notebook usage from baseline to 3-month follow-up. No changes seen in Caregiver Strain Index, Rivermead Behavioural Memory Test, or Dysexecutive Questionnaire. 18-month follow-up showed the retention of and actual continued improvement in the behavioral changes targeted (i.e., using memory notebook and walking dog).	The level of comprehension, involvement, and commitment needed by the caregiver/facilitator may limit the larger application of the intervention to other clients/families. Errorless learning with self-generated cues facilitated by caregivers can make functional behavioral changes in everyday activities.

Campbell, L., Wilson, F. C., McCann, J., Kernahan, G., & Rogers, R. G. (2007). Single case experimental design study of Carer Facilitated Errorless Learning in a patient with severe memory impairment following TBI. *NeuroRehabilitation, 22*, 325–333.

(continued)

Author/Year	Study Objectives	Level/Design/ Participants	Intervention and Outcome Measures	Results	Study Limitations	Implications for Occupational Therapy
Ehlhardt et al. (2005)	Develop and evaluate an instructional package (TEACH–M) that facilitates learning and retention of a sequence of steps for using a simple e-mail interface by learners with memory and executive function impairments	IV—Single-subject experimental design; multiple baseline across participants *Participants:* 9, reduced to 4 (2 already could do task, 1 refused, 1 disqualified, 1 refused after 4 treatments because of lack of success), persons with acquired brain injury in chronic phase of recovery. Recruited from local transitional living programs and support groups. Age range: 36–58 years; age at injury ranged from 16–28 years. All were in coma for 1 to 4 months after injury. All 5 had severe cognitive impairments; none were employed and all received assistance with basic activities of daily living and instrumental activities of daily living. None had prior experience with e-mail and, as a group, very little computer experience. Reported to have significant difficulty in learning new, multi-step procedures.	TEACH–M is theoretically based and has these components: 1) task analysis; 2) errorless learning; 3) assess performance initially and ongoing; 4) regularly review previously learned skills; 5) high rates of correct practice trials; 6) metacognitive strategy training in which the prediction technique can be used to encourage active processing of the material. A simplified e-mail interface was developed that allowed the participants to read and reply to e-mail from 4 hypothetical partners (not a live Internet connection). *Outcome measures:* ▪ Number of correct e-mail steps completed in sequence ▪ Number of correct e-mail steps completed, regardless of sequence ▪ Number of training sessions required to reach criterion for mastery without prompts.	A functional relationship between the independent variable and dependent variables was demonstrated with replication of the treatment effect across all 4 participants. The number of sessions required for mastery for 3 consecutive measurements ranged from 7–15 treatments, with a group mean of 11 (~4 to nearly 9 hours). 3 of the 4 participants maintained the treatment effects at the 1-month follow-up. Generalization of effects to an altered interface was observed in all 4 participants. The participants were enthusiastic about the program, especially the teacher modeling of the steps and the fact that treatment sessions were held 4 to 5 times per week.	Threats to external validity include 1) the fact that the e-mail interface was specially designed, simplified program; 2) the high number of treatment sessions per week, which may not be practical in rehabilitation settings; 3) the first author designed, implemented, and evaluated the treatment package so it is unknown whether other therapists would have the same effect; and 4) there were only 4 participants, who may or may not be representative of the traumatic brain injury (TBI) population. There was no statistical or graphical analysis of data; no data reported.	Direct instruction, as personified by the TEACH–M procedure, was effective for 4 participants. Occupational therapy practitioners could use the TEACH–M as a model to review/evaluate their teaching methodology for persons with TBI who have severe learning disabilities. Occupational therapy researchers could use this study as a model for documenting the effectiveness of particular occupational therapy treatments.

Ehlhardt, L. A., Sohlberg, M. M., Glang, A., & Albin, R. (2005). TEACH–M: A pilot study evaluating an instructional sequence for persons with impaired memory and executive functions. *Brain Injury, 19,* 569–583.

| Kirsch et al. (2004) | Describe development of a generic, in-house alphanumeric paging system; test the hypothesis that alphanumeric cues would increase use of a daily planner for recording critical therapy activities or assignments that the participant had been asked to discuss with a family member each evening | IV—Single-case experimental ABA' design

Participant: Male in mid-30s with severe traumatic brain injury (TBI), postsurgical removal of large subdural hematoma in the right frontoparietal area. Came to neurorehabilitation on day 30 and was rated Level V on the Rancho Los Amigos Cognitive Scale | *Intervention: Control (A & A')*: Each treatment day, participant was reminded to record summary information or therapeutic instructions in his daily planner at the conclusion of each therapy session to discuss with family in the evening, or to remind about evening homework assignments or about anything he should remember to bring from home for the next day's therapy.

Experimental (B):
All procedures were identical, with addition of the pager that sent cues 5 min before the end of each therapy session to remind him to record the information. The pager was set daily for the particular schedule. Duration ~5 months.

Outcome measures:
Percentage of entries that corresponded directly to a scheduled activity the participant had attended during a treatment day. Non therapy activities or nonrecurring appointments were excluded. | The mean percentage for entries during nonintervention baseline (A) trials was 22.38%, for intervention trials (B) 93.7%, and for nonintervention return-to-baseline trials (A') 49.22%. Qualitatively, the entries during the B phase were more relevant, more elaborate, and consistently labeled with the initials or name of the therapy session to which they pertained than in the A or A' phases. | The design offers few controls for intervening variables. Since only 1 subject was used, the results may not generalize to others. No statistical analysis of data and no information concerning validity or reliability of outcome measures. The evaluator probably was not blind to phase assignment. | In this one case, the alphanumeric paging system improved the prospective memory performance as compared to pre- and postbaseline periods. This would suggest that alphanumeric pagers could be a useful memory orthotic. More study is required. The components of the pager system are listed in the article. |

Kirsch, N. L., Shenton, M., & Rowan, J. (2004). A generic, 'in-house,' alphanumeric paging system for prospective activity impairments after traumatic brain injury. *Brain Injury, 18*, 725–734.

(continued)

EVIDENCE TABLE. LEVEL IV (EXPERIMENTAL SINGLE-CASE STUDY[1]) FOR FOCUSED QUESTION 4 (cont.)

Author/Year	Study Objectives	Level/Design/ Participants	Intervention and Outcome Measures	Results	Study Limitations	Implications for Occupational Therapy
McKerracher et al. (2005)	Compare the standard memory notebook format of Solhberg & Mateer (2001) with the modified format described by Donaghy & Williams (1998)	IV—Single-case, experimental ABAB design *Participant:* 46-year-old male, attending an outpatient brain injury rehabilitation unit. He had sustained a mild traumatic brain injury (TBI) 1 year previously and a more severe head injury 2 years earlier. His attention/ concentration problems endangered his safety. He was anxious and depressed. Resistant to use of a memory aid until he underwent a period of reality testing.	*Condition A:* A typical diary format suggested by Solhberg & Mateer consisting of 4 sections: 1) weekly timetable; 2) "to do" section; 3) memory log (a record of the day's events); 4) transport notes (details of transport to rehab unit). Follows the format of most standard personal organizers. Trained to use in 3 stages: 1) acquisition (how to use it); 2) application (where and when to use it); 3) adaptation (how to update it. *Condition B:* Modified diary suggested by Donaghy & Williams contains a pair of pages for each day of the week. Essential differences between formats were that the standard diary contained a weekly timetable and a separate to-do list; the modified diary contained a daily timetable and a daily to-do list on adjacent pages.	Significantly better performance on a series of prospective memory tasks for the "modified" notebook. During the 4 weeks of standard diary use, the participant carried out 1/20 prospective tasks; during the 4 weeks of use of the modified diary, he carried out 15/20 tasks. There was no change in memory impairment or mood during the experimental period.	Only 1 subject, so the result may not be generalizable; no statistical analysis of data; no information about the reliability of outcome measures. Evaluators probably not blind to the condition assignment.	This study suggests to occupational therapy practitioners that the modified version of a memory notebook suggested by Donaghy & Williams may be more useful than the standard format suggested by Solhberg & Mateer. More research is required before a definitive recommendation can be made. In this case, the participant preferred the notebook to an electronic memory orthoses because of the latter's complexity, unfamiliarity, and cost.

McKerracher, G., Powell, T., & Oyebode, J. (2005). A single-case experimental design comparing two memory notebook formats for a man with memory problems caused by traumatic brain injury. *Neuropsychological Rehabilitation, 15,* 115–128.

Each condition consisted of 1 training day and 2 weeks of use. On each training day, 5 10-minute training sessions (at the end of 5 therapies).

Outcome measures: 5 prospective, meaningful memory tasks each week Number of tasks successfully completed was collected from the staff at the end of each week.

| Raskin & Sohlberg (1996) | Evaluate more clearly the possible effect prospective memory training might have on prospective memory performance in naturalistic, nonclinical settings and on retrospective memory functions; to replicate the effects noted in earlier descriptive accounts in an experimentally controlled paradigm; to address some methodological challenges | IV—CABAB single-case experimental design, counterbalanced across 2 subjects. *Participants:* 2 men, ages 25 and 27 years, selected from list of those needing cognitive rehabilitation, but who could not afford it; chosen because they met all inclusion criteria, including prospective memory ability of <10 minutes and >1 year postinjury. They were not participating in any other therapy. | One baseline condition (C; 2 weeks) and two treatment conditions: A for prospective memory training; B for retrospective memory training. Each subject started with either A or B. *Condition A:* Subject asked to remember to carry out simple, one-step tasks in a specified number of minutes. *Condition B:* Retrospective memory drill. Series of retrospective memory tasks analogous to those in condition A. Time interval | Both subjects experienced an overall increase in the length of their prospective memory ability over the course of the training from 1 to 2 minutes at baseline to 5 to 6 minutes. *PROMS:* Improved above baseline for both subjects under both A and B2 conditions, but not under the B1 condition. Neither subject completed the generalization telephone task during baseline, but did partially complete the task during condition A and B2. Both subjects improved in their ability to successfully | Despite careful design of the study to control for intervening variables, one such threat to internal validity was evident. That is, carryover effects were evident on the B2 condition; the 1st subject had experienced two A conditions before the B2, while the 2nd subject had experienced only one A condition before B2. Statistical analysis was sparse. External validity cannot be assumed because of few subjects. Reliability of measurement was not reported. The scorer was probably not blind to assignment, although for | Because lack of prospective memory for intentions, more than lack of retrospective memory for information, keeps a patient with traumatic brain injury dependent on others for initiation of activities of daily living and safety, treatment to improve this function is important. This study gave some weak evidence that prospective memory can be improved through practice and feedback and is an important focus of therapy. These ideas are important for occupational therapy practitioners to consider. The best |

(continued)

Author/Year	Study Objectives	Level/Design/ Participants	Intervention and Outcome Measures	Results	Study Limitations	Implications for Occupational Therapy
Raskin & Sohlberg (1996) (*cont.*)			between task performance and query matched the increasing time intervals in Condition A. *Outcome measures:* ■ Prospective Memory Screening (PROMS), administered 5 times during phase C and at the end of each other phase ■ Accuracy of task performance and percentage of trials completed accurately each week ■ Two generalization probes ■ Social validation interview.	complete intended future tasks in their own environment. At baseline, 1st subject scored 6/20 while 2nd subject scored 0. At the end of the experiment, 1st subject scored 15/20 and 2nd scored 10/20. McNemar test for change indicates that these changes were significant (*p* < .01) improvements. Social validation: Both subjects said they preferred the prospective memory training; they enjoyed it and found it useful.	other neurological tests (not reported in this review) the administrator was blind to the study.	method of improving prospective memory is not known, but the procedures used in this study could be a jumping-off point to start such therapy. Occupational therapy researchers should join the neuropsychologists in studying treatment for prospective memory, since it is important for independent occupational functioning, and therefore falls within the realm of occupational therapy.

Raskin, S. A., & Sohlberg, M. M. (1996). The efficacy of prospective memory training in two adults with brain injury. *Journal of Head Trauma Rehabilitation, 11*(3), 32–51.

| Stapleton et al. (2007) | Evaluate the effectiveness of a "reminders" function on a mobile phone as a compensatory memory aid for persons with traumatic brain injury (TBI) | IV—Single-subject ABAB reversal design

$N = 5$ participants at a rehabilitation center at least 1 year postinjury, reported to have everyday memory problems and living with a caregiver | *Intervention:* Participants were provided with mobile phones that were programmed with individualized reminder messages using the reminders function. A combination of fading verbal prompts, errorless learning, and operant conditioning were employed to teach participants to use the mobile phone as a memory aid.

Outcome measures:
■ Speed and capacity of language processing
■ Rivermead Behavioral Memory Test (RBMT)
■ Tower Test (executive functioning)
■ Measure of everyday memory success in achieving target behaviors | An increase in target behaviors was noted for two participants, and did not return to baseline when the phone was removed. Those who did not benefit scored within the severe impairment range on the RBMT, were significantly impaired on the Tower Test and required 24-hour care. | Small sample size; responses of the caregivers following changes were not recorded | Mobile phones, a common device in today's society, hold promise to be used as memory aids for individuals with mild to moderate impairments who do not require 24-hour care or have executive functioning difficulties. Learning of occupational routines can be facilitated through a combination of fading verbal prompts, errorless learning, and operant conditioning using a common device. |

Stapleton, S., Adams, M., & Atterton, L. (2007). A mobile phone as a memory aid for individuals with traumatic brain injury: A preliminary investigation. *Brain Injury, 21,* 401–411.

(continued)

EVIDENCE TABLE. LEVEL IV (EXPERIMENTAL SINGLE-CASE STUDY[1]) FOR FOCUSED QUESTION 4 (*cont.*)

Author/Year	Study Objectives	Level/Design/Participants	Intervention and Outcome Measures	Results	Study Limitations	Implications for Occupational Therapy
Van den Broek et al. (2000)	Examine whether brain-injured patients could learn to use the Voice Organizer as a memory aid and utilize it to reduce prospective memory errors in their daily routine; determine whether successful use of the aid led to beneficial changes in patients' affect.	IV—ABA single-case experimental design *Participants:* 5 participants were included; however, only 1 of those had traumatic brain injury (TBI). Only his treatment and results will be reported. He was a 25-year-old man 21 months postinjury; scored 2 on the Rivermead Behavioural Memory Test (RBMT), indicating severe impairment of everyday memory.	Voice Organizer (Model #5300 by Voice Powered Technology International, Inc.), which presents current time, day, and date. Voice activated. *Phase A:* 3 weeks, during which 2 prospective tasks were assessed in the home without Voice Organizer. *Phase B:* 3 weeks, including training to use the Voice Organizer and use of it to recall the tasks *Outcome measures:* ▪ Positive & Negative Affect Schedule (PANAS) ▪ Message-Passing Task ▪ Domestic Tasks	The patient with TBI scored 0/24 during both A phases on the Message-Passing Task, but 16/24 during the B phase. He scored 0/12 for the domestic tasks in both A phases, but 10/12 for the B phase. He showed no significant improvement or deterioration on PANAS during the A or B phases.	Few controls for intervening variables; too few subjects (only 1 subject with TBI), so the result may not be generalizable; no statistical analysis of data; no information about the reliability of outcome measures. Evaluators probably not blind to the condition assignment.	The patient with TBI improved immediately on his ability to remember to do certain tasks with the use of the Voice Organizer. Although the research design is weak, the outcome with this one patient suggests that this aid may be useful and something to try in occupational therapy practice. Occupational therapy clinical researchers need to establish the efficacy of practical use of this aid to improve everyday performance of prospective tasks for long-term use.

Van den Broek, M. D., Downes, J., Johnson, Z., Dayus, B., & Hilton, N. (2000). Evaluation of an electronic memory aid in the neuropsychological rehabilitation of prospective memory deficits. *Brain Injury, 14,* 455–462.

[1]These studies describe the treatment procedures in detail, and readers are referred to the original sources for detailed guidance for treatment application.

EVIDENCE TABLE. LEVEL V (ANECDOTAL CASE REPORTS) FOR QUESTION 4.

What is the evidence for the effect of interventions to address cognitive/perceptual functions (attention, memory, executive functions) on the occupational performance for persons with traumatic brain injury?

Author/Year	Study Objectives	Level/Design/Participants	Intervention and Outcome Measures	Results	Study Limitations	Implications for Occupational Therapy
Clegg & Rowe (1996)	Illustrate the effectiveness of a method of teaching word-processing skills through two case studies	Level—V, case reports *Case 1:* 16-year-old-boy with brain damage after stroke—not included in this review *Case 2:* 17-year-old with traumatic brain injury	*Intervention:* One-on-one teaching method determined from a detailed task analysis of basic computer use and word processing using Microsoft Word. Five levels of achievement were identified, each with 4 to 7 skills required to achieve success. Errorless learning methods were used whenever possible. Adaptive devices determined by the occupational therapist were provided. Case #2 received 3—4 hours of training per week for 6 months. *Outcome measure:* Speed of performance (measured manually).	*Results:* After 2 months, Case #2 acquired basic level skills (Level 2); his letter-finding speed improved to near normal. After 6 months, he had acquired Level 3 skills and was moving toward Level 4.	Case reports present interesting ideas, but cannot establish the intervention as the cause of change observed because there are no controls for threats to internal validity. The uniqueness of the subject precludes external validation or generalization to other patients.	This report offers no trustworthy evidence that the interventions described caused the outcomes reported. The outcome was very modest in light of the extent (and cost) of therapy involved.

Clegg, F. M., & Rowe, A. L. (1996). A structured method for teaching word-processing skills to people with brain injury. *British Journal of Therapy and Rehabilitation, 3,* 553–558.

(continued)

EVIDENCE TABLE. LEVEL V (ANECDOTAL CASE REPORTS) FOR QUESTION 4 (*cont.*)

Author/Year	Study Objectives	Level/Design/ Participants	Intervention and Outcome Measures	Results	Study Limitations	Implications for Occupational Therapy
Gorman et al. (2003)	Illustrate the effectiveness of the ISAAC system in assisting 2 patients with generalization of rehabilitation to their home environments	Level—V, case reports *Participants: Case 1:* Anoxic brain injury secondary to myocardial infarction (not reported in this review) *Case 2:* 31-year-old male with traumatic brain injury with significant cognitive impairment	The ISAAC system is a small, individualized, wearable cognitive prosthetic assistive technology system. It enables presentation of each patient's individualized prompts and procedural content. It is used to initiate behavior, to provide basic structure to the patient's day, and to provide needed information to carry out an activity. Performance-based training is provided to learn to use the device. In Case 2, ISAAC was authored to provide checklists for morning and evening routines. When he completed the routine, he checked off each item by tapping the checkbox on the touch screen. He used it for 1 year. *Outcome measures:* FIM used to measure change in client performance but outcome measures were not reported by authors.	After 4 months of treatment, Case 2 met his goal of independence at home and his safety restrictions were lifted. FIM scores increased to 6 (modified independence) using external strategies, including the ISAAC system. His performance, using the ISAAC continued to improve during the 1 year of use. After 1 year, his routines were established and internalized and his personal safety was no longer an issue. ISAAC was discontinued.	Case reports present interesting ideas, but cannot establish the intervention as the cause of change observed because there are no controls for threats to internal validity. The uniqueness of the subject precludes external validation or generalization to other patients.	This report offers no trustworthy evidence that the interventions described caused the outcomes reported.

Gorman, P., Dayle, R., Hood, C-A., & Rumrell, L. (2003). Effectiveness of the ISAAC cognitive prosthetic system for improving rehabilitation outcomes with neurofunctional impairment. *NeuroRehabilitation, 18,* 57–67.

| Kim et al. (1999) | Describe the trial of a palmtop computer as a memory aid in a patient with traumatic brain injury | Level—V, case report

Participant: A 22-year-old man with deficits in prospective memory and executive function; 8 weeks postinjury; 4 weeks into in-patient rehabilitation; needed maximal cues for all aspects of his schedule | A palmtop computer (PSION Series 3a) was used as an electronic cueing device through use of the alarm application. When the alarm rang, the schedule information for that time filled the screen.

Outcome measures:
On-time attendance at therapy and on-time asking for medications as scheduled. | With this intervention, the patient demonstrated an immediate improvement in the ability to attend every therapy and ask for every medication on his schedule. | This report offers no trustworthy evidence that the interventions described caused the outcomes reported.

Case reports present interesting ideas, but cannot establish the intervention as the cause of change observed because there are no controls for threats to internal validity. The uniqueness of the subject precludes external validation or generalization to other patients. |

Kim, H. J., Burke, D. T., Dowds, M. M., & George, J. (1999). Utility of a microcomputer as an external memory aid for a memory-impaired head injury patient during in-patient rehabilitation. *Brain Injury, 13,* 147–150.

| Landa-Gonzalez (2001) | Examine the effectiveness of a multicontextual, community reentry occupational therapy program directed at awareness training and compensation for cognitive problems after traumatic brain injury | Level—V, case report

Participant: 34-year-old man; post-TBI, he had substantial memory and executive function impairments and poor insight about his functional limitations. He required constant supervision in a highly structured environment for his daily activities. | Metacognitive training, exploration and use of effective processing strategies, task gradations, and practice of functional activities in multiple environmental contexts. Treatment carried out at home and in his community (real-world environment). Strategies included self-prediction, self-monitoring, role reversal, use of checklists. 6 months duration.

Outcome measures:
■ Canadian Occupational Performance Measure (COPM)
■ Kohlman Evaluation of Living Skills (KELS)
■ Self-rating awareness checklist. | Client's awareness level, occupational function, and satisfaction with performance improved while level of attendant care decreased. KELS: He needed assistance with 10 skills at baseline, but only 3 at discharge (budgeting for food, budgeting monthly income, use of phone and book). COPM: He gained 1.5 to 2 points for each performance score and 1.5 to 3 points for each satisfaction score. He predicted task performance more accurately and closer to actual performance. Gains made in treatment were maintained 8 weeks after discharge. | This article offers suggestions, but no real evidence, that the interventions used in the study may be effective for persons with severe memory, executive function, or awareness impairments. The outcome was very modest in light of the extent (and cost) of therapy involved.

Case reports present interesting ideas, but cannot establish the intervention as the cause of change observed because there are no controls for threats to internal validity. The uniqueness of the subject precludes external validation or generalization to other patients. |

Landa-Gonzalez, B. (2001). Multicontextual occupational therapy intervention: A case study of traumatic brain injury. *Occupational Therapy International, 8*(1), 49–62.

(continued)

EVIDENCE TABLE. LEVEL V (ANECDOTAL CASE REPORTS) FOR QUESTION 4 (cont.)

Author/Year	Study Objectives	Level/Design/ Participants	Intervention and Outcome Measures	Results	Study Limitations	Implications for Occupational Therapy
Schwartz (1995)	Apply the decision-making and dynamic assessment models of occupational therapy in the home setting and to apply one or more of the following treatment methods: saturational cueing with behavioral chaining and positive reinforcement; coordinated team approach that included patient, family or significant others, and therapists; and environmental adaptations	Level—V, case reports In Case 1, therapy began 2 years post injury. In Cases 2 and 3, therapy began 1 year postinjury. Case 1 was a 50-year-old man with short-term memory loss, among other impairments. Case 2 was a 30-year-old man with severe executive function impairment. Case 3 had brain damage secondary to a rare blood disease and is not included in this review.	The treatment technique applied to each patient depended on the skill to be learned and the patient's learning style. *Case 1:* Increase independence in basic hygiene and grooming skills. Treatment: Reinforcement of specific behavioral sequences and education of home health attendants and wife about how to provide consistent routine and decrease assistance. *Case 2:* Improve initiation of morning bathing, dressing, and grooming routine. Treatment: Tape recorder with personalized recording of the behavioral chain to shower, shave, brush teeth, shampoo, and take medications.	*Case 1:* After 3 months, he became independent in tooth brushing and shaving daily. *Case 2:* 2 years after initiation of the tape-recorded messages, he followed his morning routine with only a checklist in the bathroom. He was unable to transfer these skills to a different context.	Case reports present interesting ideas, but cannot establish the intervention as the cause of change observed because there are no controls for threats to internal validity. The uniqueness of the subjects precludes external validation or generalization to other patients. Study did not include formal outcome measures.	This report offers no trustworthy evidence that the interventions described caused the outcomes reported. The outcome was very modest in light of the extent (and cost) of therapy involved.

Schwartz, S. M. (1995). Adults with traumatic brain injury: Three case studies of cognitive rehabilitation in the home setting. *American Journal of Occupational Therapy, 49,* 655–667.

| Wade & Troy (2001) | Evaluate whether a mobile phone was an effective memory aid by comparing self-initiated performance in remembering to carry out target tasks both prior to and with the mobile phone | Level—V, case reports

Participants: 5 persons with significant impairment of everyday memory who needed to carry out activities independently. Ages ranged from 18 to 51 years. Time since injury ranged from 1 to 15 years. | Standard mobile phones activated by computer sent reminder messages regarding 1 to 7 target tasks. If the message was not answered, the computer repeated attempts at regular intervals. Patients confirmed completion of tasks by keying their personalized number into the phone. Therapy applied at home.

Outcome measures: Individualized diaries for the patient and/or caregiver to record how frequently the identified targets were remembered independently for 6 weeks before introduction of the phone and for a variable period during phone use. | *Case 1:* 3 targets chosen; at baseline remembered 6%, with phone remembered 100%; maintained after removal of phone.
Case 2: 7 targets chosen; at baseline remembered 62%, with phone remembered 100%; phone use discontinued due to client making outgoing calls.
Case 3: 1 target chosen; at baseline remembered 48% of time, with phone, remembered 92%.
Case 4: 4 targets chosen; at baseline remembered 43%, with phone remembered 100%.
Case 5: 3 targets chosen; at baseline remembered 3% of time, with phone remembered 81%.
Cases 3, 4 and 5 continued to use the phone. | Case reports present interesting ideas, but cannot establish the intervention as the cause of change observed because there are no controls for threats to internal validity.

This report offers no trustworthy evidence that the interventions described caused the outcomes reported. |

Wade. T. K., & Troy, J. C. (2001). Mobile phones as a new memory aid: A preliminary investigation using case studies. *Brain Injury, 15,* 305–320.

Appendix E. Recommendations for Occupational Therapy Interventions for Clients With Traumatic Brain Injury: Supporting Evidence

Overall Recovery

Early and aggressive general rehabilitative intervention to reduce length of stay and improve short-term functional outcomes (B)

I - Cullen, N., Bayley, M., Bayona, N., Hilditch, M., & Aubut, J. (2007). Management of heterotopic ossification and venous thromboembolism following acquired brain injury. *Brain Injury, 21*, 215–230.

I - Turner-Stokes, L., Disler, P. B., Nair, A., & Wade, D. T. (2005). Multi-disciplinary rehabilitation for acquired brain injury in adults of working age. *Cochrane Database of Systematic Reviews*, Issue 3. Art. No.: CD004170. DOI: 10.1002/14651858. CD004170.pub2.

I - Zhu, X. L., Poon, W. S., Chan, C. C., & Chan, S. S. (2007). Does intensive rehabilitation improve the functional outcome of patients with traumatic brain injury (TBI)? A randomized controlled trial. *Brain Injury, 21*, 681–690.

I - Zhu, X. L., Poon, W. S., Chan, C. H., & Chan, S. H. (2001). Does intensive rehabilitation improve the functional outcome of patients with traumatic brain injury? Interim result of a randomized controlled trial. *British Journal of Neurosurgery, 15*, 464–473.

Challenging therapeutic interventions requiring mental manipulation to reorganize brain function (I)

V - Laatsch, Jobe, Sychra, Lin, & Blend, 1997; Laatsch, Thulborn, Krisky, Shobat, & Sweeney, 2004; Page & Levine, 2003; Scheibel et al., 2003, 2004; Tillerson & Miller, 2002

V - Scheibel, R. S., Pearson, D. A., Faria, L. P., Kotrla, K. J., Aylward, E., Bachevalier, J., et al. (2003). An fMRI study of executive functioning after severe diffuse TBI. *Brain Injury, 17*, 919–930.

Continued outpatient therapy sustains early gains (C)

II - Goranson, T. E., Graves, R. E., Allison, D., & LaFreniere, R. (2003). Community integration following multidisciplinary rehabilitation for traumatic brain injury. *Brain Injury, 17*, 759–774.

Short-term intervention for individuals with MTBI (I)

I - Paniak, C., Toller-Lobe, G., Durand, A., & Nagy, J. (1998). A randomized trial of two treatments for mild traumatic brain injury. *Brain Injury, 12*, 1011–1023.

I - Paniak, C., Toller-Lobe, G., Reynolds, S., Melnyk, A., & Nagy, J. (2000). A randomized trial of two treatments for mild traumatic brain injury: 1 year follow-up. *Brain Injury, 14*, 219–226.

Note. See Table 6 for definitions of A, B, C, D, and I. Levels of evidence are defined in Appendix C.

Family intervention (I)

I - Boschen, K., Gargaro, J., Gan, C., Gerber, G., & Brandys, C. (2007). Family interventions after acquired brain injury and other chronic conditions: A critical appraisal of the quality of the evidence. *NeuroRehabilitation, 22*, 19–41.

Post-acute functional-based rehabilitation (B)

IV - Parish, L., & Oddy, M. (2007). Efficacy of rehabilitation for functional skills more than 10 years after extremely severe brain injury. *Neuropsychological Rehabilitation, 17*, 230–243.

Interventions Focused on Client Factors/Impairments

Constraint-induced movement therapy (A)

Articles from brain injury/hemiparesis

III - Cho, Y. W., Jang, S. H., Lee, Z. I., Song, J. C., Lee, H. K., & Lee, H. Y. (2005). Effect and appropriate restriction period of constraint-induced movement therapy in hemiparetic patients with brain injury: A brief report. *NeuroRehabilitation, 20*, 71–74.

III - Shaw, S. E., Morris, D. M., Uswatte, G., McKay, S., Meythaler, J. M., & Taub, E. (2005). Constraint-induced movement therapy for recovery of upper-limb function following traumatic brain injury. *Journal of Rehabilitation Research and Development, 42*, 769–778.

IV - Page, S., & Levine, P. (2003). Forced use after TBI: Promoting plasticity and function through practice. *Brain Injury, 17*, 675–684.

Articles from stroke/hemiparesis

I - Lin, K.-C., Wu, C. Y., Wei, T. H., Lee, C. Y., & Liu, J. S. (2007). Effects of modified constraint-induced movement therapy on reach-to-grasp movements and functional performance after chronic stroke: A randomized controlled study. *Clinical Rehabilitation, 21*, 1075–1086.

I - Page, S. J., Levine, P., Leonard, A., Szaflarski, J. P., & Kissela, B. M. (2008). Modified constraint-induced therapy in chronic stroke: Results of a single-blinded randomized controlled trial. *Physical Therapy, 88*, 1–8.

I - Ro, T., Noser, E., Boake, C., Johnson, R., Gaber, M., Speroni, A., et al. (2006). Functional reorganization and recovery after constraint-induced movement therapy in subacute stroke: Case reports. *Neurocase, 12*, 50–60.

I - Sterr, A., Elbert, T., Berthold, I., Kolbel, S., Rockstroh, B., & Taub, E. (2002). Longer versus shorter daily constraint-induced movement therapy of chronic hemiparesis: An exploratory study. *Archives of Physical Medicine, 83*, 1374–1377.

I - Underwood, J., Clark, P. C., Blanton, S., Aycock, D. M., & Wolf, S. L. (2006). Pain, fatigue, and intensity of practice in people with stroke who are receiving constraint-induced movement therapy. *Physical Therapy, 86*, 1241–1250.

I - Wittenberg, G. F., Chen, R., Ishii, K., Bushara, K. O., Eckloff, S., Croarkin, E., et al. (2003). Constraint-induced therapy in stroke: Magnetic-stimulation motor maps and cerebral activation. *Neurorehabilitation and Neural Repair, 17*, 48–57.

I - Wolf, S. L., Winstein, C. J., Miller, J. P., Taub, E., Uswatte, G., Morris, D., et al. (2006). Effect of constraint-induced movement therapy on upper extremity function 3 to 9 months after stroke: The EXCITE randomized clinical trial. *JAMA, 296*, 2095–2104.

I - Wolf, S. L., Winstein, C. J., Miller, J. P., Thompson, P. A., Taub, E., Uswatte, G., et al. (2008). Retention of upper limb function in stroke survivors who have received constraint-induced movement therapy: The EXCITE randomized trial. *Lancet Neurology, 7*(1), 33–40.

I - Wu, C. Y., Chen, C. L., Tsai, W. C., Lin, K. C., & Chou, S. H. (2007). A randomized controlled trial of modified constraint-induced movement therapy for elderly stroke survivors: Changes in motor impairment, daily functioning, and quality of life. *Archives of Physical Medicine and Rehabilitation, 88*, 273–278.

I - Wu, C. Y., Lin, K. C., Chen, H. C., Chen, I. H., & Hong, W. H. (2007). Effects of modified constraint-induced movement therapy on movement kinematics and daily function in patients with stroke: A kinematic study of motor control mechanisms. *Neurorehabilitation and Neural Repair, 21,* 460–466.

II - Taub, E., Uswatte, G., King, D. K., Morris, D., Crago, J. E., & Chatterjee, A. (2006). A placebo-controlled trial of constraint-induced movement therapy for upper extremity after stroke. *Stroke, 37,* 1045–1049.

II - Uswatte, G., Taub, E., Morris, D., Barman, J., & Crago, J. (2006). Contribution of the shaping and restraint components of constraint-induced movement therapy to treatment outcome. *NeuroRehabilitation, 21,* 147–156.

III - Brogardh, C., & Sjölund, B. H. (2006). Constraint-induced movement therapy in patients with stroke: A pilot study on effects of small group training and of extended mitt use. *Clinical Rehabilitation, 20,* 218–227.

III - Flinn, N. A., Schamburg, S., Fetrow, J. M., & Flanigan, J. (2005). The effect of constraint-induced movement treatment on occupational performance and satisfaction in stroke survivors. *OTJR: Occupation, Participation, and Health, 25,* 119–127.

III - Fritz, S. L., Light, K. E., Clifford, S. N., Patterson, T. S., Behrman, A. L., & Davis, S. B. (2006). Descriptive characteristics as potential predictors of outcomes following constraint-induced movement therapy for people after stroke. *Physical Therapy, 86,* 825–832.

III - Liepert, J. (2006). Motor cortex excitability in stroke before and after constraint-induced movement therapy. *Cognitive and Behavioral Neurology, 19,* 41–47.

III - Liepert, J., Bauder, H., Wolfgang, H. R., Miltner, W. H., Taub, E., & Weiller, C. (2000). Treatment-induced cortical reorganization after stroke in humans. *Stroke, 31,* 1210–1216.

III - Page, S. J., & Levine, P. (2006). Back from the brink: Electromyography-triggered stimulation combined with modified constraint-induced movement

therapy in chronic stroke. *Archives of Physical Medicine and Rehabilitation, 87,* 27–31.

III - Szaflarski, J. P., Page, S. P., Kissela, B. M., Lee, J-H., Levine, P., & Strakowski, S. M. (2006). Cortical reorganization following modified constraint-induced movement therapy: A study of 4 patients with chronic stroke. *Archives of Physical Medicine and Rehabilitation, 87,* 1052–1058.

IV - Liepert, J., Hamzei, F., & Weiller, C. (2004). Lesion-induced and training-induced brain reorganization. *Restorative Neurology and Neuroscience, 22,* 269–277.

Serial casting of ankle plantar contractures (A)

I - Marshall, S., Teasell, R., Bayona, N., Lippert, C., Chundamala, J., Villamere, J., et al. (2007). Motor impairment rehabilitation post acquired brain injury. *Brain Injury, 21,* 133–160.

Serial casting of upper-extremity contractures (B)

I - Marshall, S., Teasell, R., Bayona, N., Lippert, C., Chundamala, J., Villamere, J., et al. (2007). Motor impairment rehabilitation post acquired brain injury. *Brain Injury, 21,* 133–160.

II - Hill, J. (1994). The effects of casting on upper-extremity motor disorders after brain injury. *American Journal of Occupational Therapy, 48,* 219–224.

III - Pohl, M., Ruckriem, S., Mehrholz, J., Ritschel, D., Strik, H., & Pause, M. R. (2002). Effectiveness of serial casting in patients with severe cerebral spasticity: A comparison study. *Archives of Physical Medicine and Rehabilitation, 83,* 784–790.

Purposeful activities for fine motor recovery (B)

I - Neistadt, M. E. (1994). The effects of different treatment activities on functional fine motor coordination in adults with brain injury. *American Journal of Occupational Therapy, 48,* 877–882.

Sensory stimulation or coma arousal programs (I)

I - Johnson, D. A., Roethig-Johnson, K., & Richards, D. (1993). Biochemical and physiological parameters of recovery in acute severe head injury: Responses to multisensory stimulation. *Brain Injury, 7,* 491–499.

I - Lombardi, F., Taricco, M., De Tanti, A., Telaro, E., & Liberati, A. (2002). Sensory stimulation of brain-injured individuals in coma or vegetative state: Results of a Cochrane systematic review. *Clinical Rehabilitation, 16,* 464–472.

II - Davis, A. E., & Gimenez, A. (2003). Cognitive–behavioral recovery in comatose patients following auditory sensory stimulation. *Journal of Neuroscience Nursing, 35,* 202–209, 214.

II - Mitchell, S., Bradley, V. A., Welch, J. L., & Britton, P. G. (1990). Coma arousal procedure: A therapeutic intervention in the treatment of head injury. *Brain Injury, 4,* 273–279.

IV - Wilson, S. L., Brock, D., Powell, G. E., Thwaites, H., & Elliott, K. (1996). Constructing arousal profiles for vegetative state patients—A preliminary study. *Brain Injury, 10,* 105–113.

IV - Wilson, S. L., Powell, G. E., Brock, D., & Thwaites, H. (1996). Vegetative state and responses to sensory stimulation: An analysis of 24 cases. *Brain Injury, 10,* 807–818.

V - Watson, M., & Horn, S. (1991). "The ten pound note test": Suggestions for eliciting improved responses in the severely brain-injured patient. *Brain Injury, 5,* 421–424.

Cognitive–behavioral therapy for insomnia (I)

IV - Ouellet, M. C., & Morin, C. M. (2007). Efficacy of cognitive–behavioral therapy for insomnia associated with traumatic brain injury: A single-case experimental design. *Archives of Physical Medicine and Rehabilitation, 88,* 1581–1592.

Continuous passive motion for heterotopic ossification in lower extremity (I)

I - Cullen, N., Bayley, M., Bayona, N., Hilditch, M., & Aubut, J. (2007). Management of heterotopic ossification and venous thromboembolism following acquired brain injury. *Brain Injury, 21,* 215–230.

Calendars for temporal reorientation (I)

I - Watanabe, T. K., Black, K. L., Zafonte, R. D., Millis, S. R., & Mann, N. R. (1998). Do calendars enhance posttraumatic temporal orientation?: A pilot study. *Brain Injury, 12,* 81–85.

Telerehabilitation for cognitive impairments (I)

IV - Tam, S-F., Man, W. K., Hui-Chan, C. W. Y., Lau, A., Yip, B., & Cheung, W. (2003). Evaluating the efficacy of tele-cognitive rehabilitation for functional performance in three case studies. *Occupational Therapy International, 10*(1), 20–38.

Nocturnal hand splinting to improve range of motion, pain, or function is not effective (D)

II - Lannin, N. A., Horsley, S. A., Herbert, R., McCluskey, A., & Cusick, A. (2003). Splinting the hand in the functional position after brain impairment: A randomized, controlled trial. *Archives of Physical Medicine and Rehabilitation, 84,* 297–302.

Interventions Focused on Performance Skills

Errorless learning (A)

I - Kessels, R. P. C., & de Haan, E. H. F. (2003). Implicit learning in memory rehabilitation: A meta-analysis on errorless learning and vanishing cue methods. *Journal of Clinical and Experimental Neuropsychology, 25,* 805–814.

V - Bieman-Copland, S., & Dywan, J. (2000). Achieving rehabilitative gains in anosognosia after TBI. *Brain and Cognition, 44,* 1–5.

V - Campbell, L., Wilson, F. C., McCann, J., Kernahan, G., & Rogers, R. G. (2007). Single-case experimental design study of Carer Facilitated Errorless Learning in a patient with severe memory impairment following TBI. *NeuroRehabilitation, 22,* 325–333.

Compensatory approaches to cognitive rehabilitation (A)

I - Cicerone, K. D., Dahlberg, C., Kalmar, K., Langenbahn, D. M., Malec, J. F., Berquist, T. F., et al. (2000). Evidence-based cognitive rehabilitation: Recommendations for clinical practice. *Archives of Physical Medicine and Rehabilitation, 81*, 1596–1615.

I - Cicerone, K. D., Dahlberg, C., Malec, J. F., Langenbahn, D. M., Felicetti, T., Kneipp, S., et al. (2005). Evidence-based cognitive rehabilitation: Updated review of the literature from 1998 through 2002. *Archives of Physical Medicine and Rehabilitation, 86*, 1681–1692.

Memory rehabilitation utilizing restorative (visualization, mnemonics), compensatory (internal mnemonics, external aids), and external change/adapt environment strategies for clients with mild-to-moderate impairments (A)

I - Loya, G. J. (1999). *Efficacy of memory rehabilitation among adolescent and adult TBI survivors: A meta-analysis.* Unpublished doctoral dissertation, University of Nebraska, Lincoln.

II - Freeman, M. R., Mittenberg, W., Dicowden, M., & Bat-ami, M. (1992). Executive and compensatory memory retraining in traumatic brain injury. *Brain Injury, 6*, 65–70.

III - Quemada, J. I., Cespedes, J. M. M., Ezkerra, J., Ballesteros, J., Ibarra, N., & Urruticoechea, I. (2003). Outcome of memory rehabilitation in traumatic brain injury assessed by neuropsychological tests and questionnaires. *Journal of Head Trauma Rehabilitation, 18*, 532–540.

Computerized memory orthoses for prospective memory (A)

I - Rees, L., Marshall, S., Hartridge, C., Mackie, D., & Weiser, M. (2007). Cognitive interventions post acquired brain injury. *Brain Injury, 21*, 161–200.

II - Burke, D. T., Leeb, S. B., Hinman, R. T., Lupton, E. C., Burke, J., Schneider, J. C., et al. (2001). Using talking lights to assist brain-injured patients with a daily inpatient therapeutic schedule. *Journal of Head Trauma Rehabilitation, 16*, 284–291.

II - Wright, P., Rogers, N., Hall, C., Wilson, B., Evans, J., & Emslie, H. (2001). Enhancing an appointment diary on a pocket computer for use by people after brain injury. *International Journal of Rehabilitation Research, 24*, 299–308.

II - Wright, P., Rogers, N., Hall, C., Wilson, B., Evans, J., Emslie, H., & Bartram, C. (2001). Comparison of pocket-computer memory aids for people with brain injury. *Brain Injury, 15*, 787-800.

III - Gentry, T., Wallace, J., Kvarfordt, C., & Lynch, K. B. (2008). Personal digital assistants as cognitive aids for individuals with severe traumatic brain injury: A community-based trial. *Brain Injury, 22*, 19–24.

IV - Van den Broek, M. D., Downes, J., Johnson, Z., Dayus, B., & Hilton, N. (2000). Evaluation of an electronic memory aid in the neuropsychological rehabilitation of prospective memory deficits. *Brain Injury, 14*, 455-462.

Awareness training embedded in functional task performance (A)

I - Goverover, Y., Johnston, M. V., Toglia, J., & DeLuca, J. (2007). Treatment to improve self-awareness in persons with acquired brain injury. *Brain Injury, 21*, 913–923.

I - Ownsworth, T., Fleming, J., Shum, D., Kuipers, P., & Strong, J. (2008). Comparison of individualized, group and combined intervention formats in a randomized controlled trial for facilitating goal attainment and improving psychosocial function following acquired brain injury. *Journal of Rehabilitation Medicine, 40*, 81–88.

IV - Ownsworth, T., Fleming, J., Desbois, J., Strong, J., & Kuipers, P. (2006). A metacognitive contextual intervention to enhance error awareness and functional outcome following traumatic brain injury: A single-case experimental design. *Journal of the International Neuropsychological Society, 12*, 54-63.

V - Landa-Gonzales, B. (2001). Multicontextual occupational therapy intervention: A case study of traumatic brain injury. *Occupational Therapy International, 8,* 49–62.

Group-based cognitive rehabilitation (A)

I - Ownsworth, T., Fleming, J., Shum, D., Kuipers, P., & Strong, J. (2008). Comparison of individualized, group, and combined intervention formats in a randomized controlled trial for facilitating goal attainment and improving psychosocial function following acquired brain injury. *Journal of Rehabilitation Medicine, 40,* 81–88.

I - Thickpenny-Davis, K. L., & Barker-Collo, S. L. (2007). Evaluation of a structured group format memory rehabilitation program for adults following brain injury. *Journal of Head Trauma Rehabilitation, 22,* 303–313.

III - Braverman, S. E., Spector, J., Warden, D. L., Wilson, B. C., Ellis, T. E., Bamdad, M. J., et al. (1999). A multidisciplinary TBI inpatient rehabilitation programme for active duty service members as part of a randomized clinical trial. *Brain Injury, 13,* 405–415.

Social skills training (B)

I - Dahlberg, C. A., Cusick, C. P., Hawley, L. A., Newman, J. K., Morey, C. E., Harrison-Felix, C. L., et al. (2007). Treatment efficacy of social communication skills training after traumatic brain injury: A randomized treatment and deferred treatment controlled trial. *Archives of Physical Medicine and Rehabilitation, 88,* 1561–1573.

V - Gutman, S. A., & Leger, D. L. (1997). Enhancement of one-to-one interpersonal skills necessary to initiate and maintain intimate relationships: A frame of reference for adults having sustained traumatic brain injury. *Occupational Therapy in Mental Health, 13,* 51–67.

V - Sladyk, K. (1992). Case Report: Traumatic brain injury, behavioral disorder, and group treatment. *American Journal of Occupational Therapy, 46,* 267–270.

V - Yuen, H. K. (1997). Positive talk training in an adult with traumatic brain injury. *American Journal of Occupational Therapy, 51,* 780–783.

Establishment of goals valued by the client combined with compensatory training and environmental adaptation (B)

I - Ownsworth, T., Fleming, J., Shum, D., Kuipers, P., & Strong, J. (2008). Comparison of individualized, group, and combined intervention formats in a randomized controlled trial for facilitating goal attainment and improving psychosocial function following acquired brain injury. *Journal of Rehabilitation Medicine, 40,* 81–88.

II - Goranson, T. E., Graves, R. E., Allison, D., & LaFreniere, R. (2003). Community integration following multidisciplinary rehabilitation for traumatic brain injury. *Brain Injury, 17,* 759–774.

III - Mills, V. M., Nesbeda, T., Katz, D. I., & Alexander, M. P. (1992). Outcomes for traumatically brain-injured patients following post-acute rehabilitation programmes. *Brain Injury, 6,* 219–228.

III - Trombly, C. A., Radomski, M. V., Trexel, C., & Burnett-Smith, S. E. (2002). Occupational therapy and achievement of self-identified goals by adults with acquired brain injury: Phase II. *American Journal of Occupational Therapy, 56,* 489–498.

V - Walker, J. P. (2002). Case Study: Functional outcome: A case for mild traumatic brain injury. *Brain Injury, 16,* 611–625.

Pager systems for memory and planning problems (B)

I - Wilson, B. A., Emslie, H. C., Quirk, K., & Evans, J. J. (2001). Reducing everyday memory and planning problems by means of a paging system: A randomized control crossover design. *Journal of Neurology, Neurosurgery, and Psychiatry, 70,* 477–482.

Treating the client within environments that are graded to reduce structure and to increase distractions equal to real-life situations (I)

III - Hayden, M. E., Moreault, A. M., LeBlanc, J., & Plenger, P. M. (2000). Reducing level of handicap in traumatic brain injury: An environmentally based model of treatment. *Brain Injury, 15,* 1000–1021.

V - Kowalske, K., Plenger, P. M., Lusby, B., & Hayden, M. E. (2000). Vocational reentry following TBI: An enablement model. *Journal of Head Trauma Rehabilitation, 15,* 989–999.

PDA to remind client about therapy goals (B)

I - Hart, T., Hawkey, K., & Whyte, J. (2002). Use of a portable voice organizer to remember therapy goals in traumatic brain injury rehabilitation: A within-subjects trial. *Journal of Head Trauma Rehabilitation, 17,* 556–570.

Mobile phones as compensatory memory aids (B)

IV - Stapleton, S., Adams, M., & Atterton, L. (2007). A mobile phone as a memory aid for individuals with traumatic brain injury: A preliminary investigation. *Brain Injury, 21,* 401–411.

V - Wade, T. K., & Troy, J. C. (2001). Mobile phones as a new memory aid: A preliminary investigation using case studies. *Brain Injury, 15,* 305–320.

Goal management training (C)

I - Levine, B., Robertson, I. H., Clare, L., Carter, G., Hong, J., Wilson, B. A., et al. (2000). Rehabilitation of executive functioning: An experimental–clinical validation of Goal Management Training. *Journal of the International Neuropsychological Society, 6,* 299–312.

Behavioral approach using positive reinforcement (C)

III - McMorrow, M. J., Braunling-McMorrow, D., & Smith, S. (1998). Evaluation of functional outcomes following proactive behavioral–residential treatment. *Journal of Rehabilitation Outcomes Measurement, 2,* 22–30.

III - Murrey, G. J., & Starzinski, D. (2004). An inpatient neurobehavioral rehabilitation programme for persons with traumatic brain injury: Overview of and outcome data for the Minnesota Neurorehabilitation Hospital. *Brain Injury, 18,* 519–531.

IV - Schlund, M. W., & Pace, G. (1999). Relations between traumatic brain injury and the environment:

Feedback reduces maladaptive behaviour exhibited by three persons with traumatic brain injury. *Brain Injury, 13,* 889–897.

V - Fluharty, G., & Glassman, N. (2001). Case Study: Use of antecedent control to improve the outcome of rehabilitation for a client with frontal lobe injury and intolerance for auditory and tactile stimuli. *Brain Injury, 15,* 995–1002.

V - Rothwell, N. A., LaVigna, G. W., & Willis, T. J. (1999). A non-aversive rehabilitation approach for people with severe behavioural problems resulting from brain injury. *Brain Injury, 13,* 521–533.

Environmental cues for performance of ADLs and IADLs (B)

I - Manly, T., Hawkins, K., Evans, J., Woldt, K., & Robertson, I. H. (2002). Rehabilitation of executive function: Facilitation of effective goal management on complex tasks using periodic auditory alerts. *Neuropsychologia, 40,* 271–281.

V - Gorman, P., Dayle, R., Hood, C-A., & Rumrell, L. (2003). Effectiveness of the ISAAC cognitive prosthetic system for improving rehabilitation outcomes with neurofunctional impairment. *NeuroRehabilitation, 18,* 57–67.

V - Kim, H. J., Burke, D. T., Dowds, M. M., & George, J. (1999). Utility of a microcomputer as an external memory aid for a memory-impaired head injury patient during in-patient rehabilitation. *Brain Injury, 13,* 147–150.

V - Landa-Gonzales, B. (2001). Multicontextual occupational therapy intervention: A case study of traumatic brain injury. *Occupational Therapy International, 8,* 49–62.

V - Schwartz, S. M. (1995). Adults with traumatic brain injury: Three case studies of cognitive rehabilitation in the home setting. *American Journal of Occupational Therapy, 49,* 655–667.

Attention remediation programs for clients in the chronic phase of recovery (B)

I - Novack, T. A., Caldwell, S. G., Duke, L. W., Bergquist, T. F., & Gage, R. G. (1996). Focused versus unstructured intervention for attention deficits after traumatic brain injury. *Journal of Head Trauma Rehabilitation, 11,* 52–60.

I - Park, N. W., & Ingles, J. L. (2001). Effectiveness of attention rehabilitation after an acquired brain injury: A meta-analysis. *Neuropsychology, 15,* 199–210. [Also published in 2000 in *Brain and Cognition, 44,* 1–18.]

Attention processing therapy (C)

I - Sohlberg, M. M., McLaughlin, K. A., Pavese, A., Heidrich, A., & Posner, M. I. (2000). Evaluation of attention process training and brain injury education in persons with acquired brain injury. *Journal of Clinical and Experimental Neuropsychology, 22,* 656–676.

Prospective memory training (I)

IV - Raskin, S. A., & Sohlberg, M. M. (1996). The efficacy of prospective memory training in two adults with brain injury. *Journal of Head Trauma Rehabilitation, 11,* 32–51.

Positive talk training (I)

V - Yuen, H. K. (1997). Positive talk training in an adult with traumatic brain injury. *American Journal of Occupational Therapy, 51,* 780–783.

Organizational supports to reduce everyday memory problems (I)

V - Turkstra, L. S., & Flora, T. L. (2002). Compensating for executive function impairments after TBI: A single-case study of functional intervention. *Journal of Communication Disorders, 35,* 467–482.

Multidisciplinary cognitive rehabilitation (I)

I - Salazar, A. M., Warden, D. L., Schwab, K., Spector, J., Braverman, S., Waler, J., et al. (2000). Cognitive rehabilitation for traumatic brain injury: A randomized trial. *JAMA, 283,* 3075–3081.

I - Turner-Stokes, L., Disler, P. B., Nair, A., & Wade, D. T. (2005). Multi-disciplinary rehabilitation for acquired brain injury in adults of working age.

Cochrane Database of Systematic Reviews, Issue 3. Art. No.: CD004170. DOI: 10.1002/14651858. CD004170.pub2.

III - Braverman, S. E., Spector, J., Warden, D. L., Wilson, B. C., Ellis, T. E., Bamdad, M. J., et al. (1999). A multidisciplinary TBI inpatient rehabilitation programme for active duty service members as part of a randomized clinical trial. *Brain Injury, 13,* 405–415.

III - Ho, M. R., & Bennett, T. L. (1997). Efficacy of neuropsychological rehabilitation for mild–moderate traumatic brain injury. *Archives of Clinical Neuropsychology, 12,* 1–11.

III - Mills, V. M., Nesbeda, T., Katz, D. I., & Alexander, M. P. (1992). Outcomes for traumatically brain-injured patients following post-acute rehabilitation programmes. *Brain Injury, 6,* 219–228.

TEACH–M approach for using a simple e-mail interface (I)

IV - Ehlhardt, L. A., Sohlberg, M. M., Glang, A., & Albin, R. (2005). TEACH–M: A pilot study evaluating an instructional sequence for persons with impaired memory and executive functions. *Brain Injury, 19,* 569–583.

Self-determination model to address integrated self-awareness (I)

V - DeHope, E., & Finegan, J. (1999). The self-determination model: An approach to develop awareness for survivors of traumatic brain injury. *NeuroRehabilitation, 13,* 3–12.

Intervention focused on perception of emotion on psychosocial functioning (I)

I - Bornhofen, C., & McDonald, S. (2008). Treating deficits in emotional perception following traumatic brain injury. *Neuropsychological Rehabilitation, 18,* 22–44.

Gross motor activities for attention (I)

V - Shimelman, A., & Hinojosa, J. (1995). Gross motor activity and attention in three adults with brain injury. *American Journal of Occupational Therapy*, *49*, 973–979.

Sustained attention training for hemi-attention disorder (I)

V - Wilson, F. C., & Manly, T. (2003). Sustained attention training and errorless learning facilitates self-care functioning in chronic ipsilesional neglect following severe traumatic brain injury. *Neuropsychological Rehabilitation, 13,* 537–548.

Web-based interactive assistance for performance of targeted functional activity (I)

IV - Kirsch, N. L., Shenton, M., Spirl, E., Rowan, J., Simpson, R., Schreckengost, D., et al. (2004). Web-based assistive technology interventions for cognitive impairments after traumatic brain injury: A selective review and two case studies. *Rehabilitation Psychology, 49,* 200–212.

Modified memory diary with a pair of pages for each day of the week (i.e., timetable and to-do list) (I)

IV - McKerracher, G., Powell, T., & Oyebode, J. (2005). A single-case experimental design comparing two memory notebook formats for a man with memory problems caused by traumatic brain injury. *Neuropsychological Rehabilitation, 15,* 115–128.

Use of an alphanumeric pager system to increase memory notebook use (I)

IV - Kirsch, N. L., Shenton, M., & Rowan, J. (2004). A generic, 'in-house,' alphanumeric paging system for prospective activity impairments after traumatic brain injury. *Brain Injury, 18,* 725–734.

Computer-related activities designed to enhance participation in desired social roles (I)

V - Gutman, S. A. (2000). Using a computer as an environmental facilitator to promote post-head injury social role resumption: A case report. *Occupational Therapy in Mental Health, 15,* 71–89.

Game format to teach information about TBI (I)

IV - Zhou, J., Chittum, R., Johnston, K., Poppen, R., Guercio, J., & McMorrow, M. J. (1996). The utilization of a game format to increase knowledge of residuals among people with acquired brain injury. *Journal of Head Trauma Rehabilitation, 11,* 51–61.

Role-playing to achieve friendships and intimate relationships (I)

V - Gutman, S. A., & Leger, D. L. (1997). Enhancement of one-to-one interpersonal skills necessary to initiate and maintain intimate relationships: A frame of reference for adults having sustained traumatic brain injury. *Occupational Therapy in Mental Health, 13,* 51–67.

Cognitive groups to achieve return to employment (I)

III - Parente, R., & Stapleton, M. (1999). Development of a cognitive strategies group for vocational training after traumatic brain injury. *NeuroRehabilitation, 13,* 13–20.

Drills and computerized practice training are not effective for improving attention or memory (D)

I - Rees, L., Marshall, S., Hartridge, C., Mackie, D., & Weiser, M. (2007). Cognitive interventions post acquired brain injury. *Brain Injury, 21,* 161–200.

II - Tam, S-F., & Man, W-K. (2004). Evaluating computer-assisted memory retraining programmes for people with post-head injury amnesia. *Brain Injury, 18,* 461–470.

Interventions Focused on Occupational Performance Areas or Participation

Functional–experiential treatment for older clients with TBI and independent living goals (B)

I - Vanderploeg, R. D., Schwab, K., Walker, W. C., Fraser, J. A., Sigford, B. J., Date, E. S., et al. (2008). Rehabilitation of traumatic brain injury in active duty military personnel and veterans: Defense and Veter-

Appendix E. Recommendations for Occupational Therapy Interventions for Clients With Traumatic Brain Injury: Supporting Evidence

229

ans' Brain Injury Center randomized controlled trial of two rehabilitation approaches. *Archives of Physical Medicine and Rehabilitation, 89,* 2227–2238.

Written contracts to achieve short-term goals (B)

I - Powell, J., Heslin, J., & Greenwood, R. (2002). Community-based rehabilitation after severe traumatic brain injury: A randomized controlled trial. *Journal of Neurology, Neurosurgery, and Psychiatry, 72,* 193–202.

Life skills training to increase community participation (B)

II - Wheeler, S. D., Lane, S. J., & McMahon, B. T. (2007). Community participation and life satisfaction following intensive, community-based rehabilitation using a life skills training approach. *OTJR: Occupation, Participation, and Health, 27,* 13–22.

III - Malec, J. F. (2001). Impact of comprehensive day treatment on societal participation for persons with acquired brain injury. *Archives of Physical Medicine and Rehabilitation, 82,* 885–895.

Intensive cognitive rehabilitation to return to work for military personnel (B)

I - Salazar, A. M., Warden, D. L., Schwab, K., Spector, J., Braverman, S., Waler, J., et al. (2000). Cognitive rehabilitation for traumatic brain injury: A randomized trial. *JAMA, 283,* 3075–3081.

I - Vanderploeg, R. D., Schwab, K., Walker, W. C., Fraser, J. A., Sigford, B. J., Date, E. S., et al. (2008). Rehabilitation of traumatic brain injury in active duty military personnel and veterans: Defense and Veterans' Brain Injury Center randomized controlled trial of two rehabilitation approaches. *Archives of Physical Medicine and Rehabilitation, 89,* 2227–2238.

III - Braverman, S. E., Spector, J., Warden, D. L., Wilson, B. C., Ellis, T. E., Bamdad, M. J., et al. (1999). A multidisciplinary TBI inpatient rehabilitation programme for active duty service members as part of a randomized clinical trial. *Brain Injury, 13,* 405–415.

Electronic aids for daily living (I)

III - Boman, I-L., Tham, K., Granqvist, A., Bartfai, A., & Hemmingsson, H. (2007). Using electronic aids to daily living after acquired brain injury: A study of the learning process and the usability. *Disability and Rehabilitation: Assistive Technology, 2,* 23–33.

Wrist-worn electronic device for community navigation (I)

II - Sohlberg, M. M., Fickas, S., Hung, P., & Fortier, A. (2007). A comparison of four prompt modes for route finding for community travellers with severe cognitive impairments. *Brain Injury, 21,* 531–538.

■ ■ ■

References

Abreu, B. C., & Peloquin, S. M. (2005). The quad-raphonic approach: A holistic rehabilitation model for brain injury. In N. Katz (Ed.), *Cognition and occupation across the life span* (2nd ed., pp. 73–112). Bethesda, MD: AOTA Press.

Abreu, B. C., Seale, G., Scheibel, R. S., Huddleston, H., Zhang, L., & Ottenbacher, K. J. (2001). Levels of self-awareness after acute brain injury: How patients' and rehabilitation specialists' perceptions compare. *Archives of Physical Medicine and Rehabilitation, 82,* 49–56.

Acimovic, M. L., & Keatley, M. A. (1991, October). *Cognitive brain injury descriptor scale: Automated program evaluation.* Paper presented at the meeting of the Colorado Head Injury Foundation, Boulder.

Agency for Healthcare Research and Quality, U.S. Preventive Services Task Force. (2009). *Standard recommendation language.* Retrieved February 14, 2009, from http://www.ahrq.gov/clinic/uspstf/standard.htm

Alderman, N., Knight, C., & Morgan, C. (1997). Use of a modified version of the Overt Aggression Scale in the measurement and assessment of aggressive behaviours following brain injury. *Brain Injury, 11,* 503–523.

Alderson, A. L., Novack, T. A., & Dowler, R. (2003). Reliable serial measurement of cognitive processes in rehabilitation: The Cognitive Log. *Archives of Physical Medicine and Rehabilitation, 84,* 668–672.

Allen, C. K. (1985). *Occupational therapy for psychiatric diseases: Measurement and management of cognitive disabilities.* Boston: Little, Brown.

Allen, C. K. (1993). Creating a need-satisfying, safe environment: Management and maintenance approaches. In C. B. Royeen (Ed.), *AOTA Self-Study Series: Cognitive rehabilitation* (Lesson 11). Rockville, MD: American Occupational Therapy Association.

American Occupational Therapy Association. (1979). Uniform terminology for occupational therapy. *Occupational Therapy News, 35*(11), 1–8.

American Occupational Therapy Association. (1989). Uniform terminology for occupational therapy (2nd ed.). *American Journal of Occupational Therapy, 43,* 808–815.

American Occupational Therapy Association. (1994). Uniform terminology for occupational therapy (3rd ed.). *American Journal of Occupational Therapy, 48,* 1047–1054.

American Occupational Therapy Association. (2002). Occupational therapy practice framework: Domain and process. *American Journal of Occupational Therapy, 56,* 609–639.

American Occupational Therapy Association. (2004). Guidelines for supervision, roles, and responsibilities during the delivery of therapy services. *American Journal of Occupational Therapy, 58,* 663–667.

American Occupational Therapy Association. (2005). Standards of practice for occupational therapy. *American Journal of Occupational Therapy, 59,* 663–665.

American Occupational Therapy Association. (2006). Policy 1.44: Categories of occupational therapy personnel. In *Policy manual* (2008 ed., pp. 33–34). Bethesda, MD: Author.

American Occupational Therapy Association. (2007a). Accreditation standards for a doctoral-degree-level educational program for the occupational therapist. *American Journal of Occupational Therapy, 61,* 641–651.

American Occupational Therapy Association. (2007b). Accreditation standards for a master's-degree-level educational program for the occupational therapist. *American Journal of Occupational Therapy, 61,* 652–661.

American Occupational Therapy Association. (2007c). Accreditation standards for an educational program for the occupational therapy assistant. *American Journal of Occupational Therapy, 61,* 662–671.

American Occupational Therapy Association. (2008a). Guidelines for documentation of occupational therapy. *American Journal of Occupational Therapy, 62,* 684–689.

American Occupational Therapy Association. (2008b). Occupational therapy practice framework: Domain and process (2nd cd.). *American Journal of Occupational Therapy, 62,* 625–688.

Ansell, B. J., & Keenan, J. E. (1989). The Western Neurosensory Stimulation Profile: A tool for assessing slow-to-recover head-injured patients. *Archives of Physical Medicine and Rehabilitation, 70,* 104–108.

Arnadottir, G. (1990). *The brain and behavior: Assessing cortical dysfunction through activities of daily living.* St. Louis, MO: Mosby.

Ashman, T. A., Gordon, W. A., Cantor, J. B., & Hibbard, M. R. (2006). Neurobehavioral consequences of traumatic brain injury. *Mount Sinai Journal of Medicine, 73,* 999–1005.

Averbuch, S., & Katz, N. (2005). Cognitive rehabilitation: A retraining model for clients with neurological disabilities. In N. Katz (Ed.), *Cognitive and occupation across the life span: Models for intervention in occupational therapy* (2nd ed., pp. 113–138). Bethesda, MD: AOTA Press.

Avery-Smith, W. (1996). Eating dysfunction position paper. *American Journal of Occupational Therapy, 50,* 746–847.

Avery-Smith, W., & Dellarosa, D. M. (1994). Approaches to treating dysphagia in patients with brain injury. *American Journal of Occupational Therapy, 48,* 235–239.

Banovac, K., & Speed, J., (2008). *Heterotopic ossification.* Retrieved July 1, 2008, from http://www.emedicine.com/pmr/topic51.htm

Berg, J. (1997). Playing the outcomes game. *OT Week, 11*(22), 12–15.

Bergman, M. M. (2000). Successful mastery with a cognitive orthotic in people with traumatic brain injury. *Applied Neuropsychology, 7,* 76–82.

Berthier, M. L., Kulisevsky, J. J., Gironell, A., & López, O. L. (2001). Obsessive–compulsive disorder and traumatic brain injury: Behavioral, cognitive, and neuroimaging findings. *Neuropsychiatry, Neuropsychology, and Behavioral Neurology, 14,* 23–31.

Bieman-Copeland, S., & Dywan, J. (2000). Achieving rehabilitative gains in anosognosia after TBI. *Brain and Cognition, 44,* 1–5.

Black, K. L., Hanks, R. A., Wood, D. L., Zafonte, R. D., Cullen, N., Cifu, D. X., et al. (2002). Blunt versus penetrating violent traumatic brain injury: Frequency and factors associated with secondary conditions and complications. *Journal of Head Trauma Rehabilitation, 17,* 489–496.

Blundon, G., & Smits, E. (2000). Cognitive rehabilitation: A pilot survey of therapeutic modalities used by Canadian occupational therapists with survivors of traumatic brain injury. *Canadian Journal of Occupational Therapy, 67,* 184–196.

Boake, C. (1996). Supervision Rating Scale: A measure of functional outcome from brain injury. *Archives of Physical Medicine and Rehabilitation, 77,* 765–772.

Bogner, J. A., Corrigan, J. D., Fugate, L., Mysiw, W. J., & Clinchot, D. (2001). Role of agitation in prediction of outcomes after traumatic brain injury. *American Journal of Physical Medicine and Rehabilitation, 80,* 636–644.

Bohannon, R. W., & Smith, M. B. (1987). Interrater reliability of a Modified Ashworth Scale of muscle spasticity. *Physical Therapy, 67,* 206–207.

Boman, I-L., Tham, K., Granqvist, A., Bartfai, A., & Hemmingsson, H. (2007). Using electronic aids to daily living after acquired brain injury: A study of the learning process and the usability. *Disability and Rehabilitation: Assistive Technology, 2,* 23–33.

Book, D. (2002). Disorders of brain function. In C. M. Porth (Ed.), *Pathophysiology: Concepts of altered health states* (6th ed., pp. 1159–1199). Philadelphia: Lippincott Williams & Wilkins.

Borgaro, S. R., & Prigatano, G. P. (2003). Modification of the Patient Competency Rating Scale for use on an acute neurorehabiliation unit: The PCRS–NR. *Brain Injury, 17,* 847–853.

Bornhofen, C., & McDonald, S. (2008). Treating deficits in emotional perception following traumatic brain injury. *Neuropsychological Rehabilitation, 18,* 22–44.

Boschen, K., Gargaro, J., Gan, C., Gerber, G., & Brandys, C. (2007). Family interventions after acquired brain injury and other chronic conditions: A critical appraisal of the quality of the evidence. *NeuroRehabilitation, 22,* 19–41.

Boyd, T. M., & Sautter, S. W. (1993). Route-finding: A measure of everyday executive functioning in the head-injured adult. *Applied Cognitive Psychology, 7,* 171–181.

Brain Injury Association of America. (n.d.). Causes of traumatic brain injury. In *Causes of brain injury* (para. 4). Retrieved December 28, 2007, from www.biausa.org/Pages/causes_of_brain_injury.html

Branswell, D., Hartry, A., Hoornbeek, S., Johansen, A., Johnson, L., Schultz, J., et al. (1992). *The Profile of Executive Control System.* Puyallup, WA: Association for Neuropsychological Research and Development.

Braverman, S. E., Spector, J., Warden, D. L., Wilson, B. C., Ellis, T. E., Bamdad, M. J., et al. (1999). A multidisciplinary TBI inpatient rehabilitation programme for active duty service members as part of a randomized clinical trial. *Brain Injury, 13,* 405–415.

Brogardh, C., & Sjölund, B. H. (2006). Constraint-induced movement therapy in patients with stroke: A pilot study on effects of small group training and of extended mitt use. *Clinical Rehabilitation, 20,* 218–227.

Brown, A. W., Leibson, C. L., Malec, J. F., Perkins, P. K., Diehl, N. N., & Larson, D. R. (2004). Long-term survival after traumatic brain injury: A population-based analysis. *NeuroRehabilitation, 19,* 37–43.

Bulger, E. M., Nathens, A. B., Rivara, F. P., Moore, M., MacKenzie, E. J., & Jurkovich, G. J. (2002). Management of severe head injury: Institutional variations in care and effect on outcome. *Critical Care Medicine, 30,* 1870–1876.

Burgess, P. W., Alderman, N., Forbes, C., Costello, A., Coates, L. M., Dawson, D. R., et al. (2006). The case for the development and use of "ecologically valid" measures of executive function in experimental and clinical neuropsychology. *Journal of the International Neuropsychological Society, 12,* 194–209.

Burke, D. T., Leeb, S. B., Hinman, R. T., Lupton, E. C., Burke, J., Schneider, J. C., et al. (2001). Using Talking Lights to assist brain-injured patients with daily inpatient therapeutic schedule. *Journal of Head Trauma Rehabilitation, 16,* 284–291.

Burleigh, S., Farber, R., & Gillard, M. (1998). Community integration and life satisfaction after traumatic brain injury: Long-term findings. *American Journal of Occupational Therapy, 52,* 45–52.

Callaway, L., Sloan, S., & Winkler, D. (2005). Maintaining and developing friendships following severe traumatic brain injury: Principles of occupational therapy practice. *Australian Occupational Therapy Journal, 52,* 257–260.

Cameron, C. M., Purdie, D. M., Kliewer, E. V., & McClure, R. J. (2008). Ten-year outcomes following traumatic brain injury: A population-based cohort. *Brain Injury, 22,* 437–449.

Campbell, L., Wilson, F. C., McCann, J., Kernahan, G., & Rogers, R. G. (2007). Single case experimental design study of Carer Facilitated Errorless Learning in a patient with severe memory impairment following TBI. *NeuroRehabilitation, 22,* 325–333.

Cantor, J. B., Ashman, T., Gordon, W., Ginsberg, A., Engmann, C., Egan, M., et al. (2008). Fatigue after traumatic brain injury and its impact on participation and quality of life. *Journal of Head Trauma Rehabilitation, 23,* 41–51.

Carr, J. H., Shepherd, R. B., Nordholm, L., & Lynne, D. (1985). Investigation of a New Motor Assessment Scale for stroke patients. *Physical Therapy, 65,* 175–180.

Carroll, D. (1965). A quantitative test of upper extremity function. *Journal of Chronic Diseases, 18,* 479–491.

Center for Outcomes Measurement in Brain Injury. (2000). *Home page.* Retrieved August 27, 2007, from http://www.tbims.org/combi/index.html

Centers for Disease Control and Prevention. (1999). *Traumatic brain injury in the United States: A report to Congress.* Retrieved August 1, 2007, from http://www.cdc.gov/ncipc/tbi/tbi_congress/TBI_in_the_US.PDF

Centers for Disease Control and Prevention. (2003). *Traumatic brain injury.* Retrieved August 1, 2007, from www.cdc.gov/ncipc/factsheets/tbi.htm

Centers for Disease Control and Prevention. (2006). *Traumatic brain injury in the United States: Emergency department visits, hospitalizations, and deaths.* Retrieved August 1, 2007, from http://www.cdc.gov/ncipc/pub-res/TBI_in_US_04/TBI%20in%20the%20US_Jan_2006.pdf

Cho, Y. W., Jang, S. H., Lee, Z. I., Song, J. C., Lee, H. K., & Lee, H. Y. (2005). Effect and appropriate restriction period of constraint-induced movement therapy in hemiparetic patients with brain injury: A brief report. *NeuroRehabilitation, 20,* 71–74.

Cicerone, K. D. (2007). Cognitive rehabilitation. In N. D. Zasler, D. I. Katz, & R. D. Zafonte (Eds.), *Brain injury medicine: Principles and practice* (pp. 765–777). New York: Demos.

Cicerone, K. D., Dahlberg, C., Kalmar, K., Langenbahn, D. M., Malec, J. F., Berquist, T. F., et al. (2000). Evidence-based cognitive rehabilitation: Recommendations for clinical practice. *Archives of Physical Medicine and Rehabilitation, 81,* 1596–1615.

Cicerone, K. D., Dahlberg, C., Malec, J. F., Langenbahn, D. M., Felicetti, T., Kneipp, S., et al. (2005). Evidence-based cognitive rehabilitation: Updated review of the literature from 1998 through 2002. *Archives of Physical Medicine and Rehabilitation, 86,* 1681–1692.

Cicerone, K. D., Mott, T., Azulay, J., & Friel, J. C. (2004). Community integration and satisfaction with

functioning after intensive cognitive rehabilitation for traumatic brain injury. *Archives of Physical Medicine and Rehabilitation, 85,* 943–950.

Clegg, F. M., & Rowe, A. L. (1996). A structured method for teaching word-processing skills to people with brain injury. *British Journal of Therapy and Rehabilitation, 3,* 553–558.

Clinchot, D. M., Bogner, J., Mysiw, W. J., Fugate, L., & Corrigan, J. (1998). Defining sleep disturbance after brain injury. *American Journal of Physical Medicine and Rehabilitation, 77,* 291–295.

Coetzer, B. R. (2004). Obsessive–compulsive disorder following brain injury: A review. *International Journal of Psychiatric Medicine, 34,* 363–377.

Coetzer, R., & Rushe, R. (2005). Post-acute rehabilitation following traumatic brain injury: Are both early and later improved outcomes possible? *International Journal of Rehabilitation Research, 28,* 361–363.

Colantonio, A., Ratcliff, G., Chase, S., & Vernich, L. (2004). Aging with traumatic brain injury: Long-term health conditions. *International Journal of Rehabilitation Research, 27,* 209–214.

Colarusso, R. P., & Hammill, D. D. (2002). *Motor-Free Visual Perception Test (MVPT–3).* Austin, TX: Pro-Ed.

Cope, N., & Hall, K. (1982). Head injury rehabilitation: Benefit of early intervention. *Archives of Physical Medicine and Rehabilitation, 63,* 433–437.

Corral, L., Ventura, J. L., Herrero, J. I., Monfort, J. L., Juncadella, M., Gabarrós, A., et al. (2007). Improvement in GOS and GOSE scores 6 and 12 months after severe traumatic brain injury. *Brain Injury, 21,* 1225–1231.

Corrigan, J. D. (1989). Development of a scale for assessment of agitation following traumatic brain injury. *Journal of Clinical and Experimental Neuropsychology, 11,* 261–277.

Corrigan, J. D., Smith-Knapp, K., & Granger, C. V. (1998). Outcomes in the first 5 years after traumatic brain injury. *Archives of Physical Medicine and Rehabilitation, 79,* 298–305.

Corrigan, J. D., Whiteneck, G., & Mellick, D. (2004). Perceived needs following traumatic brain injury. *Journal of Head Trauma Rehabilitation, 19,* 205–216.

Cullen, N., Bayley, M., Bayona, N., Hilditch, M., & Aubut, J. (2007). Management of heterotopic ossification and venous thromboembolism following acquired brain injury. *Brain Injury, 21,* 215–230.

Cullen, N., Chundamala, J., Bayley, M., & Jutai, J. (2007). The efficacy of acquired brain injury rehabilitation. *Brain Injury, 21,* 113–132.

Cusick, C. P., Gerhart, K. A., & Mellick, D. C. (2000). Participant-proxy reliability in traumatic brain injury outcome research. *Journal of Head Trauma Rehabilitation, 15,* 739–749.

Dahlberg, C. A., Cusick, C. P., Hawley, L. A., Newman, J. K., Morey, C. E., Harrison-Felix, C. L., et al. (2007). Treatment efficacy of social communication skills training after traumatic brain injury: A randomized treatment and deferred treatment controlled trial. *Archives of Physical Medicine and Rehabilitation, 88,* 1561–1573.

Davis, A. E., & Gimenez, A. (2003). Cognitive–behavioral recovery in comatose patients following auditory sensory stimulation. *Journal of Neuroscience Nursing, 35,* 202–209, 214.

Dawson, D. R. (2002). Commentary: A multidisciplinary community-based rehabilitation programme improved social functioning in severe traumatic brain injury. *Evidence-Based Mental Health, 5,* 84.

Dawson, D. R., & Chipman, M. (1995). The disablement experienced by traumatically brain-injured adults living in the community. *Brain Injury, 9,* 339–353.

DeHope, E., & Finegan, J. (1999). The self-determination model: An approach to develop awareness for survivors of traumatic brain injury. *NeuroRehabilitation, 13,* 3–12.

Diehl, M., Willis, S. L., & Schaie, W. (1995). Everyday problem solving in older adults: Observational

assessments and cognitive correlates. *Psychology and Aging, 10,* 478–491.

Dietz, J., Beeman, C., & Thorn, D. (1993). *Test of Orientation for Rehabilitation Patients.* San Antonio, TX: Psychological Corporation.

Dijkers, M. P. (2004). Quality of life after traumatic brain injury: A review of research approaches and findings. *Archives of Physical Medicine and Rehabilitation, 85*(Suppl. 2), S21–S35.

Dikmen, S., Machamer, J., Miller, B., Doctor, J., & Temkin, N. (2001). Functional status examination: A new instrument for assessing outcome in traumatic brain injury. *Journal of Neurotrauma, 18,* 127–140.

Donaghy, S., & Williams, W. (1998). A new protocol for training severely impaired patients in the usage of memory journals. *Brain Injury, 12,* 1061–1076.

Dunn, W., McClain, L. H., Brown, C., & Youngstrom, M. J. (1998). The ecology of human performance. In M. E. Neistadt & E. B. Crepeau (Eds.), *Willard and Spackman's occupational therapy* (9th ed., pp. 525–535). Philadelphia: Lippincott Williams & Wilkins.

Egan, J., Worrall, L., & Oxenham, D. (2005). An Internet training intervention for people with traumatic brain injury: Barriers and outcomes. *Brain Injury, 19,* 555–568.

Ehlhardt, L. A., Sohlberg, M. M., Glang, A., & Albin, R. (2005). TEACH–M: A pilot study evaluating an instructional sequence for persons with impaired memory and executive functions. *Brain Injury, 19,* 569–583.

Ergh, T. C., Rapport, L. J., Coleman, R. D., & Hanks, R. A. (2002). Predictors of caregiver and family functioning following traumatic brain injury: Social support moderates caregiver distress. *Journal of Head Trauma Rehabilitation, 17,* 155–174.

Eslinger, P. J., Zappalà, G., Chakara, F., & Barrett, A. M. (2007). Cognitive impairments after TBI. In N. D. Zasler, D. I. Katz, & R. D. Zafonte (Eds.), *Brain injury medicine: Principles and practice* (pp. 779–790). New York: Demos.

Evans, R. W. (1996). The postconcussion syndrome and the sequelae of mild head injury. In R. W. Evans (Ed.), *Neurology and trauma* (pp. 28–52). Philadelphia: W. B. Saunders.

Fisher, A. G. (1993a). Functional measures: Part 1: What is function, what should we measure, and how should we measure it? *American Journal of Occupational Therapy, 46,* 183–185.

Fisher, A. G. (1993b). Functional measures: Part 2: Selecting the right test, minimizing the limitations. *American Journal of Occupational Therapy, 46,* 278–281.

Flinn, N. A., Schamburg, S., Fetrow, J. M., & Flanigan, J. (2005). The effect of constraint-induced movement treatment on occupational performance and satisfaction in stroke survivors. *OTJR: Occupation, Participation, and Health, 25,* 119–127.

Fluharty, G., & Glassman, N. (2001). Case Study: Use of antecedent control to improve the outcome of rehabilitation for a client with frontal lobe injury and intolerance for auditory and tactile stimuli. *Brain Injury, 15,* 995–1002.

Fraas, M., Balz, M., & DeGrauw, W. (2007). Meeting the long-term needs of adults with acquired brain injury through community-based programming. *Brain Injury, 21,* 1267–1281.

Freeman, M. R., Mittenberg, W., Dicowden, M., & Bat-ami, M. (1992). Executive and compensatory memory retraining in traumatic brain injury. *Brain Injury, 6,* 65–70.

Friedemann-Sánchez, G., Sayer, N. A., & Pickett, T. (2008). Provider perspectives on rehabilitation of patients with polytrauma. *Archives of Physical Medicine and Rehabilitation, 89,* 171–178.

Fritz, S. L., Light, K. E., Clifford, S. N., Patterson, T. S., Behrman, A. L., & Davis, S. B. (2006). Descriptive characteristics as potential predictors of outcomes following constraint-induced movement therapy for people after stroke. *Physical Therapy, 86,* 825–832.

Frosch, M. P., Anthony, D. C., & DeGirolami, U. (2005). The central nervous system. In V. Jumar, A. K.

Abbas, & N. Fausto (Eds.), *Robbins and Cotran pathologic basis of disease* (pp. 1347–1419). Philadelphia: Elsevier/Saunders.

Fugl-Meyer, A. R., Jääskö, L., Leyman, I., Olsson, S., & Steglind, S. (1975). The post-stroke hemiplegic patient, I: A method for evaluation of physical performance. *Scandinavian Journal of Rehabilitation Medicine, 7,* 13–31.

Gentry, T., Wallace, J., Kvarfordt, C., & Lynch, K. B. (2008). Personal digital assistants as cognitive aids for individuals with severe traumatic brain injury: A community-based trial. *Brain Injury, 22,* 19–24.

Giacino, J. T., Kalmar, K., & Whyte, J. (2004). The JFK Coma Recovery Scale–Revised: Measurement characteristics and diagnostic utility. *Archives of Physical Medicine and Rehabilitation, 85,* 2020–2029.

Giacino, J. T., Katz, D. I., & Schiff, N. (2007). Assessment and rehabilitative management of individuals with disorders of consciousness. In N. D. Zasler, D. I. Katz, & R. D. Zafonte (Eds.), *Brain injury medicine: Principles and practice* (pp. 423–439). New York: Demos.

Giles, G. M. (2005). A neurofunctional approach to rehabilitation following severe brain injury. In N. Katz (Ed.), *Cognition and occupation across the life span: Models for intervention in occupational therapy* (2nd ed., pp. 139–165). Bethesda, MD: AOTA Press.

Giles, G. M., & Mohr, J. D. (2007). Overview and inter-rater reliability of an incident-based rating scale for aggressive behaviour following traumatic brain injury: The Overt Aggression Scale–Modified for Neurorehabiltation–Extended (OAS–MNR–E). *Brain Injury, 21,* 505–511.

Gilson, B. S., Gilson, J. S., Bergner, M., Bobbitt, R. A., Kressel, S., Pollard, W. E., et al. (1975). The Sickness Impact Profile: Development of an outcome measure of health care. *American Journal of Public Health, 65,* 1304–1310.

Gilworth, G., Eyres, S., Carey, A., Bhakta, B., & Tennant, A. (2008). Working with a brain injury:

Personal experiences of returning to work following a mild or moderate brain injury. *Journal of Rehabilitation Medicine, 40,* 334–339.

Golisz, K. M. (2006). Introduction and overview. In K. M. Golisz (Ed.), *Neurorehabilitation for traumatic brain injury* (Neurorehabilitation Self-Paced Clinical Course Series, G. M. Giles, Series Senior Ed., pp. 1–16). Bethesda, MD: American Occupational Therapy Association.

Goranson, T. E., Graves, R. E., Allison, D., & LaFreniere, R. (2003). Community integration following multidisciplinary rehabilitation for traumatic brain injury. *Brain Injury, 17,* 759–774.

Gorman, P., Dayle, R., Hood, C-A., & Rumrell, L. (2003). Effectiveness of the ISAAC cognitive prosthetic system for improving rehabilitation outcomes with neurofunctional impairment. *NeuroRehabilitation, 18,* 57–67.

Goverover, Y. (2004). Categorization, deductive reasoning, and self-awareness: Association to everyday competence in persons with acute brain injury. *Journal of Clinical and Experimental Neuropsychology, 26,* 737–749.

Goverover, Y., Johnston, M. V., Toglia, J., & DeLuca, J. (2007). Treatment to improve self-awareness in persons with acquired brain injury. *Brain Injury, 21,* 913–923.

Graham, D. I. (1999). Pathophysiological aspects of injury and mechanisms of recovery. In M. Rosenthal, E. R. Griffith, J. S. Kreutzer, & B. Pentland (Eds.), *Rehabilitation of the adult and child with traumatic brain injury* (3rd ed., pp. 19–41). Philadelphia: F. A. Davis.

Granger, C. V., Hamilton, B. B., Linacre, J. M., Heinemann, A. W., & Wright, B. D. (1993). Performance profiles of the Functional Independence Measures. *American Journal of Physical Medicine and Rehabilitation, 72,* 35–44.

Grigorenko, E. L., & Sternberg, R. J. (1998). Dynamic testing. *Psychological Bulletin, 124,* 75–111.

Gutman, S. A. (2000). Using a computer as an environmental facilitator to promote post–head injury social role resumption: A case report. *Occupational Therapy in Mental Health, 15,* 71–89.

Gutman, S. A., & Leger, D. L. (1997). Enhancement of one-to-one interpersonal skills necessary to initiate and maintain intimate relationships: A frame of reference for adults having sustained traumatic brain injury. *Occupational Therapy in Mental Health, 13,* 51–67.

Haaland, K. Y., Temkin, N., Randahl, G., & Dikmen, S. (1994). Recovery of simple motor skills after head injury. *Journal of Clinical and Experimental Neuropsychology, 16,* 448–456.

Hagen, C. (1998). *The Rancho Los Amigos Levels of Cognitive Functioning: The revised levels* (3rd ed.). Downey, CA: Los Amigos Research and Educational Institute.

Hagen, C., Malkmus, D., & Durham, P. (1972). *Levels of Cognitive Functioning.* Downey, CA: Rancho Los Amigos Hospital.

Häggström, A., & Lund, M. L. (2008). The complexity of participation in daily life: A qualitative study of the experiences of persons with acquired brain injury. *Journal of Rehabilitation Medicine, 40,* 89–95.

Hall, K. M. (1997). The Functional Assessment Measure (FAM). *Journal of Rehabilitation Outcomes, 1,* 63–65.

Hall, K. M., Mann, N., High, W. M., Wright, J. M., Kreutzer, J. S., & Wood, D. (1996). Functional measures after traumatic brain injury: Ceiling effects of FIM, FIM+FAM, DRS, and CIQ. *Journal of Head Trauma Rehabilitation, 11,* 27–39.

Halper, A. S., Cherney, L. R., Cichowski, K., & Zhang, M. (1999). Dysphagia after head trauma: The effect of cognitive–communicative impairments on functional outcomes. *Journal of Head Trauma Rehabilitation, 14,* 486–496.

Hammond, F. M., Hart, T., Bushnik, T., Corrigan, J. D., & Sasser, H. (2004). Change and predictors of change in communication, cognition, and social function between 1 and 5 years after traumatic brain injury. *Journal of Head Trauma Rehabilitation, 19,* 314–328.

Hanks, R. A., Wood, D. L., Millis, S., Harrison-Felix, C., Pierce, C. A., Rosenthal, M., et al. (2003). Violent traumatic brain injury: Occurrence, patient characteristics, and risk factors from the Traumatic Brain Injury Model Systems Project. *Archives of Physical Medicine and Rehabilitation, 84,* 249–254.

Harrison-Felix, C., Whiteneck, G., DeVivo, M., Hammond, F. M., & Jha, A. (2004). Mortality following rehabilitation in the Traumatic Brain Injury Model Systems of Care. *NeuroRehabilitation, 19,* 45–54.

Hart, R. P., Levenson, J. L., Sessler, C. N., Best, A. M., Schwartz, S. M., & Rutherford, L. E. (1996). Validation of a cognitive test for delirium in medical ICU patients. *Psychosomatics, 37,* 533–546.

Hart, T., Hawkey, K., & Whyte, J. (2002). Use of a portable voice organizer to remember therapy goals in traumatic brain injury rehabilitation: A within-subjects trial. *Journal of Head Trauma Rehabilitation, 17,* 556–570.

Hawkins, M. L., Lewis, F. D., & Medeiros, R. S. (2005). Impact of length of stay on functional outcomes of TBI patients. *American Surgery, 71,* 920–929.

Hayden, M. E., Moreault, A. M., LeBlanc, J., & Plenger, P. M. (2000). Reducing level of handicap in traumatic brain injury: An environmentally based model of treatment. *Journal of Head Trauma Rehabilitation, 15,* 1000–1021.

Helm-Estabrooks, N., & Hotz, G. (1991). *Brief Test of Head Injury.* Chicago: Riverside.

High, W. M., Roebuck-Spencer, T., Sander, A. M., Struchen, M. A., & Sherer, M. (2006). Early versus later admission to postacute rehabilitation: Impact on functional outcome after traumatic brain injury. *Archives of Physical Medicine and Rehabilitation, 87,* 334–342.

Hill, J. (1994). The effects of casting on upper-extremity motor disorders after brain injury. *American Journal of Occupational Therapy, 48,* 219–224.

Hillier, S. (2003). Community-based rehabilitation improves function of patients with traumatic brain injury. *Australian Journal of Physiotherapy, 49,* 277.

Ho, M. R., & Bennett, T. L. (1997). Efficacy of neuropsychological rehabilitation for mild–moderate traumatic brain injury. *Archives of Clinical Neuropsychology, 12,* 1–11.

Holm, M. B. (2000). Eleanor Clarke Slagle Lecture—Our mandate for the new millennium: Evidence-based practice. *American Journal of Occupational Therapy, 54,* 575–585 .

Hudak, A. M., Caesar, R. R., Frol, A. B., Krueger, K., Harper, C. R., Temkin, N. R., et al. (2005). Functional outcome scales in traumatic brain injury: A comparison of the Glasgow Outcome Scale (Extended) and the Functional Status Examination. *Journal of Neurotrauma, 22,* 1319–1326.

Incoccia, C., Formisano, R., Muscato, P., Reali, G., & Zoccolotti. P. (2004). Reaction and movement times in individuals with chronic traumatic brain injury with good motor recovery. *Cortex, 40,* 111–115.

Ivanco, T. L., & Greenough, W. T. (2000). Physiological consequences of morphologically detectable synaptic plasticity: Potential uses for examining recovery following damage. *Neuropharmacology, 39,* 765–776.

Iverson, G. L., Lange, R. T., Gaetz, M., & Zasler, N. D. (2007). Mild TBI. In N. D. Zasler, D. I. Katz, & R. D. Zafonte (Eds.), *Brain injury medicine: Principles and practice* (pp. 333–371). New York: Demos.

Ivins, B. J., Schwab, K. A., Warden, D., Harvey, L. T., Hoilien, M. A., Powell, C. O., et al. (2003). Traumatic brain injury in U.S. Army paratroopers: Prevalence and character. *Journal of Trauma, 55,* 617–621.

Jackson, W. T., Novack, T. A., & Dowler, R. N. (1998). Effective serial measurement of cognitive orientation in rehabilitation: The Orientation Log. *Archives of Physical Medicine and Rehabilitation, 79,* 718–720.

Jenkinson, N., Ownsworth, T., & Shum, D. (2007). Utility of the Canadian Occupational Performance Measure in community-based brain injury rehabilitation. *Brain Injury, 21,* 1283–1294.

Jennett, B., & Bond, M. (1975). Assessment of outcome after severe brain damage. *Lancet, 1,* 480–484.

Johansson, B. B. (2003). Environmental influence on recovery after brain lesions—Experimental and clinical data. *Journal of Rehabilitation Medicine, 41*(Suppl.), 11–16.

Johnson, D. A., Roethig-Johnson, K., & Richards, D. (1993). Biochemical and physiological parameters of recovery in acute severe head injury: Responses to multisensory stimulation. *Brain Injury, 7,* 491–499.

Kane, L. (2006). The acute inpatient rehabilitation phase of recovery. In K. M. Golisz (Ed.), *Neurorehabilitation for traumatic brain injury* (Neurorehabilitation Self-Paced Clinical Course Series, G. M. Giles, Series Senior Ed., pp. 47–92). Bethesda, MD: American Occupational Therapy Association.

Katz, D. I., Zasler, N. D., & Zafonte, R. D. (2007). Clinical continuum of care and natural history. In N. D. Zasler, D. I. Katz, & R. D. Zafonte (Eds.), *Brain injury medicine: Principles and practice* (pp. 3–13). New York: Demos.

Katz, N., & Hartman-Maeir, A. (2005). Higher-level cognitive functions: Awareness and executive functions enabling engagement in occupation. In N. Katz (Ed.), *Cognition and occupation across the life span* (2nd ed., pp. 3–25). Bethesda, MD: AOTA Press.

Katz, N., Itzkopvich, M., Elazar, B., Averbuch, S., & Rahmani, L. (1990). *Lowenstein Occupational Therapy Cognitive Assessment (LOTCA).* Pequannock, NJ: Maddak, Inc.

Kay, T. (1986). *The unseen injury—Minor head trauma.* Framingham, MA: National Head Injury Foundation.

Kearns, Y. (2005). Coma stimulation: What, why, and how? *Physical Disabilities Special Interest Section Quarterly, 28*(1), 1–3.

Kessels, R. P. C., & de Haan, E. H. F. (2003). Implicit learning in memory rehabilitation: A meta-analysis on errorless learning and vanishing cue methods. *Journal of Clinical and Experimental Neuropsychology, 25,* 805–814.

Kiernan, R. J., Mueller, J., & Langston, J. W. (1983). *The Neurobehavioral Cognitive Status Screening Examination.* San Francisco: Northern California Neurobehavioral Group.

Kim, H. J., Burke, D. T., Dowds, M. M., & George, J. (1999). Utility of a microcomputer as an external memory aid for a memory-impaired head injury patient during in-patient rehabilitation. *Brain Injury, 13,* 147–150.

Kirsch, N. L., Shenton, M., & Rowan, J. (2004). A generic, 'in-house,' alphanumeric paging system for prospective activity impairments after traumatic brain injury. *Brain Injury, 18,* 725–734.

Kirsch, N. L., Shenton, M., Spirl, E., Rowan, J., Simpson, R., Schreckengost, D., et al. (2004). Web-based assistive technology interventions for cognitive impairments after traumatic brain injury: A selective review and two case studies. *Rehabilitation Psychology, 49,* 200–212.

Klinger, L. (2005). Occupational adaptation: Perspectives of people with traumatic brain injury. *Journal of Occupational Science, 12*(1), 9–16.

Kneipp, S., & Rubin, A. (2007). Community re-entry issues and long-term care. In N. D. Zasler, D. I. Katz, & R. D. Zafonte (Eds.), *Brain injury medicine: Principles and practice* (pp. 1085–1104). New York: Demos.

Knight, C., Alderman, N., & Burgess, P. W. (2002). Development of a simplified version of the Multiple Errands Test for use in hospital settings. *Neuropsychological Rehabilitation, 12,* 231–255.

Kohlman-Thomson, L. (1992). *Kohlman Evaluation of Living Skills* (3rd ed.). Rockville, MD: American Occupational Therapy Association.

Kolb, B. (2003). Overview of cortical plasticity and recovery from brain injury. *Physical Medicine and Rehabilitation Clinics of North America, 14,* S7–S25.

Kowalske, K., Plenger, P. M., Lusby, B., & Hayden, M. E. (2000). Vocational reentry following TBI: An enablement model. *Journal of Head Trauma Rehabilitation, 15,* 989–999.

Kreutzer, J., & Marwitz, J. (1989). *The Family Needs Questionnaire*. Richmond, VA: National Resource Center for Traumatic Brain Injury.

Kreutzer, J., Seel, R., & Marwitz, J. (1999). *The Neurobehavioral Functioning Inventory*. San Antonio, TX: Psychological Corporation.

Laatsch, L., Jobe, T., Sychra, J., Lin, Q., & Blend, M. (1997). Impact of cognitive rehabilitation therapy on neuropsychological impairments as measured by brain perfusion SPECT: A longitudinal study. *Brain Injury, 11,* 851–863.

Laatsch, L. K., Thulborn, K. R., Krisky, C. M., Shobat, D. M., & Sweeney, J. A. (2004). Investigating the neurobiological basis of cognitive rehabilitation therapy with fMRI. *Brain Injury, 18,* 957–974.

Landa-Gonzales, B. (2001). Multicontextual occupational therapy intervention: A case study of traumatic brain injury. *Occupational Therapy International, 8,* 49–62.

Langmore, S. E. (1991). Managing the complications of aspiration in dysphagic adults. *Seminars in Speech and Language, 12,* 199–208.

Lannin, N. A., Horsley, S. A., Herbert, R., McCluskey, A., & Cusick, A. (2003). Splinting the hand in the functional position after brain impairment: A randomized, controlled trial. *Archives of Physical Medicine and Rehabilitation, 84,* 297–302.

Law, M. (Ed.). (2002). *Evidence-based rehabilitation: A guide to practice*. Thorofare, NJ: Slack.

Law, M., Baptiste, S., McColl, M. A., Carswell, A., Polatajko, H., & Pollock, N. (1998). *Canadian Occupational Performance Measure* (3rd ed.). Toronto: Canadian Association of Occupational Therapists.

Law, M., & Baum, C. (1998). Evidence-based occupational therapy. *Canadian Journal of Occupational Therapy, 65,* 131–135.

Leon-Carrion, J., Dominguez-Morales, M. R., Barroso, J. M., & Martin, Y. (2005). Driving with cognitive deficits: Neurorehabilitation and legal measures are needed for driving again after severe traumatic brain injury. *Brain Injury, 19,* 213–219.

Lequerica, A. H., Rapport, L. J., Loeher, K., Axelrod, B. N., Vangel, S. J., & Hanks, R. A. (2007). Agitation in acquired brain injury: Impact on acute rehabilitation therapies. *Journal of Head Trauma Rehabilitation, 22,* 177–183.

Levin, H. S. (2003). Neuroplasticity following non-penetrating traumatic brain injury. *Brain Injury, 17,* 665–674.

Levin, H. S., O'Donnell, V. M., & Grossman, R. G. (1979). The Galveston Orientation and Amnesia Test: A practical scale to assess cognition after head injury. *Journal of Nervous and Mental Disorders, 167,* 675–684.

Levine, B., Robertson, I. H., Clare, L., Carter, G., Hong, J., Wilson, B. A., et al. (2000). Rehabilitation of executive functioning: An experimental–clinical validation of Goal Management Training. *Journal of the International Neuropsychological Society, 6,* 299–312.

Lezak, M. D., Howieson, D. B., & Loring, D. W. (2004). *Neuropsychological assessment* (4th ed.). New York: Oxford University Press.

Liepert, J. (2006). Motor cortex excitability in stroke before and after constraint-induced movement therapy. *Cognitive and Behavioral Neurology, 19,* 41–47.

Liepert, J., Bauder, H., Wolfgang, H. R., Miltner, W. H., Taub, E., & Weiller, C. (2000). Treatment-induced cortical reorganization after stroke in humans. *Stroke, 31,* 1210–1216.

Liepert, J., Hamzei, F., & Weiller, C. (2004). Lesion-induced and training-induced brain reorganization. *Restorative Neurology and Neuroscience, 22,* 269–277.

Lin, K.-C., Wu, C. Y., Wei, T. H., Lee, C. Y., & Liu, J. S. (2007). Effects of modified constraint-induced movement therapy on reach-to-grasp movements and functional performance after chronic stroke: A randomized controlled study. *Clinical Rehabilitation, 21,* 1075–1086.

Loeb, P. A. (1996). *Independent Living Scales*. San Antonio, TX: Psychological Corporation.

Lombard, L., & Zafonte, R. (2005). Agitation after traumatic brain injury: Considerations and treatment options. *American Journal of Physical Medicine and Rehabilitation, 84,* 797–812.

Lombardi, F., Taricco, M., De Tanti, A., Telaro, E., & Liberati, A. (2002). Sensory stimulation of brain-injured individuals in coma or vegetative state: Results of a Cochrane systematic review. *Clinical Rehabilitation, 16,* 464–472. *See also* Lombardi, F., Taricco, M., De Tanti, A., Telaro, E., & Liberati, A. (2004). Sensory stimulation of brain-injured individuals in coma or vegetative state (Cochrane Review). In *The Cochrane Library, 4.* Chichester, UK: Wiley.

Loya, G. J. (1999). *Efficacy of memory rehabilitation among adolescent and adult TBI survivors: A meta-analysis.* Unpublished doctoral dissertation, University of Nebraska, Lincoln.

Lundqvist, A., Alinder, J., & Rönnberg, J. (2008). Factors influencing driving 10 years after brain injury. *Brain Injury, 22,* 295–304.

Luria, A. (1973). *The working brain* (B. Haigh, Trans.). New York: Basic Books.

Lyle, R. C. (1981). A performance test for assessment of upper limb function in physical rehabilitation treatment and research. *International Journal of Rehabilitation Research, 4,* 483-492.

Mackay, L. E., Bernstein, B. A., Chapman, P. E., Morgan, A. S., & Milazzo, L. S. (1992). Early intervention in severe head injury: Long-term benefits of a formalized program. *Archives of Physical Medicine and Rehabilitation, 73,* 635–641.

MacLachlan, M., DeSilva, M. J., Devane, D., Desmond, D., Gallagher, P., Schnyder, U., et al. (2007). Psychosocial interventions for the prevention of disability following traumatic physical injury (Protocol). *Cochrane Database of Systematic Reviews, 1,* CD006422.

Mahoney, F., & Barthel, D. (1965). Functional evaluation: The Barthel Index. *Maryland State Medical Journal, 14,* 56–61.

Malec, J. F. (2001). Impact of comprehensive day treatment on societal participation for persons with acquired brain injury. *Archives of Physical Medicine and Rehabilitation, 82,* 885–895.

Malec, J. F. (2005). *The Mayo–Portland Adaptability Inventory.* Retrieved August 27, 2007, from http://www.tbims.org/combi/mpai

Malec, J. F., Buffington, A. L. H., Moessner, A. M., & Degiorgio, L. (2000). A medical/vocational case coordination system for persons with brain injury: An evaluation of employment outcomes. *Archives of Physical Medicine and Rehabilitation, 81,* 1007–1015.

Manly, T., Hawkins, K., Evans, J., Woldt, K., & Robertson, I. H. (2002). Rehabilitation of executive function: Facilitation of effective goal management on complex tasks using periodic auditory alerts. *Neuropsychologia, 40,* 271–281.

Marshall, S., Teasell, R., Bayona, N., Lippert, C., Chundamala, J., Villamere, J., et al. (2007). Motor impairment rehabilitation post acquired brain injury. *Brain Injury, 21,* 133–160.

Mayer, N. H., Whyte, J., Wannstedt, G., & Ellis, C. A. (2008). Comparative impact of 2 botulinum toxin injection techniques for elbow flexor hypertonia. *Archives of Physical Medicine and Rehabilitation, 89,* 982–987.

Mayrose, J., & Jehle, D. V. (2002). Vehicle weight and fatality risk for sport utility vehicle-versus-passenger car crashes. *Journal of Trauma, 53,* 751–753.

McAllister, T. W., & Arciniegas, D. (2002). Evaluation and treatment of postconcussive symptoms. *NeuroRehabilitation, 17,* 265–283.

McCabe, P., Lippert, C., Weiser, M., Hilditch, M., Hartridge, C., & Villamere, J. (2007). Community reintegration following acquired brain injury. *Brain Injury, 21,* 231–257.

McDonald, B. C., Flashman, L. A., & Saykin, A. J. (2002). Executive dysfunction following traumatic brain injury: Neural substrates and treatment strategies. *NeuroRehabilitation, 17,* 333–344.

McKerracher, G., Powell, T., & Oyebode, J. (2005). A single-case experimental design comparing two memory notebook formats for a man with memory problems caused by traumatic brain injury. *Neuropsychological Rehabilitation, 15,* 115–128.

McMillan, T., & Herbert, C. (2004). Further recovery in a potential treatment withdrawal case 10 years after brain injury. *Brain Injury, 18,* 935–940.

McMorrow, M. J., Braunling-McMorrow, D., & Smith, S. (1998). Evaluation of functional outcomes following proactive behavioral–residential treatment. *Journal of Rehabilitation Outcomes Measurement, 2,* 22–30.

McNeny, R. (2006). The client in coma. In K. M. Golisz (Ed.), *Neurorehabilitation for traumatic brain injury* (Neurorehabilitation Self-Paced Clinical Course Series, G. M. Giles, Series Senior Ed., pp. 17–46). Bethesda, MD: American Occupational Therapy Association.

McNeny, R. (2007). Therapy for activities of daily living: Theoretical and practical perspectives. In N. D. Zasler, D. I. Katz, & R. D. Zafonte (Eds.), *Brain injury medicine: Principles and practice* (pp. 947–959). New York: Demos.

Mellick, D., Walker, N., Brooks, C. A., & Whiteneck, G. (1999). Incorporating the cognitive independence domain into CHART. *Journal of Rehabilitation Outcomes Measures, 3,* 12–21.

Michon, J. A. (1985). A critical view of driver behavior models: What do we know, what should we do? In L. Evans & R. C. Schwing (Eds.), *Human behavior and traffic safety* (pp. 485–520). New York: Plenum Press.

Millis, S. R., Rosenthal, M., Novack, T. A., Sherer, M., Nick, T. G., Kreutzer, J. S., et al. (2001). Long-term neuropsychological outcome after traumatic brain injury. *Journal of Head Trauma Rehabilitation, 16,* 343–355.

Mills, V. M., Nesbeda, T., Katz, D. I., & Alexander, M. P. (1992). Outcomes for traumatically brain-injured patients following post-acute rehabilitation programmes. *Brain Injury, 6,* 219–228.

Minkel, J. L. (1996). Assistive technology and outcome measurement: Where do we begin? *Technology and Disability, 5,* 285–288.

Mitchell, S., Bradley, V. A., Welch, J. L., & Britton, P. G. (1990). Coma arousal procedure: A therapeutic intervention in the treatment of head injury. *Brain Injury, 4,* 273–279.

Moyers, P., & Dale, L. (2007). *The guide to occupational therapy practice* (2nd ed.). Bethesda, MD: AOTA Press.

Murrey, G. J., & Starzinski, D. (2004). An inpatient neurobehavioral rehabilitation programme for persons with traumatic brain injury: Overview of and outcome data for the Minnesota Neurorehabilitation Hospital. *Brain Injury, 18,* 519–531.

Mysiw, W. J., Fugate, L. P., & Clinchot, D. M. (2007). Assessment, early rehabilitation, and tertiary prevention. In N. D. Zasler, D. I. Katz, & R. D. Zafonte (Eds.), *Brain injury medicine: Principles and practice* (pp. 283–301). New York: Demos.

Nakase-Richardson, R., Yablon, S. A., & Sherer, M. (2007). Prospective comparison of acute confusion severity with duration of post-traumatic amnesia in predicting employment outcome after traumatic brain injury. *Journal of Neurology, Neurosurgery, and Psychiatry, 78,* 872–876.

National Institute of Neurological Disorders and Stroke, National Institutes of Health. (2005). *Cognitive rehabilitation interventions: Moving from bench to bedside.* Retrieved December 23, 2008, from http://www.ninds.nih.gov/news_and_events/proceedings/execsumm07_19_05.htm

Neistadt, M. E. (1994). The effects of different treatment activities on functional fine motor coordination in adults with brain injury. *American Journal of Occupational Therapy, 48,* 877–882.

Novack, T. A., Caldwell, S. G., Duke, L. W., Bergquist, T. F., & Gage, R. G. (1996). Focused versus unstructured intervention for attention deficits after traumatic brain injury. *Journal of Head Trauma Rehabilitation, 11,* 52–60.

Nudo, R. J. (2003). Adaptive plasticity in motor cortex: Implications for rehabilitation after brain injury. *Journal of Rehabilitation Medicine, 41*(Suppl.), 7–10.

Nudo, R. J., & Dancause, N. (2007). Neuroscientific basis for occupational and physical therapy interventions. In N. D. Zasler, D. I. Katz, & R. D. Zafonte (Eds.), *Brain injury medicine: Principles and practice* (pp. 913–928). New York: Demos.

Oakley, F., Kielhofner, G., Barris, R., & Reichler, R. K. (1986). The Role Checklist: Development and empirical assessment of reliability. *Occupational Therapy Journal of Research, 6,* 157–170.

O'Brien, L. (2007). Achieving a successful and sustainable return to the workforce after ABI: A client-centred approach. *Brain Injury, 21,* 465–478.

O'Brien, L., & Bailey, M. (2008). Determinants of compliance with hand splinting in an acute brain-injured population. *Brain Injury, 22,* 411–418.

Olver, J. D., Ponsford, J. L., & Curran, C. A. (1996). Outcome following traumatic brain injury: A comparison between 2 and 5 years after injury. *Brain Injury, 10,* 841–848.

Ouellet, M. C., & Morin, C. M. (2007). Efficacy of cognitive–behavioral therapy for insomnia associated with traumatic brain injury: A single-case experimental design. *Archives of Physical Medicine and Rehabilitation, 88,* 1581–1592.

Ownsworth, T., Fleming, J., Desbois, J., Strong, J., & Kuipers, P. (2006). A metacognitive contextual intervention to enhance error awareness and functional outcome following traumatic brain injury: A single-case experimental design. *Journal of the International Neuropsychological Society, 12,* 54–63.

Ownsworth, T., Fleming, J., Shum, D., Kuipers, P., & Strong, J. (2008). Comparison of individualized, group, and combined intervention formats in a randomized controlled trial for facilitating goal attainment and improving psychosocial function following acquired brain injury. *Journal of Rehabilitation Medicine, 40,* 81–88.

Page, S., & Levine, P. (2003). Forced use after TBI: Promoting plasticity and function through practice. *Brain Injury, 17,* 675–684.

Page, S. J., & Levine, P. (2006). Back from the brink: Electromyography-triggered stimulation combined with modified constraint-induced movement therapy in chronic stroke. *Archives of Physical Medicine and Rehabilitation, 87,* 27–31.

Page, S. J., Levine, P., Leonard, A., Szaflarski, J. P., & Kissela, B. M. (2008). Modified constraint-induced therapy in chronic stroke: Results of a single-blinded randomized controlled trial. *Physical Therapy, 88,* 1–8.

Palmer, S., Bader, M. K., Qureshi, A., Palmer, J., Shaver, T., Borzatta, M., et al. (2001). The impact on outcomes in a community hospital setting of using the AANS Traumatic Brain Injury Guidelines. *Journal of Trauma, Injury, Infection, and Critical Care, 50,* 657–664.

Paniak, C., Toller-Lobe, G., Durand, A., & Nagy, J. (1998). A randomized trial of two treatments for mild traumatic brain injury. *Brain Injury, 12,* 1011–1023.

Paniak, C., Toller-Lobe, G., Reynolds, S., Melnyk, A., & Nagy, J. (2000). A randomized trial of two treatments for mild traumatic brain injury: 1 year follow-up. *Brain Injury, 14,* 219–226.

Parente, R., & Stapleton, M. (1999). Development of a cognitive strategies group for vocational training after traumatic brain injury. *NeuroRehabilitation, 13,* 13–20.

Parish, L., & Oddy, M. (2007). Efficacy of rehabilitation for functional skills more than 10 years after extremely severe brain injury. *Neuropsychological Rehabilitation, 17,* 230–243.

Park, N. W., & Ingles, J. L. (2001). Effectiveness of attention rehabilitation after an acquired brain injury: A meta-analysis. *Neuropsychology, 15,* 199–210. [Also published in 2000 in *Brain and Cognition, 44,* 1–18.]

Phipps, S. (2006). Community participation. In K. M. Golisz (Ed.), *Neurorehabilitation for traumatic brain injury* (Neurorehabilitation Self-Paced Clinical Course Series, G. M. Giles, Series Senior Ed., pp. 93–134). Bethesda, MD: American Occupational Therapy Association.

Phipps, S., & Richardson, P. (2007). Occupational therapy outcomes for clients with traumatic brain injury and stroke using the Canadian Occupational Performance Measure. *American Journal of Occupational Therapy, 61,* 328–334.

Pierce, C. A., & Hanks, R. A. (2006). Life satisfaction after traumatic brain injury and the World Health Organization Model of Disability. *American Journal of Physical Medicine and Rehabilitation, 85,* 889–898.

Pintar, F. A., Yoganandan, N., & Gennarelli, T. A. (2000). Airbag effectiveness on brain trauma in frontal crashes. *Annual Proceedings of the Association for Advancement of Automotive Medicine, 44,* 149–169.

Pohl, M., Ruckriem, S., Mehrholz, J., Ritschel, D., Strik, H., & Pause, M. R. (2002). Effectiveness of serial casting in patients with severe cerebral spasticity: A comparison study. *Archives of Physical Medicine and Rehabilitation, 83,* 784–790.

Poole, J. H., Dahdah, M. N., Schwab, K., Lew, H. L., Warden, D. L., & Date, E. S. (2007). Long-term outcomes after traumatic brain injury in veterans: Successes and challenges. *American Journal of Physical Medicine and Rehabilitation, 86,* 333–334.

Powell, J. H., Beckers, K., & Greenwood, R. J. (1998). Measuring progress and outcome in community rehabilitation after brain injury with a new assessment instrument—The BICRO–39 Scales. *Archives of Physical Medicine and Rehabilitation, 79,* 1213–1225.

Powell, J., Heslin, J., & Greenwood, R. (2002). Community-based rehabilitation after severe traumatic brain injury: A randomized controlled trial. *Journal of Neurology, Neurosurgery, and Psychiatry, 72,* 193–202.

Powell, J. M., Machamer, J. E., Temkin, N. R., & Dikmen, S. S. (2001). Self-report of extent of recovery and barriers to recovery after traumatic brain injury: A longitudinal study. *Archives of Physical Medicine and Rehabilitation, 82,* 1025–1030.

Prigatano, G. P., & Altman, I. M. (1990). Impaired awareness of behavioral limitations after traumatic brain injury. *Archives of Physical Medicine and Rehabilitation, 71,* 1058–1064.

Quemada, J. I., Cespedes, J. M. M., Ezkerra, J., Ballesteros, J., Ibarra, N., & Urruticoechea, I. (2003). Outcome of memory rehabilitation in traumatic brain injury assessed by neuropsychological tests and questionnaires. *Journal of Head Trauma Rehabilitation, 18,* 532–540.

Radomski, M. V. (2001). *Occupational therapy practice guidelines for adults with traumatic brain injury.* Bethesda, MD: American Occupational Therapy Association.

Rappaport, M. (2005). The Disability Rating Scale and Coma/Near Coma Scales in evaluating severe head injury. *Neuropsychological Rehabilitation, 15,* 442–453.

Rappaport, M., Dougherty, A. M., & Kelting, D. L. (1992). Evaluation of coma and vegetative states. *Archives of Physical Medicine and Rehabilitation, 73,* 628–634.

Rappaport, M., Hall, K., Hopkins, K., & Belleza, T. (1982). Disability Rating Scale for severe head trauma: Coma to community. *Archives of Physical Medicine and Rehabilitation, 63,* 118–123.

Rapport, L. J., Coleman Bryer, R., & Hanks, R. A. (2008). Driving and community integration after traumatic brain injury. *Archives of Physical Medicine and Rehabilitation, 89,* 922–930.

Raskin, S. A., & Sohlberg, M. M. (1996). The efficacy of prospective memory training in two adults with brain injury. *Journal of Head Trauma Rehabilitation, 11,* 32–51.

Rees, L., Marshall, S., Hartridge, C., Mackie, D., & Weiser, M. (2007). Cognitive interventions post acquired brain injury. *Brain Injury, 21,* 161–200.

Rehabilitation of Persons With Traumatic Brain Injury. (1998, October 26–28). *NIH Consensus Statement Online, 16,* 1–41. Retrieved August 27, 2007, from http://consensus.nih.gov/1998/1998TraumaticBrainInjury109html.htm

Ro, T., Noser, E., Boake, C., Johnson, R., Gaber, M., Speroni, A., et al. (2006). Functional reorganization and recovery after constraint-induced movement therapy in subacute stroke: Case reports. *Neurocase, 12,* 50–60.

Robertson, I. H., Ward, T., Ridgeway, V., & Nimmo-Smith, I. (1994). *The Test of Everyday Attention (TEA).* Bury St. Edmunds, UK: Thames Valley Test Company.

Robinson, B. (1983). Validation of a Caregiver Strain Index. *Journal of Gerontology, 38,* 344–348.

Rodgers, M. L., Strode, A. D., Norell, D. M., Short, R. A., Dyck, D. G., & Becker, B. (2007). Adapting multiple-family group treatment for brain and spinal cord injury intervention development and preliminary outcomes. *American Journal of Physical Medicine and Rehabilitation, 86,* 482–492.

Roth, R. M., Isquith, P. K., & Gioia, G. A. (2005). *Behavior Rating Inventory of Executive Function–Adult Version.* Lutz, FL: Psychological Assessment Resources.

Rothwell, N. A., LaVigna, G. W., & Willis, T. J. (1999). A non-aversive rehabilitation approach for people with severe behavioural problems resulting from brain injury. *Brain Injury, 13,* 521–533.

Rotondi, A. J., Sinkule, J., Balzer, K., Harris, J., & Moldovan. R. (2007). A qualitative needs assessment of persons who have experienced traumatic brain injury and their primary family caregivers. *Journal of Head Trauma Rehabilitation, 22,* 14–25.

Ruff, R. M., Camenzuli, L., & Mueller, J. (1996). Miserable minority: Emotional risk factors that influence the outcome of a mild traumatic brain injury. *Brain Injury, 10,* 551–565.

Rutland-Brown, W., Langlois, J. A., Thomas, K. E., & Xi, Y. L. (2006). Incidence of traumatic brain injury in the United States, 2003. *Journal of Head Trauma Rehabilitation, 21,* 544–548.

Sabari, J. (2008). *Occupational therapy practice guidelines for adults with stroke.* Bethesda, MD: AOTA Press.

Sackett, D. L., Rosenberg, W. M., Muir Gray, J. A., Haynes, R. B., & Richardson, W. S. (1996). Evidence-based medicine: What it is and what it isn't. *British Medical Journal, 312,* 71–72.

Salazar, A. M., Warden, D. L., Schwab, K., Spector, J., Braverman, S., Waler, J., et al. (2000). Cognitive rehabilitation for traumatic brain injury: A randomized trial. *JAMA, 283,* 3075–3081.

Sayer, N. A., Chiros, C. E., Sigford, B., Scott, S., Clothier, B., Pickett, T., et al. (2008). Characteristics and rehabilitation outcomes among patients with blast and other injuries sustained during the global war on terror. *Archives of Physical Medicine and Rehabilitation, 89,* 163–170.

Sbordone, R. J., Liter, J., & Pettler-Jennings, P. (1995). Recovery of function following severe traumatic brain injury: A retrospective 10-year follow-up. *Brain Injury, 9,* 285–299.

Scheibel, R. S., Pearson, D. A., Faria, L. P., Kotrla, K. J., Aylward, E., Bachevalier, J., et al. (2003). An fMRI study of executive functioning after severe diffuse TBI. *Brain Injury, 17,* 919–930.

Scheibel, R. S., Pearson, D. A., Faria, L. P., Kotrla, K. J., Aylward, E., Bachevalier, J., et al. (2004). Erratum: An fMRI study of executive functioning after severe diffuse TBI. *Brain Injury, 18,* 219–220.

Schlund, M. W., & Pace, G. (1999). Relations between traumatic brain injury and the environment: Feedback reduces maladaptive behaviour exhibited by three persons with traumatic brain injury. *Brain Injury, 13,* 889–897.

Schwab, K. A., Warden, D., Lux, W. E., Shupenko, L. A., & Zitnay, G. (2007). Defense and Veterans' Brain Injury Center: Peacetime and wartime missions [Guest Editorial]. *Journal of Rehabilitation Research and Development, 44,* xiii–xxii.

Schwartz, S. M. (1995). Adults with traumatic brain injury: Three case studies of cognitive rehabilitation in the home setting. *American Journal of Occupational Therapy, 49,* 655–667.

Shallice, T., & Burgess, P. (1991). Deficits in strategy application following frontal lobe damage in man. *Brain, 114,* 727–741.

Shavelle, R. M., Strauss, D. J., Day, S. M., & Ojdana, K. A. (2007). Life expectancy. In N. D. Zasler, D. I. Katz, & R. D. Zafonte (Eds.), *Brain injury medicine:*

Principles and practice (pp. 247–261). New York: Demos.

Shaw, S. E., Morris, D. M., Uswatte, G., McKay, S., Meythaler, J. M., & Taub, E. (2005). Constraint-induced movement therapy for recovery of upper-limb function following traumatic brain injury. *Journal of Rehabilitation Research and Development, 42,* 769–778.

Sherer, M., Bergloff, P., Boake, C., High, W., & Levin, E. (1998). The Awareness Questionnaire: Factor structure and internal consistency. *Brain Injury, 12,* 63–68.

Sherer, M., Nakase-Thompson, R., Yablon, S. A., & Gontkovsky, S. T. (2005). Multidimensional assessment for acute confusion after TBI. *Archives of Physical Medicine and Rehabilitation, 86,* 896–904.

Shimelman, A., & Hinojosa, J. (1995). Gross motor activity and attention in three adults with brain injury. *American Journal of Occupational Therapy, 49,* 973–979.

Siegel, J. H., Loo, G., Dischinger, P. C., Burgess, A. R., Wang, S. C., Schneider, L. W., et al. (2001). Factors influencing the patterns of injuries and outcomes in car-versus-car crashes compared to sport utility, van, or pick-up truck versus car crashes: Crash Injury Research Engineering Network Study. *Journal of Trauma, 51,* 975–990.

Sigford, B. J. (2008). "To care for him who shall have borne the battle and for his widow and his orphan" (Abraham Lincoln): The Department of Veterans' Affairs Polytrauma System of Care. *Archives of Physical Medicine and Rehabilitation, 89,* 160–162.

Sirois, M. J., Lavoie, A., & Dionne, C. E. (2004). Impact of transfer delay to rehabilitation in patients with severe trauma. *Archives of Physical Medicine and Rehabilitation, 85,* 184–191.

Sladyk, K. (1992). Case Report: Traumatic brain injury, behavioral disorder, and group treatment. *American Journal of Occupational Therapy, 46,* 267–270.

Smith, D. H., Meaney, D. F., & Shull, W. H. (2003). Diffuse axonal injury in head trauma. *Journal of Head Trauma Rehabilitation, 18,* 307–316.

Sohlberg, M. M., Fickas, S., Hung, P., & Fortier, A. (2007). A comparison of four prompt modes for route finding for community travellers with severe cognitive impairments. *Brain Injury, 21,* 531–538.

Sohlberg, M. M., & Mateer, C. A. (2001). *Cognitive rehabilitation: An integrative neuropsychological approach.* New York: Guilford Press.

Sohlberg, M. M., McLaughlin, K. A., Pavese, A., Heidrich, A., & Posner, M. I. (2000). Evaluation of attention process training and brain injury education in persons with acquired brain injury. *Journal of Clinical and Experimental Neuropsychology, 22,* 656–676.

Stapleton, S., Adams, M., & Atterton, L. (2007). A mobile phone as a memory aid for individuals with traumatic brain injury: A preliminary investigation. *Brain Injury, 21,* 401–411.

Sterr, A., Elbert, T., Berthold, I., Kolbel, S., Rockstroh, B., & Taub, E. (2002). Longer versus shorter daily constraint-induced movement therapy of chronic hemiparesis: An exploratory study. *Archives of Physical Medicine, 83,* 1374–1377.

Sterr, A., & Freivogel, S. (2003). Motor improvement following intensive training in low-functioning chronic hemiparesis. *Neurology, 61,* 842–844.

Stewart, T. C., Girotti, M. J., Nikore, V., & Williamson, J. (2003). Effect of airbag deployment on head injuries in severe passenger motor vehicle crashes in Ontario, Canada. *Journal of Trauma, 54,* 266–272.

Stuss, D. T., Binns, M. A., Carruth, F. G., Levine, B., Brandys, C. E., Moulton, R. J., et al. (1999). The acute period of recovery from traumatic brain injury: Posttraumatic amnesia or posttraumatic confusional state. *Journal of Neurosurgery, 90,* 635–643.

Sullivan, K. J. (2007). Therapy interventions for mobility impairments and motor skill acquisition after TBI. In N. D. Zasler, D. I. Katz, & R. D. Zafonte (Eds.), *Brain injury medicine: Principles and practice* (pp. 929–946). New York: Demos.

Szaflarski, J. P., Page, S. P., Kissela, B. M., Lee, J-H., Levine, P., & Strakowski, S. M. (2006). Cortical reorganization following modified constraint-induced movement therapy: A study of 4 patients with chronic stroke. *Archives of Physical Medicine and Rehabilitation, 87,* 1052–1058.

Tam, S-F., & Man, W-K. (2004). Evaluating computer-assisted memory retraining programmes for people with post-head injury amnesia. *Brain Injury, 18,* 461–470.

Tam, S-F., Man, W. K., Hui-Chan, C. W. Y., Lau, A., Yip, B., & Cheung, W. (2003). Evaluating the efficacy of tele-cognitive rehabilitation for functional performance in three case studies. *Occupational Therapy International, 10*(1), 20–38.

Tamietto, M., Torrini, G., Adenzato, M., Pietrapiana, P., Rago, R., & Perino, C. (2006). To drive or not to drive (after TBI)? A review of the literature and its implications for rehabilitation and future research. *NeuroRehabilitation, 21,* 81–92.

Taub, E., Crago, J. E., & Uswatte, G. (1998). Constraint-induced movement therapy: A new approach to treatment in physical rehabilitation. *Rehabilitation Psychology, 43,* 152–170.

Taub, E., Uswatte, G., King, D. K., Morris, D., Crago, J. E., & Chatterjee, A. (2006). A placebo-controlled trial of constraint-induced movement therapy for upper extremity after stroke. *Stroke, 37,* 1045–1049.

Taub, E., Uswatte, G., Mark, V. W., & Morris, D. M. (2006). The learned nonuse phenomenon: Implications for rehabilitation. *Europa Medicophysica, 42,* 241–255.

Teasdale, G., & Jennett, B. (1974). Assessment of coma and impaired consciousness: A practical scale. *Lancet, 2,* 81–84.

Teasell, R., Bayona, N., Marshall, S., Cullen, N., Bayley, M., Chundamala, J., et al. (2007). A systematic review of the rehabilitation of moderate to severe acquired brain injuries. *Brain Injury, 21,* 107–112.

Temkin, N. R., Machamer, J. E., & Dikmen, S. S. (2003). Correlates of functional status 3–5 years after traumatic brain injury with CT abnormalities. *Journal of Neurotrauma, 20,* 229–241.

Terré, R., & Mearin, F. (2007). Prospective evaluation of oro-pharyngeal dysphagia after severe traumatic brain injury. *Brain Injury, 21,* 1411–1417.

Testa, J. A., Malec, J. F., Moessner, A. M., & Brown, A. W. (2006). Predicting family functioning after TBI: Impact of neurobehavioral factors. *Journal of Head Trauma Rehabilitation, 21,* 236–247.

Thickpenny-Davis, K. L., & Barker-Collo, S. L. (2007). Evaluation of a structured group format memory rehabilitation program for adults following brain injury. *Journal of Head Trauma Rehabilitation, 22,* 303–313.

Tickle-Degnen, L. (2000). Monitoring and documenting evidence during assessment and intervention. *American Journal of Occupational Therapy, 54,* 434–436.

Tickle-Degnen, L., & Bedell, G. (2003). Heterarchy and hierarchy: A critical appraisal of the "levels of evidence" as a tool for clinical decision making. *American Journal of Occupational Therapy, 57,* 234–237.

Tillerson, J. L., & Miller, G. W. (2002). Forced limb use and recovery following brain injury. *The Neuroscientist, 8,* 574–585.

Toglia, J. P. (1993). *The Contextual Memory Test.* Tucson, AZ: Therapy Skill Builders.

Toglia, J. P. (1994). *Toglia Category Assessment (TCA).* Paquannock, NJ: Maddak.

Toglia, J. P. (2005). A dynamic interactional model to cognitive–rehabilitation. In N. Katz (Ed.), *Cognition and occupation across the life span* (2nd ed., pp. 29–72). Bethesda, MD: AOTA Press.

Toglia, J. P., Golisz, K. M., & Goverover, Y. (2008). Cognitive–perceptual evaluation and intervention. In E. B. Creapeau, B. Schell, & E. Cohn (Eds.), *Willard and Spackman's occupational therapy* (11th ed. pp. 740–777). Philadelphia: Lippincott Williams & Wilkins.

Toglia, J., & Kirk, U. (2000). Understanding awareness deficits following brain injury. *NeuroRehabilitation, 15,* 57–70.

Townsend, E. A., & Wilcock, A. A. (2004). Occupational justice. In C. H. Christiansen & E. A. Townsend (Eds.), *Introduction to occupation: The art and science of living* (pp. 243–273). Upper Saddle River, NJ: Prentice Hall.

Traumatic Brain Injury Act of 1996, P.L. 144-166.

Traumatic Brain Injury Model Systems of Care. (2008). *TBIMS presentation*. Retrieved on February 14, 2009, from: http://www.tbindsc.org/

Trombly, C. A. (1995). Occupation: Purposefulness and meaningfulness as therapeutic mechanisms. *American Journal of Occupational Therapy, 49,* 960–972.

Trombly, C. A., Radomski, M. V., & Davis, E. S. (1998). Achievement of self-identified goals by adults with traumatic brain injury: Phase I. *American Journal of Occupational Therapy, 52,* 810–818.

Trombly, C. A., Radomski, M. V., Trexel, C., & Burnett-Smith, S. E. (2002). Occupational therapy and achievement of self-identified goals by adults with acquired brain injury. Phase II. *American Journal of Occupational Therapy, 56,* 489–498.

Trzepacz, P. T., Mittal, D., Torres, R., Kanary, K., Norton, J., & Jimerson, N. (2001). Validation of the Delirium Rating Scale–Revised: Comparison with the Delirium Rating Scale and the Cognitive Test for Delirium. *Journal of Neuropsychiatry and Clinical Neuroscience, 13,* 229–242.

Turkstra, L. S., & Flora, T. L. (2002). Compensating for executive function impairments after TBI: A single-case study of functional intervention. *Journal of Communication Disorders, 35,* 467–482.

Turner-Stokes, L., Disler, P. B., Nair, A., & Wade, D. T. (2005). Multi-disciplinary rehabilitation for acquired brain injury in adults of working age. *Cochrane Database of Systematic Reviews, 3,* CD004170. DOI: 10.1002/14651858.CD004170.pub2.

Underwood, J., Clark, P. C., Blanton, S., Aycock, D. M., & Wolf, S. L. (2006). Pain, fatigue, and intensity of practice in people with stroke who are receiving constraint-induced movement therapy. *Physical Therapy, 86,* 1241–1250.

Uniform Data System for Medical Rehabilitation. (1997). *Guide for the Uniform Data Set for Medical Rehabilitation (including the FIM™ instrument), Version 5.1.* Buffalo: State University of New York at Buffalo.

Uswatte, G., Taub, E., Morris, D., Barman, J., & Crago, J. (2006). Contribution of the shaping and restraint components of constraint-induced movement therapy to treatment outcome. *NeuroRehabilitation, 21,* 147–156.

van Baalen, B., Odding, E., & Stam, H. J. (2008). Cognitive status at discharge from the hospital determines discharge destination in traumatic brain injury patients. *Brain Injury, 22,* 25–32.

Van den Broek, M. D., Downes, J., Johnson, Z., Dayus, B., & Hilton, N. (2000). Evaluation of an electronic memory aid in the neuropsychological rehabilitation of prospective memory deficits. *Brain Injury, 14,* 455–462.

Vanderploeg, R. D., Schwab, K., Walker, W. C., Fraser, J. A., Sigford, B. J., Date, E. S., et al. (2008). Rehabilitation of traumatic brain injury in active duty military personnel and veterans: Defense and Veterans' Brain Injury Center randomized controlled trial of two rehabilitation approaches. *Archives of Physical Medicine and Rehabilitation, 89,* 2227–2238.

Wade, T. K., & Troy, J. C. (2001). Mobile phones as a new memory aid: A preliminary investigation using case studies. *Brain Injury, 15,* 305–320.

Wagner, A. K. (2007). Conducting research in TBI: Current concepts and issues. In N. D. Zasler, D. I. Katz, & R. D. Zafonte (Eds.), *Brain injury medicine: Principles and practice* (pp. 33–42). New York: Demos.

Wagner, A. K., Sasser, H. C., Hammond, F. C., Wiercisiewski, D., & Alexander, J. (2000). Intentional traumatic brain injury: Epidemiology, risk factors, and associations with injury severity and mortality. *Journal of Trauma Injury, Infection, and Critical Care, 49,* 404–410.

Walker, J. P. (2002). Case Study: Functional outcome: A case for mild traumatic brain injury. *Brain Injury, 16,* 611–625.

Walker, W. C., Marwitz, J. H., Kreutzer, J. S., Hart, T., & Novack, T. A. (2006). Occupational categories and return to work after traumatic brain injury: A multicenter study. *Archives of Physical Medicine and Rehabilitation, 87,* 1576–1582.

Walker, W. C., & Pickett, T. C. (2007). Motor impairment after severe traumatic brain injury: A longitudinal multicenter study. *Journal of Rehabilitation Research and Development, 44,* 975–982.

Warren, M. (1998). *Brain Injury Visual Assessment Battery for Adults.* Lenexa, KS: visABILITIES Rehab Services.

Watanabe, T. K., Black, K. L., Zafonte, R. D., Millis, S. R., & Mann, N. R. (1998). Do calendars enhance posttraumatic temporal orientation? A pilot study. *Brain Injury, 12,* 81–85.

Watson, M., & Horn, S. (1991). "The ten pound note test": Suggestions for eliciting improved responses in the severely brain-injured patient. *Brain Injury, 5,* 421–424.

Wheeler, S. D., Lane, S. J., & McMahon, B. T. (2007). Community participation and life satisfaction following intensive, community-based rehabilitation using a life skills training approach. *OTJR: Occupation, Participation, and Health, 27,* 13–22.

Whiteneck, G. G., Charlifue, S. W., Gerhart, K. A., Overhosler, J. D., & Richardson, G. N. (1992). Quantifying handicap: A new measure of long-term rehabilitation outcomes. *Archives of Physical Medicine and Rehabilitation, 73,* 519–526.

Whiteneck, G. G., Gerhart, K. A., & Cusick, C. P. (2004). Identifying environmental factors that influence the outcomes of people with traumatic brain injury. *Journal of Head Trauma Rehabilitation, 19,* 191–204.

Whiteneck, G., Harrison-Felix, C., Mellick, D., Brooks, C., Charlifue, S., & Gerhart, K. (2004). Quantifying environmental factors: A measure of physical, attitudinal, service, productivity, and policy barriers. *Archives of Physical Medicine and Rehabilitation, 85,* 1324–1335.

Wijdicks, E. F. M., Bamlet, W. R., Maramattom, B. V., Manno, E. M., & McClelland, R. L. (2005). Validation of a new coma scale: The FOUR score. *Annals of Neurology, 58,* 585–593.

Will, B., Galani, R., Kelche, C., & Rosenzweig, M. R. (2004). Recovery from brain injury in animals: Relative efficacy of environmental enrichment, physical exercise, or formal training (1990–2002). *Progress in Neurobiology, 72,* 167–182.

Willer, B., Ottenbacher, K. J., & Coad, M. L. (1994). The Community Integration Questionnaire: A comparative examination. *American Journal of Physical Medicine and Rehabilitation, 73,* 103–111.

Wilson, B. A., Alderman, N., Burgess, P., Emslie, H., & Evans, J. (1996). *Behavioural Assessment of the Dysexecutive Syndrome.* Bury St. Edmunds, UK: Thames Valley Test Company.

Wilson, B. A., Clare, L., Baddeley, A., Watson, P., & Tate, R. (1998). *The Rivermead Behavioral Memory Test–Extended Version (RBMT–E).* Bury St. Edmunds, UK: Thames Valley Test Company.

Wilson, B. A., Emslie, H. C., Quirk, K., & Evans, J. J. (2001). Reducing everyday memory and planning problems by means of a paging system: A randomized control crossover design. *Journal of Neurology, Neurosurgery, and Psychiatry, 70,* 477–482.

Wilson, B. A., & Watson, P. C. (1996). A practical framework for understanding compensatory behaviour in people with organic memory impairment. *Membranes, 4,* 456–486.

Wilson, F. C., & Manly, T. (2003). Sustained attention training and errorless learning facilitates self-care functioning in chronic ipsilesional neglect following severe traumatic brain injury. *Neuropsychological Rehabilitation, 13,* 537–548.

Wilson, J. T., Pettigrew, L. E., & Teasdale, G. M. (1998). Structured interviews for the Glasgow Outcome Scale and the Extended Glasgow Outcome Scale: Guidelines for their use. *Journal of Neurotrauma, 15,* 573–585.

Wilson, S. L., Brock, D., Powell, G. E., Thwaites, H., & Elliott, K. (1996). Constructing arousal profiles for vegetative state patients—A preliminary study. *Brain Injury, 10,* 105–113.

Wilson, S. L., Powell, G. E., Brock, D., & Thwaites, H. (1996). Vegetative state and responses to sensory stimulation: An analysis of 24 cases. *Brain Injury, 10,* 807–818.

Wittenberg, G. F., Chen, R., Ishii, K., Bushara, K. O., Eckloff, S., Croarkin, E., et al. (2003). Constraint-induced therapy in stroke: Magnetic-stimulation motor maps and cerebral activation. *Neurorehabilitation and Neural Repair, 17,* 48–57.

Wolf, S. L., Winstein, C. J., Miller, J. P., Taub, E., Uswatte, G., Morris, D., et al. (2006). Effect of constraint-induced movement therapy on upper extremity function 3 to 9 months after stroke: The EXCITE randomized clinical trial. *JAMA, 296,* 2095–2104.

Wolf, S. L., Winstein, C. J., Miller, J. P., Thompson, P. A., Taub, E., Uswatte, G., et al. (2008). Retention of upper limb function in stroke survivors who have received constraint-induced movement therapy: The EXCITE randomized trial. *Lancet Neurology, 7,* 33–40.

World Health Organization. (2001). *International classification of functioning, disability, and health.* Geneva, Switzerland: Author.

Wright, P., Rogers, N., Hall, C., Wilson, B., Evans, J., & Emslie, H. (2001a). Enhancing an appointment diary on a pocket computer for use by people after brain injury. *International Journal of Rehabilitation Research, 24,* 299–308.

Wright, P., Rogers, N., Hall, C., Wilson, B., Evans, J., Emslie, H., et al. (2001b). Comparison of pocket-computer memory aids for people with brain injury. *Brain Injury, 15,* 787–800.

Wu, C. Y., Chen, C. L., Tsai, W. C., Lin, K. C., & Chou, S. H. (2007). A randomized controlled trial of modified constraint-induced movement therapy for elderly stroke survivors: Changes in motor impairment, daily functioning, and quality of life. *Archives of Physical Medicine and Rehabilitation, 88,* 273–278.

Wu, C. Y., Lin, K. C., Chen, H. C., Chen, I. H., & Hong, W. H. (2007). Effects of modified constraint-induced movement therapy on movement kinematics and daily function in patients with stroke: A kinematic study of motor control mechanisms. *Neurorehabilitation and Neural Repair, 21,* 460–466.

Ylvisaker, M., & Feeney, T. (2001). What I really want is a girlfriend: Meaningful social interaction after traumatic brain injury. *Brain Injury Source, 5,* 12–17.

Yuen, H. K. (1997). Positive talk training in an adult with traumatic brain injury. *American Journal of Occupational Therapy, 51,* 780–783.

Zhou, J., Chittum, R., Johnston, K., Poppen, R., Guercio, J., & McMorrow, M. J. (1996). The utilization of a game format to increase knowledge of residuals among people with acquired brain injury. *Journal of Head Trauma Rehabilitation, 11,* 51–61.

Zhu, X. L., Poon, W. S., Chan, C. C., & Chan, S. S. (2007). Does intensive rehabilitation improve the functional outcome of patients with traumatic brain injury (TBI)? A randomized controlled trial. *Brain Injury, 21,* 681–690.

Zhu, X. L., Poon, W. S., Chan, C. H., & Chan, S. H. (2001). Does intensive rehabilitation improve the functional outcome of patients with traumatic brain injury? Interim result of a randomized controlled trial. *British Journal of Neurosurgery, 15,* 464–473.